Male Alopecia

Ralph M. Trüeb • Won-Soo Lee

Male Alopecia

Guide to Successful Management

Springer

Ralph M. Trüeb
Center for Dermatology and
Hair Diseases
Wallisellen-Zurich
Switzerland

Won-Soo Lee
Department of Dermatology
Yonsei University Wonju
College of Medicine
Wonju
Kangwon-Do
Korea
Republic of (South Korea)

ISBN 978-3-319-34974-9 ISBN 978-3-319-03233-7 (eBook)
DOI 10.1007/978-3-319-03233-7
Springer Cham Heidelberg New York Dordrecht London

Softcover reprint of the hardcover 1st edition 2014

Printed on acid-free paper

Springer is part of Springer Science+Business Media (www.springer.com)

Preface

Do you not see that I am too tall and comely to look on?
And yet the same fate awaits my hair,
and I bear with resignation the aging of my locks in youth.
Be assured that nothing is more pleasing than beauty,
but nothing shorter-lived.

Domitian (51–96 AD) on the condition of his hair.
From: Suetonius, The Lives of the Caesars

Male alopecia is a common complaint, with androgenetic alopecia representing by far the most frequent cause of hair loss in men. First signs may occur in adolescence, leading to a patterned, non-scarring, age-dependent progressive loss of scalp hair. Due to the frequency and the often significant impairment of life quality perceived by affected individuals, hair loss cures have been experimented on for centuries. What is remarkable about their history is that despite the more recent genuine advances in effective medical treatments, hair cosmetics, and surgical procedures, phony hair loss solutions continue to be marketed today with an amazing success. Therefore, competent diagnosis and treatment are particularly important in dealing with hair loss.

Evidence-based medicine (EBM) aims for the ideal that healthcare professionals should make conscientious, explicit, and judicious use of the best available evidence gained from the scientific method. However, EBM guidelines do not remove the problem of extrapolation to different populations or longer timeframes. Even if top-quality studies are available, questions remain as to how far and to which populations the results may be generalized. Certain patient populations have been under-researched, such as children, the elderly and ethnic minorities. Ultimately, EBM applies to groups of people, and knowledge gained from clinical research does not directly answer the primary clinical question of what is best for the individual patient. The limited success rate of EBM-guided treatments of male alopecia points to a more important complexity of the problem. One must remain open-minded for the possibility of other causes or a multitude of cause relationships underlying the hair loss problem, such as inflammatory phenomena and scarring; external factors, such as smoking and UV radiation, nutritional factors, medications; age-related phenomena; and ultimately the problems of comorbidities and multimorbidity in the elderly. Therefore, EBM should not preclude clinicians from using their personal experience in deciding how to treat each patient in an individual manner.

Good medical practice means integrating expert opinion with the best available external evidence from EBM. While mainstream scientist are working on gene polymorphisms diagnostics for prediction of risk, prevention, diagnosis, and targeted treatment development for male alopecia, on stem cell technologies, and on bioengineering of the hair follicle, health-care providers are becoming increasingly aware of a more holistic approach to the problem of hair loss. Ultimately, combination regimens and adjuvant treatments may act synergistic to enhance hair growth and quality.

The aim of this monograph is to provide specialists as was well as primary care physicians with interest in hair with the practical know-how for successful management of male alopecia.

Wallisellen, Switzerland Ralph M. Trüeb
Wonju, South Korea Won-Soo Lee

Authors

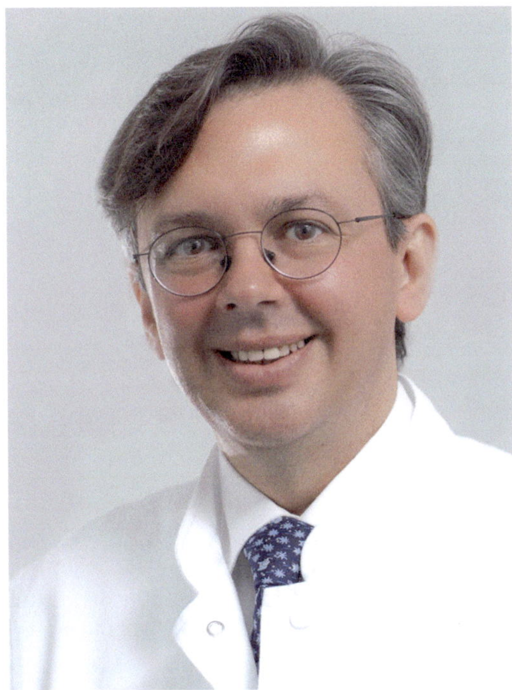

Ανέγνων, έγνων, κατέγνων

Ralph M. Trüeb is professor of dermatology. He received his MD and Swiss Board Certification for Dermatology and Venerology as well as for Allergology and Clinical Immunology from the University of Zurich, Switzerland. In 1994–1995 he spent a year at the University of Texas Southwestern Medical Center at Dallas with Rick Sontheimer and at the Howard Hughes Medical Institute in Dallas with Bruce Beutler to complete his Fellowship in Immunodermatology. After 20 years of tenure at the Department of Dermatology, University Hospital of Zurich, where he established and was head of the Hair Consultation Clinic, he established in 2010 his private Center for Dermatology and Hair Diseases in Zurich–Wallisellen. He is past president of the European Hair Research Society (2008–2011) and founding president of the Swiss Skin and Hair Foundation (2011). His clinical research interests focus on hair loss, inflammatory phenomena, hair aging and antiaging, and patient expectation management. He is currently author of 172 peer-reviewed scientific publications and author or editor of 5 textbooks on hair.

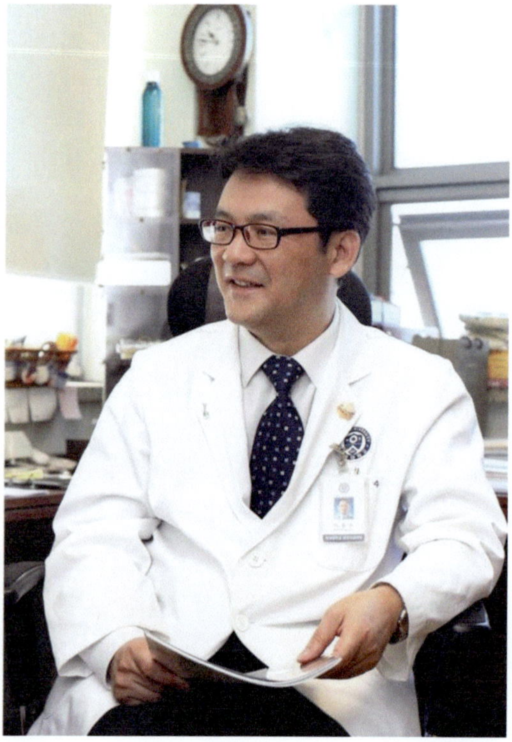

Won-Soo Lee is a professor and chairman of Dermatology at the Yonsei University Wonju College of Medicine in Wonju, Korea. He is a director of Institute of Hair and Cosmetic Medicine, a research institute he founded to perform clinical and experimental research in association with the pharmaceutical and cosmetic industry. His research interests include hair loss, hair photoaging, integral hair lipid, hair cosmetology, and hair neurobiology. He has received 15 national and international awards and honors. He has published more than 180 scientific and medical articles in peer-reviewed journals including the *Journal of the American Academy of Dermatology*, *Archives of Dermatology*, *British Journal of Dermatology*, and *Journal of Investigative Dermatology*. He is a secretary general of the Korean Hair Research Society and a congress president of the 2014 8th World Congress for Hair Research on Jeju Island, Korea. He is a past secretary general of the Korean Society of Cosmetic Dermatology. He received his medical degree from the Yonsei University School of Medicine in Seoul, Korea, in 1985. He completed a dermatology residency at the Severance Hospital, Yonsei University, in 1989. He received his PhD from the Yonsei University in 1992. Won-Soo Lee has contributed Sects. 3.1.1, 3.1.2, 3.1.3, 3.1.4, 3.1.7, 3.1.8, 3.1.9, 3.1.10, 3.1.11, and 3.2.6 of the book.

Acknowledgement

In the sick room, ten cents' worth of human understanding equals ten dollars' worth of medical science.

Martin H. Fischer (1879–1962)

We would like to acknowledge the many patients who over the years have taught us more about their hair loss and its successful management than any academic authority.

Contents

1 Introduction

Hair is the first thing. And teeth the second. Hair and teeth. A man got those two things he's got it all.

James Brown (1933–2006)

The face, including the cranial hair, represents an area of our body with a high impact on our social interactions. It is strongly associated with individual identity, and it communicates to others immediately information on our age, gender, individual, and group identity. Since our craniofacial presentation affects our self-perception, it has a bearing on our social behavior as well.

1.1 Symbolism of Male Hair

Hair has been significant to human civilization at all times and in all cultures in terms of symbolism for strength, sexuality, and magic. Throughout the ages people have represented through craniofacial characteristics their identities with respect to a wide range of social phenomena: religious, political, sexual, occupational, etc. Hair not only symbolizes the self but is itself a part of our body. Therefore, its condition also reflects our general health and mental status. Accordingly, any change in the appearance of our hair can be expected to have a major impact on the way we are perceived, on our self-perception, and ultimately on our well-being.

More specifically, the male expresses his ideologies and status in his hair. The biblical story of Samson and Delilah (Judges 16) shows how important a man's hairstyle can be. Short or long, loose or taut, men's hairstyles have passed through many stages throughout history. At most times and in most cultures, men have worn their hair in styles different from women's.

> American sociologist Rose Weitz pointed out that the most prevalent cultural rule about hair is that women's and men's hair must differ from each other.

During most periods in human history when men and women wore similar hairstyles, as in the 1920s and 1960s, it has therefore generated significant social concern and approbation.

A hairstyle refers to the manner of arranging human scalp hair. Its aesthetic considerations are determined by a number of factors, such as the individual's physical attributes and desired self-image or the hairstylist's artistic intentions. Physical factors include natural hair type and growth patterns, face and head shape, and overall body proportions. Self-image may be directed toward conforming to mainstream values, identifying with distinctively groomed subgroups, or following religious rules.

Early in human civilization, voluntary cutting of one's hair has been related to spiritual expression: In Ancient Egypt, the priests of Amun-Ra shaved their heads, and wealthy men or members of the royal elite would cover their shaven heads with elaborate headdresses. Upon reaching manhood, Greek youths sacrificed their hair to the river. In ancient Rome, haircutting was a puberty ritual, with spiritual significance.

In stark contrast, the Germanic tribes Teutons and Celts refrained from haircutting in order to differentiate themselves from their shaven slaves.

R.M. Trüeb, W.-S. Lee, *Male Alopecia*,
DOI 10.1007/978-3-319-03233-7_1, © Springer International Publishing Switzerland 2014

Upon subduing the Gauls, who associated long hair with male dignity and liberty, Julius Caesar (100–44 BC) required them to cut their hair as a token of submission. That abundant hair symbolized power presented a problem for Caesar himself, since his hairline was gradually receding. First, he began growing it long in the back and combing it straight forward over his bald spot.

> Ultimately, Caesar took to wearing a laurel wreath around his head to conceal his hair loss. The trademark wreath soon became a symbol of power and authority.

Following the downfall of the Roman Empire, most of Europe adopted the hair of the Germanic peoples. During the reign of the Merovingian dynasty, King Chlodio V (395–448) was nicknamed "Le Chevelu" because he wore his hair longer than most of his predecessors. During this time, long locks were a symbol of status. Royalty wore their hair long while members of the lower classes either had short hair or shaved heads.

During the English Civil War (1642–1651), the followers of Oliver Cromwell decided to crop their hair close to their head, as an act of defiance to the curls and ringlets of the king's men. This led to the Parliamentary faction being nicknamed *Roundheads*.

In the seventeenth-century France, wearing a long wig was a sign of status, made popular by the French Kings Louis XIII (1601–1643) and Louis XIV (1638–1715). Louis XIII began wearing a wig to cover his thinning hair. Soon, members of the court followed his example, regardless of their own hair condition. Louis XIV, also known as "Le Roi-Soleil" (the Sun King), made public appearances and frequently posed for portraits in a long, dark brown wig with loose waves. Wigs became symbols of wealth and power, and the height, length, and bulk of wigs increased accordingly, with giant powdered wigs setting the trend in the French court.

In England, King Charles II (1635–1685) was restored to the throne after his exile in Versailles, France, where he had been exposed to the French fashioning of wigs. During the Restoration period following Cromwell, the English were soon not to be outdone. Charles II was popularly known as the Merry Monarch, in reference to both the liveliness and hedonism of his court and the general relief at the return to normality after over a decade of rule by Oliver Cromwell and the Puritans.

Around 1710, in the Rococo era, the long-flowing *allonge* wigs went out of fashion, and hairdos stayed close to the scalp. Except for a few locks around the forehead, the main part of the hair (natural or artificial) was brushed to the back. Later on, some people wore a pigtail modelled on the hairstyle of the Prussian soldiers, a hairstyling still fashioned today by designer Karl Lagerfeld. He is well recognized around the world for his trademark white hair, black glasses, and high starched collars.

In the Americas, upper class American colonists picked up the wig fashion, and by the late eighteenth century, wealthy people wore wigs to signify their elevated class. Not until the American War of Independence (1775–1783) and in France the subsequent Revolution (1789), the look of royalty and elevated class distinction together with wigs fell out of favor.

At the end of the eighteenth century, men of fashion began to wear short and more natural hair, sporting cropped curls and long sideburns in a classical manner much like Grecian warriors and Roman senators.

A scarcity of flour to powder the wigs in 1795, combined with the introduction of a hair powder tax to raise state revenues, brought the fashion for wigs and powder to an abrupt halt. Men protested and a new more natural hairstyle became fashionable. The *Bedford Crop* became a hairstyle favored by the Duke of Bedford, who, in protest to the tax, abandoned his wigs in favor of a short cropped and unpowdered hairstyle. He challenged his friends to do the same. His natural-looking crop was parted on the side with a dab of hair wax.

The Romantic movement also influenced a natural, unpretentious aesthetic. A dry disordered look that used very few artificial products began to rule.

Dandy prototype Beau Brummel's (1778–1840) influence cannot be discounted: His own grooming included shorter hair and a clean-shaven face. Every morning he examined his face in a dentist mirror and plucked any remaining stray hairs with tweezers. Brummel was to become an iconic figure in Regency England, and the arbiter of men's fashion. He established the mode of dress for men that rejected overly ornate fashions for one of understated, but perfectly fitted and tailored clothing. Brummell is credited with introducing, and establishing as fashion, the modern men's suit, worn with a necktie. He claimed he took 5 h a day to dress and recommended that boots be polished with champagne.

The history of the Chinese dynasties is one of repeated conquers by foreign powers, who assimilated genuine Chinese culture but repressed the autochthonous Han Chinese. Upon subduing the Ming in 1644, the Manchus (Qing Dynasty, 1644–1912) imposed the partly shaven head and pigtail upon the Han men as a sign of submission. Breaking with tradition was dramatically put into scene in Bertolucci's epic cinema film "The Last Emperor" (1987), when young Emperor Puyi (1906–1967, reign 1908–1912) cuts off his pigtail.

In the 1920s, Actor Rudolph Valentino (1895–1926) lighted up the silver screen with his defined side part and glossy jet black hair in such films as "Beyond the Rocks" (1922) and "The Young Rajah" (1922). Western men soon began to wear their hair short, and either parted on the side or in the middle or combed straight back, and used pomade, creams, and tonics to keep their hair in place.

Finally, the crew cut originated when Yale rowing team members started to cut their hair short, presumably with the intention to differentiate themselves from members of the football team, who wore their hair longer for extra padding under their thin leather helmets. During World War II, soldiers sported crew cuts to help control head lice in their tight quarters.

In his monograph on *The Unconscious Significance of Hair*, psychoanalyst Charles Berg reviewed the anthropological literature on hair and developed Freud's insights into a cross-cultural theory of hair practices.

> According to Berg, hair has practically no other significance except as a sexual symbol, and there is no normal individual without some degree of hair fetishism.

In a spiritual context, hair has been recognized to have two perceived symbolic meanings: shaven hair is a symbol of celibacy and chastity; in contrast, uncut hair is seen as a withdrawal from worldly concern and vanities. Sometimes long hair represents a concession to religion, such as in the Sikh religion, although today it has also become a symbol of identity. Ultimately, shaving the head is found in many faiths and cultures as a symbol of dedication to God, seen in ancient Buddhism and Hinduism, as well as in Christianity.

The Roman Catholic rite of admission to the clerical state by clipping or shaving the head of monks provides yet another example. In his Letter to the Corinthians, Apostle Paul indicates that it is unnatural and degrading for a man to wear long hair. A synod held at Elvira in 309 AD forbid women to associate with long-haired men, under penalty of excommunication. Therefore, any man aspiring recognition as a good Christian, as well as one simply seeking the consortium of a religiously respectable Christian woman, was provided with a motivation to trim his hair.

Today, long hair, especially in men, is often understood to signal ideological opposition to the establishment. People commonly make personality attributions that relate to intelligence, personality, social aptitudes, or deviation, based simply on appearance. Cutting the hair is understood to indicate submission to social control, whereas long hair suggests an intent to evade the rules and restrictions of society or institutions.

In the 1950s, Beat poets wore longer hairstyles, as did the urban gay culture, although long hair was far from popular. In 1960, a small *beatnik* community in Newquay, Cornwall, England, attracted attention by growing their hair to a length past the shoulders, resulting in a television interview on BBC television.

The 1960s also introduced "The Beatles," who initiated a more widespread trend toward longer hair. The social revolution of the 1960s led to a revival of unchecked hair growth, and long hair was worn as a political or countercultural symbol of protest. Specific long hairstyles, such as dreadlocks, have been part of counterculture movements seeking to define alternative cultures and lifestyles since this time. The popularity of Jamaica's reggae music and musician Bob Marley (1945–1981) prompted international interest in dreadlocks. The antiestablishment philosophy of the Rastafari, echoed in much of the reggae of the time, resonated with enthusiastic youths of all ethnicities, primarily among African-Americans and other blacks but also among counterculture whites.

Long hair remained popular among the youth rebellion throughout the liberal decade and *hippie* movement of the 1960s, culminating in the successful American rock musical "Hair" (lyrics by James Rado and Gerome Ragni, music by Galt MacDermot). It tells the story of a group of politically active, long-haired hippies living a bohemian life in New York City and fighting against conscription into the Vietnam War. After its debut in 1967 at Joseph Papp's Public Theater, the show opened on Broadway in 1968 and ran for 1,750 performances. Simultaneous productions in cities across the USA and Europe followed shortly thereafter, including a successful London production that ran for 1,997 performances. Since then, numerous productions have been staged around the world with dozens of recordings of the musical. Finally, in the 1970s, longer hairstyles would become the norm.

> In discussing long hair in males in the USA, American anthropologist Marvin K. Opler (1914–1981) felt that hairstyle is a reflection of group attitudes culturally defined rather than of individual feelings.

His investigations on male students classified as *deviant* with regard to their hair length revealed that they assigned a high value to independence and less value to recognition and conformity. In contrast, the importance placed on short hair by the armed forces of many countries reinforces the popular association of short hair with authority and discipline.

Today, longer hairstyles among men, while not as common and popular as in the 1970s, are nonetheless not uncommon, and are still quite popular among rock enthusiasts.

As opposed to long hairstyles, *skinheads* are characterized by their close-cropped or shaven heads. The skinhead originated in the 1960s among working class youths in London, England. The first skinheads were greatly influenced by the British *mods* and the Jamaican *rude boys*, in terms of fashion, lifestyle, and music. In the late 1950s, the postwar economic boom led to an increase in income among many young people. Some of these spent their earnings on new fashions popularized by American soul groups, British R&B bands, certain movie actors, and Carnaby Street clothing merchants. These youths became known as *mods*, a youth subculture noted for its consumerism and devotion to fashion and music. Mods of lesser means made do with more practical clothing styles that suited their employment circumstances and lifestyle: work boots or army boots, straight-leg jeans, button-down shirts, and suspenders. In addition to retaining mod influences, early skinheads were also interested in Jamaican rude boy styles and culture, especially the music: ska, rocksteady, and early reggae, before the tempo slowed down and lyrics became focused on topics like black nationalism and the Rastafari movement (with its dreadlocks). The rude boy subculture arose from the socially disadvantaged populace of Kingston, Jamaica, and was associated with violently discontented youths. With respect to styling, many rude boys favored sharp suits, thin ties, and pork pie or Trilby hats, showing an influence of the fashions of American jazz musicians and soul music artists. Originally, the skinhead subculture was primarily based on those elements, not politics or race but, since then, race and politics (ranging from far right to far left) have become factors by which some skinheads align themselves, though others are admittedly apolitical.

In the late 1970s, the skinhead subculture was revived after the emergence of *punk rock*.

Punk bands created fast, hard-edged music, typically with short songs, stripped-down instrumentation, and often political, antiestablishment lyrics. An associated punk subculture developed, again expressing youthful rebellion and characterized by distinctive styles of clothing and adornment and a variety of antiauthoritarian ideologies. Punk fashion, including hairstyles, varied widely, including influences from glam rock, skinheads, rude boys, greasers, and mods. Many punks used clothing as a way of making a statement. Punk fashion has been extremely commercialized, and well-established fashion designers, such as Jean Paul Gaultier, have used punk elements in their production.

Finally, the *New Romantic* movement influenced hairstyling. New Romanticism was again a popular cultural movement that began as a nightclub scene around 1979 in the United Kingdom and peaked around 1981. It can be seen as a reaction to punk, in terms of style it rejected the austerity and antifashion stance of punk. Both sexes often dressed in counter-sexual or androgynous clothing and wore cosmetics such as eyeliner and lipstick. Originally heavily influenced by David Bowie, Bryan Ferry of "Roxy Music," and Philip Oakey of "The Human League," the gender bending became particularly evident in personalities such as Pete Burns of "Dead or Alive" and Boy George of "Culture Club." Fashion was based around flamboyant, eccentric appearance and on varied looks relating to romantic themes, including frilly fop shirts in the style of the English Romantic period, Russian constructivism, Bonny Prince Charlie, French Incroyables and 1930s Cabaret, and Hollywood starlets, with any look being possible if it was adapted to be unusual and striking. Typical hairstyles included quiffs, mullets, and wedge.

In 1998, Trüeb et al. conducted a community-based survey of men in Switzerland to characterize the significance of scalp hair and self-perception of hair loss in Swiss men and to evaluate treatment of hair loss. Five hundred and eight men, aged 15–74 years, regardless of the degree of hair loss, were interviewed by telephone.

The questions addressed by the interview were as follows: degree of self-rated hair loss, time invested and products use for hair care, use of or reasons for rejecting hair growth promoting agents, relevant criteria with respect to the condition of scalp hair, and self-assessment with respect to the significance of scalp hair.

Respondents rated their hair loss on a 5-point, textual scale that ranged from "no hair loss" to "bald areas." The relevance of criteria inquired relating to the condition of hair were: trimness, adequacy, styling, and quantity of hair. Those relating to the significance of hair were as follows: personality and life style (spruceness and trendiness), occupational orientation and professional success, and male eroticism and sexual attractiveness.

Respondents were in the following age groups: 27 % age 15–27 years, 41 % age 30–49 years, and 32 % age 50–74 years.

Forty-three percent reported hair loss: 7 % reported bitemporal recession, 15 % recession of the frontal hair line, 12 % thinning of the centroparietal or vertex area, and 7 % baldness of the crown area.

With respect to the criteria relating to the condition of hair, trimness and styling were the most important, while hair length and density the least (Table 1.1).

Table 1.1 Relevant criteria to the hair among interviewed Swiss men

Criteria for hair	1 (Unimportant) (%)	2 (%)	3 (%)	4 (%)	5 (Very important) (%)	Mean
Trimness	6	3	12	24	55	4.2
Styling	13	7	21	31	28	3.5
Adequacy	19	9	22	24	26	3.3
Quantity						
Length	27	17	24	9	13	2.7
Density	35	19	21	13	12	2.5

From: Trüeb RM, de Viragh PA, and Swiss Trichology Study Group (2001) Status of scalp hair and therapy of alopecia in men in Switzerland. Praxis (Bern 1994) 90:241–248

Table 1.2 Male hair communication-types and their frequencies among interviewed Swiss men

The well-groomed male (36 %) attributes high significance to trimness, adequacy, and styling of the hair. For him, these reflect in first line personality and life style. Time invested for hair care is between 5 and 10 min daily. Other characteristics are: younger age, frontal recession.
The self-complacent male (24 %) attributes high significance to all external characteristics of hair, trimness, adequacy, styling, length and density of hair. Besides personality and life style, the condition of hair also reflects occupational orientation and professional success or male eroticism and sexual attractiveness. Time invested for hair care is >10 min daily. Use of additional hair care products and hair growth promoting agents for prevention of hair loss. Other characteristics are: usually a full head of hair, older singles, in employed status, lower income class.
The well-adapted male (20 %) attributes average significance to the external characteristics of hair. He is rather unassertive with respect to social communication characteristics of hair. The most important is not to attract attention. Other characteristics are: lesser hair or areas of baldness, higher age group, urban.
The unadjusted male (11 %) does not attribute any significance to the external characteristics of his proper hair, though he acknowledges to a high degree that the condition of hair reflects personality and life style, occupational orientation and professional success, male eroticism and sexual attractiveness. Aspects of hair care are unimportant for him, irrespective of the possible disadvantages of such an attitude. Invested time for hair care is <5 min daily, use of shampoos only. Other characteristics: middle-aged, single, in employed status.
The indifferent male (9 %) does not attribute any significance to the external characteristics of hair and does not acknowledge any communicative qualities to the condition of hair. Invested time for hair care is <5 min daily, use of shampoos only. Other characteristics: areas of baldness, middle aged, married, higher education or occupational position.

From: Trüeb RM, de Viragh PA, and Swiss Trichology Study Group (2001) Status of scalp hair and therapy of alopecia in men in Switzerland. Praxis (Bern 1994) 90:241–248

With respect to the significance of scalp hair, 23 % reported that their hair signalized personality and life style, 12 % male eroticism and sexual attractiveness, and 5 % occupational orientation and professional success.

With respect to time invested and products used for hair care, 56 % invested less than 5 min, 32 % between 5 and 10 min, 8 % between 10 and 20 min, and 2 % over 20 min daily. 64 % used shampoos only, 19 % additional styling products (gel, wax), 12 % hair conditioning products, 10 % hair spray, and 3 % hair colorants.

Of the men who reported hair loss, 26 % admitted to the use of hair growth promoting agents, 31 % rejected use of hair growth promoting agents because of no need, and 27 % because they didn't believe that they worked.

On the basis of a cluster analysis of the collected data, five "male hair communication-types" were designed (Table 1.2).

1.2 Brief History of Experiments on Hair Loss Cures

As early as can be traced in history, written documents testify endeavors shown by humanity to please by means of the hair. The literature on hair is almost as vast as the myths, legends, and superstitions that flourished around it. From the 4,000-year-old medical *papyri* of the ancient Egyptians, throughout Greek and Roman civilization down to modern times, human hair growth and color have been the object of superstition and mystery as well as cosmetic and medical interest.

The most remote representations of hair loss that could be traced dates back around 30,000 years and the story is still ongoing in our modern society.

Figure 1.1 shows four drawings taken from wall engravings in a prehistorical cave. It took about 30,000 years in order to categorized patterned hair loss in males the way we do it today.

In the history of art, male pattern baldness is represented less often in works of art than it occurs in real life. Many of the exceptions are in depictions of saints, in whom baldness may be thought to convey an element of holiness, in line with the monk's tonsured pate and the shaven heads of some Eastern religious devotees. A fine example is Rembrandt's "The Baptism of the Eunuch" (1626), in which one clearly can discern

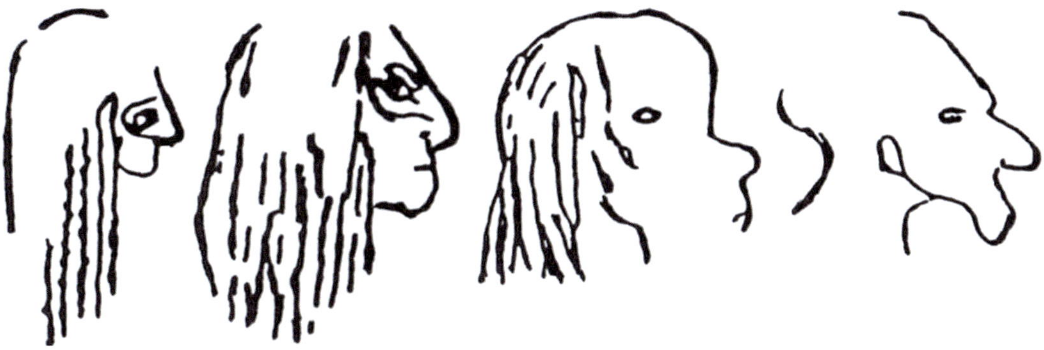

Fig. 1.1 Prehistorical cave wall engravings of patterned hair loss. From: van Neste D (2010) Aging from where to there? In: Trüeb RM, Tobin DJ (eds) Aging hair. Springer Scientific Publications, Berlin, p vii

advanced male pattern baldness in the holy man and a head full of hair in the eunuch.

Even in the nineteenth and twentieth centuries, baldness seems underrepresented, although examples can be found. Perhaps the most striking is van Gogh's portrait of deep depression, "Old Man in Sorrow," also known as "On the Threshold of Eternity," (1890). A man sits in a chair with his face buried in clenched fists. Our inability to recognize his face draws our attention to his extreme baldness, emphasized by side locks. The room is equally bare, with no carpet on the floor, and no decorations on the walls. The melancholy of the scene is emphasized by a deep blue of the man's clothing. He is, as the title tells, and as we can apprehend, "on the threshold of eternity," in other words, about to commit suicide. Hair loss is associated with depression. In a survey of 1,717 men with varying degrees of male pattern baldness, performed in four countries in 2000, hair loss was found to cause significant distress. Those with alopecia felt more worried and helpless than those without. The effects are related to the degree of hair loss and are greater in younger men. The feelings are generally mild, but some patients have intense emotional concerns about hair loss and may spend hours each day compulsively checking their scalp in the mirror, combing and re-combing their hair, and suffering considerable social anxiety and depression.

Therefore, for prevention or treatment of hair loss, countless herbal solutions, oils, lotions, magic pills, and even spiritual invocations with questionable results have been advanced at all times.

What is amazing about the history of hair loss cures is that despite the recent genuine advances in effective medical treatments, hair cosmetics, and surgical procedures, phony hair loss solutions continue to be marketed today with success.

With the advance of medical technologies, ultraviolet light-emitting lamps, electrical scalp simulators, and vacuum-cap machines have joined the repertory of treatments alleged to help stimulate the follicles to grow hair. Despite their outrageous claims, most lack scientifically measurable efficacy in preventing hair loss or promoting hair growth. But people are so concerned about their hair loss that they are prone to fall prey to all sorts of quackery.

According to ancient Greek historian Herodotus (490/480–424 BC), the Egyptian "Physician of the Head" (ιητροὶ κεφαλης), who specialized in the affections of the scalp, represented one of the oldest medical specialities.

In Ancient Egypt treatment of the scalp obtained much attention. The *papyri* of Ebers, Smith and Hearst embody an abundant *Dreckapotheke* of remedies for prevention or treatment of baldness. Most of these were accompanied by elaborate exorcisms. The Ebers *papyrus*, discovered in Luxor, Egypt, probably includes medical information drawn from the earlier described compendium of medical knowledge which was collected yet another 2,000 years earlier. It is the oldest complete medical text ever found, and it includes a written prescription for treating hair loss: a mixture of iron oxide, red lead, onions, alabaster, honey, and fat from a variety of animals including snakes, crocodiles, hippopotamuses, and lions. The mixture was to be swallowed, after first reciting magical invocations to the Sun God.

In ancient Greece, Hippocrates (460–370 BC), whom we consider the Father of Western Medicine, tried many medical solutions for his own progressive hair loss. One of his medical formulas was a mixture of opium, horseradish, pigeon droppings, beetroot, and various spices that were applied to the head.

> Despite his yearnings for preserving his own hair, Hippocrates eventually lost it to the extent that today we refer to advanced male pattern baldness as "Hippocratic baldness."

In his collection of observations called the "Aphorisms of Hippocrates," Hippocrates noted that Persian Army eunuchs guarding the king's harem never experienced hair loss. He noticed that virile "hot blooded" men went bald, but since eunuchs were castrated, they lacked "hot blood" and therefore retained their hair.

Further elaborating on the subject, Greek philosopher and scientist Aristotle (384–322 BC) declared: "Of all animals, human being are the ones which go bald most noticeably;... . ...no one goes bald before the time of sexual intercourse, ... Women do not go bald because their nature is similar to that of children:... . Eunuchs, too, do not go bald, because of their transition into the female state."

> Despite Aristotle's brilliant intellect and excellent sense for observation, today, we know that with respect to baldness, he got a few points wrong.

Among animals, the male stump-tailed macaque (*Macaca arctoides*) has been recognized and used as a model for baldness, work pioneered by biologist William Montagna (1913–1994) and continued for the study of hair growth promoting agents by Hideo Uno from the Department of Pathology, Wisconsin Regional Primate Research Center, University of Wisconsin, USA.

With respect to the time at which balding starts manifesting, in 1999, Borelli and Trüeb originally reported androgenetic alopecia with prepuberal onset in a case study. The observation was confirmed by Antonella Tosti and co-workers at the Department of Dermatology, University of Bologna, in 2005, when they reported 20 cases of androgenetic alopecia in children.

Finally, in 1977, Hamburg dermatologist Ludwig delineated patterned hair loss in his seminal publication on the classification of the types of androgenetic alopecia occurring in the female sex, while Andrew Messenger and co-workers at Royal Hallamshire Hospital in Sheffield were the first to point out that hair loss was also possible in a state of hypogonadism.

> In ancient Rome, Julius Caesar's (100–44 BC) hairline was receding as his empire was expanding. Caesar's protégée and consort, Egyptian Queen Cleopatra (69–30 BC), allegedly concocted a mixture of ground horse teeth and deer marrow to help out his receding hairline and did so to save her beloved from being ridiculed since his name *caesar* means "head of hair" in Latin.

Though there was no genuine Roman medicine, apart from superstition and Cato the Elder's (234–149 BC) recommendation to eat cabbage to keep healthy, it was in ancient Rome that Greek medicine flourished to an extent to have a profound influence on the future history of Western medicine.

Galen of Pergamon (129–200) was arguably the most accomplished of all medical researchers of antiquity, and it was only in the sixteenth century that Belgian anatomist and physician Andreas Vesalius (1514–1564) challenged his authority. Galen's understanding of medicine was principally influenced by the then-current theory of *humorism*, a now discredited theory of the makeup and workings of the human body, positing that an excess or deficiency of any of four distinct bodily fluids (blood, yellow bile, black bile, phlegm) in a person directly influences their temperament and health. Nonetheless, the idea is somewhat reminiscent of the role of our hormones. It was not until German physiologist and zoologist Arnold Adolf Berthold's (1803–1861) groundbreaking experiments, performed with chicken castration in 1949 demonstrating the role of the gonads in the development of secondary sexual characteristics of roosters, that we have begun to recognize the existence and function of the endocrine system. Very similar to Berthold's experiments on roosters, in 1942 Dr. James B. Hamilton observed that men who were castrated before puberty did not develop androgenetic alopecia and that androgenetic alopecia can be triggered in castrated men by injecting testosterone.

> Since Aristotle first noted that maleness and sexual maturity were required for balding, it was not until Hamilton's observations on men deprived of testicular androgens by castration that androgens were established beyond doubt to be prerequisites for the development of common baldness.

Byzantium represents the natural continuation of the Greco–Roman civilization from the time Constantine the Great (272–337) transferred the capital of the Roman Empire to Constantinople in 324, until 1453, when it fell to the Ottomans. Byzantium was not only a religious state of holy men; it had a bustling social life with the Byzantine people paying special attention to their appearance. The Byzantine physicians dealt especially with the speciality of dermatology and paid special attention also to the topic of cosmetics, including the condition and color of the hair.

Orabasius of Pergamum (325–403) recommended for the treatment of continual falling of hair preparations containing maidenhair (πολυτριχον in Greek, which means "many haired"), ladanum, wine, and oil of myrtle.

Alexander of Tralles (525–605) believed that the causes of hair loss were numerous, including lack of supply of nutritious substances and dense or few pores, and suggested baths and a special dietetic regime, prohibiting salt, heavy food, and excess of wine or of sex.

For the increase of hair growth, Paul of Aegina (625–690) suggested an injunction prepared from dried stomach of hare, leaves from the top of myrtle, bramble, maidenhair, and acacia, all finely chopped and sieved, with the addition of fat from bears and seals, and preserved in a lead container.

In European history, the Medieval period began in the fifth and lasted until the fifteenth century. It began with the collapse of the Western Roman Empire and merged into the early modern period. Knowledge was hard to come by in Medieval times, especially during the Dark Ages when barbarian tribes invaded western Europe. Since many of the books of the Greeks and Romans were lost, the knowledge they contained was replaced by mere speculation and superstition. Even when the universities developed with famous medical schools at Montpellier, Bologna and Salerno, lectures were rudimentary and largely referred to the authoritative scriptures of Galen that were endorsed by the Church that did not see any need to investigate any further. Although the ideas of Galen might have been debated, any new idea was judged on the debating skills of the scholar and not on scientific proof. Geoffrey Chaucer (1343–1400) gives a vivid picture of the Medieval Doctor in his "Canterbury Tales":

> A Doctor too emerged as we proceeded.
> No one alive could talk as well as he did
> On points of medicine and of surgery
> For, being grounded in astronomy
> He watched his patient's favourable star
> And, by his Natural Magic, knew what are
> The lucky hours and planetary degrees
> For making charms and effigies.
> The cause of every malady you'd got
> He knew, and whether dry, cold, moist or hot;
> He knew their seat, their humour and condition.
> He was a perfect practicing physician.
> All his apothecaries in a tribe
> Were ready with the drugs he would prescribe
> And each made money from the other's guile
> (They had been friendly for a goodish while)

He was well-versed in Aesculapius too
And what Hippocrates and Rufus knew
And Dioscurides now dead and gone,
Galen and Rhazes, Hali, Serapion.
In blood-red garments, slashed with bluish-grey
And lined with taffeta, he rode his way;
Yet he was rather close as to expenses
And kept the gold he won in pestilences. (ca. 1387)

Ignorance on the part of Medieval doctors led to numerous misunderstandings and errors. Even eminent personalities, such as Florentine professor of medicine, Taddeo Alderotti (1215–1295), who had incorporated Aristotelian natural philosophy into medical teaching and raised the status of medicine as an academic discipline, claimed, for example, that combing the hair comforts the brain.

Noteworthy are also the artistic depictions of the popular hairstyles at the time. Especially in the later half of the fifteenth century and well into the sixteenth century, the hair was shaved around the hairline or plucked at the temples and the nape of the neck, reminiscent to today's dermatologist of such pathologies as congenital triangular alopecia, ophiasis, or the more recently described frontal fibrosing alopecia (Fig. 1.2). Depictions of King Henry V of England (1387–1422) show a hairstyle particularly reminiscent of male frontal fibrosing alopecia.

The first genuine scientific studies on hair probably began when Antoni van Leeuwenhoek (1632–1723) first observed the hair shaft under the microscope, and Marcello Malpighi (1628–1694) described the anatomy of the hair follicle in his treatise *De pilii*.

And yet, nothing was understood of the biology of hair growth. In early seventeenth century, a symposium held at the *Accademia dei Fisiocratici* in Siena on *De capelli e peli* ("on hair and skin") confirmed the ancient Roman superstition that snake poison, released occasionally into the air, was detrimental to the hair. Ultimately, the physicians unanimously agreed that *miasmi pestiferi*, the ancient equivalent of today's air pollution, was the cause for hair loss.

Evidence for irrational fears of this kind can be traced until today: institutes and apothecaries offer hair analyses in relation to the environment or amalgam tooth fillings and offer treatments for detoxification.

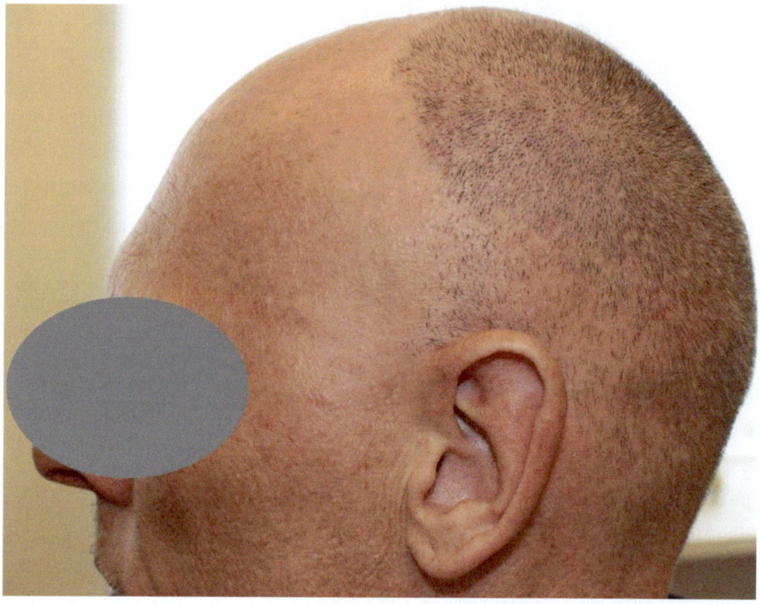

Fig. 1.2 Male frontal fibrosing alopecia, reminiscent of male hairstyle in the fifteenth century, when the hair was shaved around the hairline or plucked at the temples and the napes of the neck

A study conducted 1979 by Pierard reported diffuse alopecia related to ingestion of toxic metals in 36 of 78 patients with diffuse alopecia. Copper was involved in 17 alopecias, arsenic in 12, mercury in five, and cadmium in two. Copper intoxication was found to be related to ingestion of tap water containing a high concentration of copper salts, presumably from low pH, presence of chelating agents, or connection of electrical ground wires to copper water pipes, which caused sufficient flow of electrical current to ionize the metal.

In a study on complaints related to amalgam fillings performed by Lindberg et al. in 1994, assays of mercury in urine samples of patients indicated that exposure was far below the levels at which symptoms could be indicated by psychometric tests. On the other hand, psychological investigation indicated that the symptoms were psychosomatic. All patients had experienced important psychic traumata in close correlation with the first appearance of symptoms.

> The 1800 s were the heyday of the "snake oil" salesman. Patent medicines originated in England, where a patent was originally granted to Richard Stoughton's Elixir in 1712, but it was not until the 1906 Food and Drugs Act that there was federal regulation in the USA concerning safety and effectiveness of drugs.

For the next hundred years, bottles of hair loss cures were advertised for sale with names like (in alphabetical order): "Absalom Hair Restorer" (1879); "Acheson's Hair Generator" (1876) with the claim to restore the color to the hair, remove and prevent dandruff, cause the hair to grow, and prevent its falling out; "Adams' Hairlife," a specific for falling hair and positive cure for dandruff on the basis of sage quinine and jaborandi compound; "Professor Adler's Crown Hair Grower" (1906–1916); "Aetherian Hair Fluid" (1853–1870); "Ajax Hair Renewer"; "Alcanna". Alcanna is an Egyptian plant used to make dyes; "Alexander's Tricobaphe" (1845); "Alibert's Oleaginous Hair Tonic." Dr. Alibert was a chemist from Paris. The preparation was sold in the USA starting around 1838 allegedly prepared from a recipe from the celebrated Dr. Alibert of Paris, by one of his pupils. The term oleaginous pertained to olive oil, the actual root usage: "Bachelor's Oriental Hair Tonic" (1863); "Bachman's Teutonic Hair Grower" (1895); "Baldine Hair Renewer" (1898); "Baldpate Hair Tonic" (1914–1921) with the claim to nourish and strengthen hair follicles and promote hair growth: "Bearsch's Hair Restorative" (1872) with the claim to be a highly effective as well as harmless and agreeable liquid preparation for the restoration and preservation of the hair. To make the concoction, Bearsch would do the following:

1. Boil 1/2 peck of roasted, sliced, white onions and 10 oz of burdock root in 1 gal of white rum for about an hour, and filter it when cool.
2. Boil 1 pint of pine-tar with a gallon of water for about 15 min; when cooled, add this to the first mixture.
3. Add 1 gal of alcohol, 2 oz of cajeput oil, 1 oz of rosemary oil, 2 oz of bergamot oil, 1 oz of spirits of ammonia, 6 drams of tincture of opium, and 6 drams of tincture of castoreum.
4. Add 2 more gallons of white rum and 1 lb of glycerine.

"Brigg's Excelsior Hair Vigor" (1880); "British Oleon for the Hair" (1862); "Brownell's Hair Tonic" (1891) with the claim to be a purely herbal preparation (Maidenhair), perfectly harmless, no dye, and to grow hair on bald heads; "Professor Butler's Hair Restorative" (1880); "Cabellina Azteca" (1907); "Callitriche Hair Tonic/Restorative" (1883) with the claim to prevent the hair from falling out or turning gray and to promote the growth of hair and beautify it in general. The preparation was composed of 37 % petroleum, 30 % bay rum, 24 % glycerine, 4 % borax, and 2 % oil of bergamot; "Carney's Liquid Marrow" (1856); "St. Clair's Hair Lotion" (1896); "Cranitonic Hair Food" (1900–1915); "Crook's Hair Restorer" (1890) consisting of 2 oz of coal tar, 2 oz of soft soap, 1/2 ounce of washing soda, 2 oz of beef grease, 8 oz of beef gall, 1 1/2 ounces of water, and some suitable scent; "the Dandy Hair Tonic" (1889); "Davis' Hyperion (for the Hair)" (1851); "Emig's Hair Invigorator" (1878) with the claim of invigorating and promoting the growth of the hair of the head. The preparation was made by crushing or grinding about 1/2 bushel of white oak bark, soaking it in 7 gal of kerosene oil for about 6 weeks. After the time has elapsed, the oil was drawn off and strained, and a suitable perfume was added. "Eureka Hair Restorative" (1892); "Fish's Infallible Hair Restorative" (1859–1863); "Fletcher's Turkish Hair Tonic" (1875–1888); "Frewin's Hair Restorative" (1896 and 1901) with the claim to grow hair after 30 years baldness; "Hans Glenck's Hair Tonic" (1889) with the claim to make hair grow, prevent it from falling off, remove and prevent scurf and dandruff, preserve the hair in a healthy condition, and keep the scalp in a perfectly healthy condition. The preparation was composed of one pint of approximately 45 % grape alcohol, mixed with 2 oz of the extract of rotten apples; "Harlene" (1883). In 1912, the Parliament of the Commonwealth of Australia published a series of articles titled: *Secret Remedies – What They Cost and What They Contain*, which were analyses of patent medicines by the British Medical Association. They found Harlene to consist of 93 % water, 6 % alcohol, 5 % borax, 4 % glycerine, 1 % ammonia, and traces of other ingredients; "Hirsutine Hair and Beard Grower" (1884) with the claim to be the only infallible hair and beard grower; "Barker's Hirsutus" (1881); "Dr. Hufeland's Celebrated Hair Remedy" (1840); "Johnson's (Josiah) Hair Restorative" (1872), a compound made of 1 lb ashes of willow, 1 lb ashes of leather, one-half pound cocoanut, 4 lb butter, 2 lb tallow, and one quart white grape wine. The whole mixture was scented with bergamot or any other suitable perfume, and after the ingredients had been thoroughly mixed, the compound was boiled down to the consistency of pomatum, put up in suitable boxes, ready for market; "Kephalia" (1835); "Kreml Hair Tonic" (1928); "Dr Leon's Electric Hair Renewer" (1866); "Libbey's Indian Hair Restorative" (1866) for restoring hair lost from sickness, from a scalp diseased by morbid humors, or any unnatural heat in the head. In the case of those prematurely bald, and in many where the hair appears to have naturally fallen off through age, they may rely on a renewed, thick, and heavy growth; "Louck's Hair Restorative" (1864) compounded olive or sweet oil, tincture of *Lobelia inflata*, *Cypripedium pubescens*, and *Agrimonia Eupatoria*; "Lount's Hair Treatment" (1869) for straightening, softening, and renewing the human hair. The preparation was made by combining the oil of wild cucumber, one-half pint, with 1 gal linseed oil, 4 lb beeswax, 4 lb spermaceti, and 4 lb white rosin; "Mann's Hair Luxuriant" (1872); "Mansfield's Capillaris" (1882–1930), warranted to cure all scalp diseases, to promote luxuriant hair, and prevent dandruff. It restores hair to the bald and causes it to grow out natural color in place of gray; "Marold's Hair Tonic" (1882) made by combining 2 1/2 pounds of hop root, 3 oz of grape vine buds, and 2 oz of rosemary with 1 gal of water. The ingredients were boiled for 2 h and then filtered prior to use; "Mrs. Mason's Indian Hair Tonic" (1901); "Dr. G. S. Moore's Scientific Hair Restorer" (1903); "Nature's Hair Restorative" (1869) consisting of 1 oz of hyposulfite of soda dissolved in 13 oz of soft water, two drams of carbonate of ammonia dissolved in 13 oz of soft water, and 2 drams of sulfate of protoxide of manganese dissolved in 13 oz of soft water, made in separate vessels, and then combined and mixed together. Finally, 2 oz of pure glycerine were added; "Oil of Celsus" (1936); "Olds' Celebrated Hair Grower" (1894); "The Progress Hair Wonder" (1908); "Rowland's Macassar Oil" (1888–1953); "Sears Eau De Quinine Hair Tonic" (1902 and 1909); "Skookum Root Hair Grower" (1891); "Dr. Water's Hair Restorer" (1878) warranted to restore the hair on the baldest head in 60 days; "Worthington's Hair Lotion" (1888) claiming to be an excellent remedy for curling the hair, removing dandruff, and increasing the growth of the hair. The preparation was made by the following steps:

1. Boil 12 oz of wild indigo in 1/2 gallon of water for 1 h.
2. In another vessel, boil 24 oz of sweet-flag in 1 1/2 gallons of water for 1 h.
3. In a third vessel, boil 12 oz of wild dandelions, 8 oz of red pepper (in the pod), and 7 oz of lavender flower in 1 1/2 gallons of water for 1 h.
4. Mix the ingredients in the three vessells, and boil together until reduced to about 2 gal.
5. Add 1 quart of alcohol, to prevent fermentation.
6. Add perfume if desired.

All ingredients except the red pepper must be pulverized first.

With the advance of medical technologies in the industrial ages from 1905 on, vacuum caps, gas-filled clear glass combs, and actinic quartz ray bulbs joined the repertory of treatments alleged to help stimulate the follicles to grow hair.

Probably the first sound scientific attempt toward hair restoration was the demonstration that it was possible to transplant hair from a hair-bearing to a non-hair-bearing area in 1822 by German medical student Johann Friedrich Dieffenbach (1792–1847).

Dieffenbach's enthusiasm for tedious and technical pursuits led him to explore the regenerative capacity of transplanted hair, experimenting on himself, poking holes in his arm, and then inserting hair follicles from his head by the use of goose quills as trephines to bore out hair-bearing pieces of skin. Dieffenbach eventually summarized his findings in his doctoral thesis, *Nonnulla de Regeneratione et de Transplantatione*. But it was not until 1939 that the era of hair transplants began with the efforts of Shoji Okuda and later H. Tamura (1943) and K. Fujita (1953) who practiced in Japan. Okuda developed a circular scalpel for the purpose of transplanting hair into areas of alopecia, but his efforts did not receive the deserved attention at the time, while Tamura and Fujita worked to restore pubic hair and eyebrows, respectively.

Finally, in 1959 New York dermatologist Norman Orentreich established the theory of "donor dominance" of the hair transplant. The basis of the theory was that plugs of hair follicles taken from the occipital scalp would continue growing when moved to the balding frontal scalp because those hair follicles were genetically programmed to do so.

The concept became the foundation for the entire ensuing field of hair restoration surgery. For the following decades, dedicated surgeons all over the globe have worked on refining the method with today close to natural results.

1.3 The Modern Age

The dawn of the modern age can be placed with the clinical studies performed with topical minoxidil and oral finasteride. With respect to the study design and criteria for efficacy and safety, they have set the standards for any agent with the claim of promoting hair growth.

For the first time in 4,000 years of history, a medication has been scientifically proven to stop hair loss due to androgenetic alopecia and to promote hair growth. Minoxidil was serendipitously discovered to be a hair growth promoting agent, when patient taking the compound orally for treatment of arterial hypertensions developed generalized hypertrichosis. While minoxidil was developed for treatment of hypertension, and this feature of the drug's action was best understood, its mechanism of action on hair growth was poorly understood. Only recently, with the discovery of the mutation underlying *hypertrichotic osteochondrodysplasia* or *Cantu's syndrome* (MIM 239850), light has been shed on the molecular basis of the action of minoxidil. In Cantu's syndrome, the hypertrichosis leads to thick scalp hair extending onto the forehead and a general increase in body hair. It is caused by a mutation in the ABCC9 gene on chromosome 12p12. Interestingly, the gene codes for sulfonylurea receptor 2, involved in ATP-sensitive potassium channels, while minoxidil has been known to be a potassium-channel opener, with evidence that this effect is mediated by sulfonylurea receptor 2B. Minoxidil promotes hair growth through increasing the duration of anagen. It causes hair follicles at rest to grow and enlarges suboptimal follicles. Clinical trials were established to prove to the US Food and Drug Administration (FDA) the safety and efficacy of topical minoxidli for treatment of androgenetic alopecia, but it was not until

1988 that 2 % minoxidil lotion was approved by the FDA for treating hair loss.

In 1990, yet another medication was shown to reverse hair loss in men and to be even more effective than minoxidil in preventing baldness, oral finasteride. Finasteride is a competitive inhibitor of type 2 5α-reductase and inhibits the conversion of testosterone to dihydrotestosterone (DHT). The rationale for the use of finasteride to treat male androgenetic alopecia was based on the absence of androgenetic alopecia in men with congenital deficiency of type 2 5α-reductase and the presence of increased 5α-reductase activity and DHT levels in balding scalp. Since Aristotle first noted that "maleness" and sexual maturity were required for balding, it was not until 1942 that Hamilton's observations on men deprived of testicular androgens by castration established beyond doubt that androgens, in the form of testosterone or its metabolites, were prerequisites for development of male pattern baldness. The description of an unusual form of *incomplete male pseudohermaphroditism due to a genetic deficiency of the type 2 steroid 5α-reductase* by Imperato-McGinley et al. in 1974, implicated DHT as principal mediator of androgen-dependent hair loss: affected men, who are homozygous for mutation of the gene, do not develop androgenetic alopecia. The U.S. FDA originally approved finasteride for treatment of benign prostate hyperplasia. New clinical trials began to test the drug's safety and efficacy for treatment of male androgenetic alopecia. By 1998, 1 mg oral finasteride tablets became the second prescription drug approved by the FDA as a hair loss treatment for men.

Although testing medical interventions for efficacy had existed since the time of Avicenna's (980–1037) "The Canon of Medicine" in the eleventh century, it was only in the twentieth century that this effort evolved to impact almost all fields of health care and policy. In 1967, American physician and mathematician Alvan R. Feinstein (1925–2001) published his seminal work "Clinical Judgment", which together with Archie Cochrane's (1909–1988) celebrated book "Effectiveness and Efficiency" (1972) led to an increasing acceptance of clinical epidemiology and controlled studies during the 1970s and 1980s and prepared the way for the institutional development of evidence-based medicine (EBM) in the 1990s. EBM aims for the ideal that health-care professionals should make conscientious, explicit, and judicious use of the best available evidence gained from the scientific method to clinical decision making. It seeks to assess the strength of the evidence of risks and benefits of diagnostic tests and treatments, using techniques from science, engineering, and statistics, such as the systematic review of medical literature, meta-analysis, risk–benefit analysis, and randomized controlled trials.

As EBM guidelines on hair loss are rare, a European consensus group was recently constituted to develop guidelines for treatment of androgenetic alopecia. The European consensus group conducted a systematic literature review in Medline, Embase and Cochrane databases until August 2008. 1370 publications were found, 51 added by hand search. 85 publications fulfilled the following inclusion criteria for the guideline: prospective study with a number of patients ≥20 (no minimal patient number required in twin studies), age ≥12 years, and with confirmed diagnosis of androgenetic alopecia (diagnosis either clinically or by further diagnostic evaluations, e.g., trichogram, TrichoScan, biopsy). Objective outcome measure of efficacy described for drug therapy was mean change from baseline hair count in target area or measurement of hair growth/loss in target area by global photography.

> The guideline revealed excellent evidence levels for the therapeutic use of topical minoxidil and oral finasteride, low evidence levels for hormonal treatments (in women), and insufficient, respectively, lacking evidence for a broad panel of miscellaneous treatments available claiming effectiveness (Table 1.3).

Table 1.3 Overview of miscellaneous treatments with insufficient or lacking evidence for efficacy and proposed mechanisms of action in treatment of hair loss

Promotion of hair regrowth:	Amino acids
	Iron supplements in absence of deficiency
	Vitamins (biotin, niacin derivatives)
	Proanthocyanidines
	Millet seed (silic acid, aminoacids, vitamines, minerals)
	Marine extract and silicea component
	Chinese herbals
	Ginkgo biloba
	Aloe vera
	Ginseng
	Bergamot
	Hibiscus
	Sorphora
	Caffeine
	Melatonin
	Retinoids
	Ciclosporine
	Electromagnetic/-static field
	Low level laser
Improved perifollicular vascularisation:	Prostaglandins (viprostol, latanoprost)
	Aminexil
	Glyceroloxyesters and silicium
	Minerals
	Niacin derivatives
	Mesotherapy
DHT-inhibitory activity:	Saw palmetto
	ß-sitosterol
	Polysorbate 60
	Green tea
	Cimicifuga racemosa
Anti-inflammatory activity:	Ketoconazole
	Zinc pyrithione
	Corticosteroids
Improved hair nutrition:	Vitamines (biotin, niacin derivates)
	Trace elements (zinc, copper)
Others:	Botulinum toxin

From: Blumeyer A et al (2011) Evidence-based (S3) guideline for the treatment of androgenetic alopecia in women and in men. J Dtsch Dermatol Ges 9(Suppl 6):S1–S57

The postmodern age is heralded by the studies of Amanda Reynolds and Colin Jehoda, who, in 1999, reported that human follicle cells can be induced to grow in an incompatible host of the other sex. Reminiscent of Dieffenbach's experiments, Jahoda microdissected dermal sheath tissue from the base of his own scalp skin follicles and implanted the tissue into shallow skin wounds on the inner forearm of Reynolds, a genetically unrelated and immunologically incompatible female recipient. All the wound sites healed rapidly and lacked any overt inflammatory reaction. Remarkably, each of the sites of dermal-sheath implantation produced new follicles and hair fibers 3–5 weeks after the graft. None of the new follicles showed evidence of rejection when biopsied, and histology confirmed that the new follicles were morphologically normal. The DNA extracted from the papilla cells and analyzed had an X and Y complement and was therefore male, whereas cells taken from other regions of the same follicle and epidermis had only X chromosomes and hence were female. The reason why the graft was not rejected probably lies within the tissue itself, with the lowermost tissues of hair follicles having a special immune status. This experiment demonstrated how adult cells with inductive properties might be used in tissue and organ engineering and, more immediately, in novel treatments of hair loss.

In 1998, Angela Christiano and co-workers reported the identification of a missense mutation in the zinc finger domain of the hairless (HR) gene (arg620 to gln) on chromosome 8p21.3 underlying (congenital universal) atrichia with papular lesions (MIM 209500) and paved the way to targeted gene therapy through the identification of genes relevant to hair growth. Almost complete absence of hair associated with papular lesions over most of the body are features of the disorder. Patients are born with hair that falls out and is not replaced. Histological studies show cystic malformation of the hair follicles. Although the identification of the HR gene has been shown not to be relevant with respect to the most frequent cause of hair loss and its treatment, androgenetic alopecia, and published estimates of the prevalence of congenital atrichia with papular lesions remain surprisingly low considering

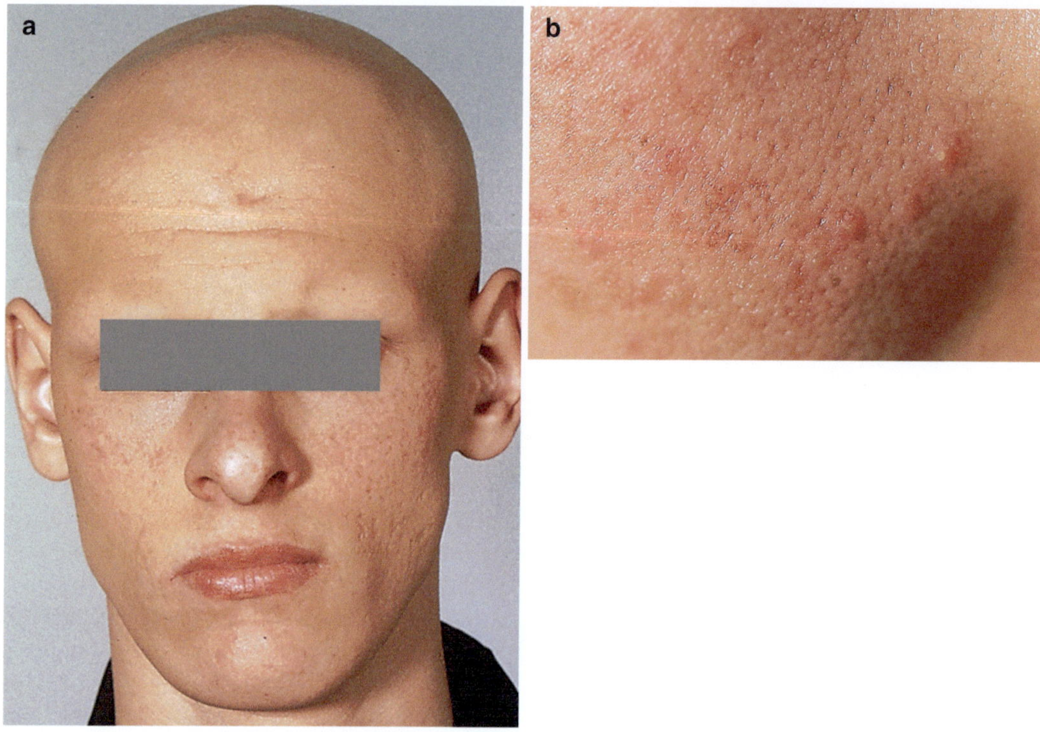

Fig. 1.3 (**a**) Patient with (congenital universal) atrichia with papular lesions, mistaken for years for (autoimmune) alopecia (areata) universalis. (**b**) Note associated papular lesions of the face

pathogenetic mutations of the HR gene have been found in distinct populations around the world. Therefore, some experts have assumed that the disorder might be more common than previously thought and frequently mistaken for the autoimmune form of alopecia (areata) universalis and suggested that infants with presumed autoimmune alopecia universalis may warrant testing for HR gene mutations, particularly before embarking on therapeutic modalities that will fail (Fig. 1.3a, b).

Ultimately, the feasibility of targeted selective gene therapy of the hair follicle was demonstrated in 1995 by Robert Hoffman and coworker. They developed a histoculture of intact hair-growing skin on sponge-gel matrices and found that liposomes can selectively target hair follicles to deliver both small and large molecules in histocultured skin. Previously they had introduced the technique of entrapping DNA in liposomes for use in gene therapy. Finally, they reported the selective targeting of the lacZ reporter gene to the hair follicles in mice after topical application of the gene entrapped in liposomes.

In summary, as early as can be traced, written documents testify endeavors shown by mankind to preserve or restore hair. Nevertheless, it is only recently that we have been witnessing substantial advances in the understanding of hair biology and its pathologic conditions. Continuous progress is being made at a high pace thanks to the impetus of a generation of astute clinical trichologists and basic scientists interested in hair biology, the powerful tools of molecular biology, and innovative technologies. Across the globe, Hair Research Societies have evolved (Australasian Hair and Wool Research Society, www.ahwrs.org.au; European Hair Research Society, www.ehrs.org; The Hair Research Society of India, www.inhrs.org; The Korean Hair Research Society, www.khrs.or.kr; The Society of Hair Research (Japan), www.tokyo-med.ac.jp/derma/shsr; North American Hair Research Society, www.nahrs.org) and regularly bring together enthusiastic scientists and clinicians for the exchange and discussion of the advances in hair research and clinics, in the fields of genetics, molecular biology, immunology, aging, neurobiology, psychosomatics, stem cells, and tissue engineering research.

At a recent meeting of the Hair Research Society of India (2012), the theme of the meeting was "To Abolish Quackery in Trichology." The congress proved worthy of its ambition, both in terms of the scientific quality and integrity of the contributions of both established authorities and young upcoming scientists and in terms of the fairness in the debates on the subject.

The consensus was that good medical practice in clinical trichology aims at:

- Understanding the hair patient on an emotional level and the medical problem on a technical level
- Delivering sound patient education and effective trichologic therapy
- Representing trichology as a discipline based on evidence from science, engineering, and statistics
- Setting standards of good medical practice in trichology
- Supporting progress in trichology through continuous medical education
- Abolishing quackery in trichology

Further Reading

Symbolism of Male Hair

Berg C (1951) The unconscious significance of hair. G. Allen and Unwin.

http://www.latimes.com/features/image/la-ig-mens-hairstyle-timeline-photos,0,7486612.photogallery

http://en.wikipedia.org/wiki/Hair_(musical)

http://en.wikipedia.org/wiki/Hairstyle

http://en.wikipedia.org/wiki/Long_hair

https://en.wikipedia.org/wiki/New_Romanticism

http://en.wikipedia.org/wiki/Punk

http://en.wikipedia.org/wiki/Skinhead

Opler M (1972) Social conceptions of deviance. In: Resnik H, Wolfgang M (eds) Sexual behaviors: social, clinical, and legal aspects. Little Brown and Co., Boston

Trüeb RM, de Viragh PA, Swiss Trichology Study Group (2001) Status of scalp hair and therapy of alopecia in men in Switzerland. Praxis (Bern 1994) 90:241–248

Weitz R (2004) Rapunzel's daughters: what Women's hair tells us about women's lives. Farrar, Straus & Giroux, New York

Brief History of Experiments on Hair Loss Cures

Aronso JK, Ramachandran M (2009) The diagnosis of art: Van Gogh and male pattern baldness. J R Soc Med 102:32–33

Borelli S, Trüeb RM (1999) Androgenetic alopecia with prepuberal onset? Dermatology 199:96

Cash TF (2001) He psychology of hair loss and its implications for patient care. Clin Dermatol 19:161–166

Fujita K (1953) Reconstruction of the eyebrows (in Japanese). La Lepro 22:364

Giacometti L (1967) Facts, legends, and myths about the scalp throughout history. Arch Dermatol 95:629–631

Girman CJ, Rhodes T, Lilly FR et al (1998) Effects of self-perceived hair loss in a community sample of men. Dermatology 197:223–229

Hamilton JB (1942) Male hormone stimulation is prerequisite and an incitement in common baldness. Am J Anat 71:451

http://www.hairraisingstories.com/

Hughes GR (1959) The cosmetic arts in ancient Egypt. J Soc Cosm Chem 10:159–163

Lambert G (1961) The conquest of baldness. The wonderful story of hair. Souvenir Press, London

Lambert G (1963) The retorts of the alchemists. The Miami News, Apr 4

Lascarotos J, Tsiamis C, Lascaratos G, Stavraineas NG (2004) The roots of cosmetic medicine: hair cosmetics in Byzantine times (AD 324–1453). Int J Dermatol 43:397–401

Lindberg NE, Lindberg E, Larsson G (1994) Psychologic factors in the etiology of amalgam illness. Acta Odontol Scand 52:219–228

Ludwig E (1977) Classification of the types of androgenetic alopecia (common baldness) occurring in the female sex. Br J Dermatol 97:247–254

Okuda S (1939) Clinical and experimental studies on transplanting of living hair (in Japanese). Jpn J Dermatol 46:135–138

Orentreich N (1959) Autografts in alopecias and other selected dermatological conditions. Ann N Y Acad Sci 83:463

Orme S, Cullen DR, Messenger AG (1999) Diffuse female hair loss: are androgens necessary? Br J Dermatol 141:521–523

Pierard G (1979) Toxic effects of metals from the environment on hair growth and structure. J Cutan Pathol 6:237–242

Rita S (2003) Aristotle's philosophy of science. Global Vision Publishing House, Delhi

Siemens HW (1952) Alopecia triangularis und Ophiasis als Schönhietsideal. Hautarzt 3:270–273

Tamura H (1943) Pubic hair transplantation. Jpn J Dermatol 53:76

Tosti A, Iorizzo M, Piraccini BM (2005) Androgenetic alopecia in children: report of 20 cases. Br J Dermatol 152:556–559

Trüeb RM (1998) Von der Hippokratischen Glatze zum Gen-Shampoo: Fortschritte der Trichologie im Jahrtausendwechsel. Akt Dermatol 24:101–107

Trüeb RM, Swiss Trichology Study Group (2001) The value of hair cosmetics and pharmaceuticals. Dermatology 202:275–282

van Neste D (2010) Aging from where to there? In: Trüeb RM, Tobin DJ (eds) Aging hair. Springer Scientific Publications, Berlin, p vii

www.hairdoc.com/book/Chapter_05_hair_loss_answers.pdf

The Modern Age

Ahmad W, Faiyaz ul Haque M, Brancolini V, Tsou HC, Ul Haque S, Lam H, Aita VM, Owen J, deBlaquiere M, Frank J, Cserhalmi-Friedman PB, Leask A, McGrath JA, Peacocke M, Ahmad M, Ott J, Christiano AM (1998) Alopecia universalis associated with a mutation in the human hairless gene. Science 279:720–724

Blumeyer A, Tosti A, Messenger A, Reygagne P, Del Marmol V, Spuls PI, Trakatelli M, Finner A, Kiesewetter F, Trüeb R, Rzany B, Blume-Peytavi U, European Dermatology Forum (EDF) (2011) Evidence-based (S3) guideline for the treatment of androgenetic alopecia in women and in men. J Dtsch Dermatol Ges 9(Suppl 6):S1–S57

Cochrane AL (1972) Effectiveness and efficiency: random reflections on health services. Nuffield Provincial Hospitals Trust, London

Feinstein AR (1967) Clinical judgement. Williams & Wilkins, Baltimore

Harakalova M, van Harssel JJT, Terhal PA, van Lieshout S, Duran K, Renkens I, Amor DJ, Wilson LC, Kirk EP, Turner CLS, Shears D, Garcia-Minaur S et al (2012) Dominant missense mutations in ABCC9 cause Cantu syndrome. Nat Genet 44:793–796

Henn W, Zlotogorski A, Lam H, Martinez-Mir A, Zaun H, Christiano AM (2002) Atrichia with papular lesions resulting from compound heterozygous mutations in the hairless gene: a lesson for differential diagnosis of alopecia universalis. J Am Acad Dermatol 47:519–523

http://en.wikipedia.org/wiki/Evidence-based_medicine

Hillmer AM, Kruse R, Betz RC, Schumacher J, Heyn U, Propping P, Nothen MM, Cichon S (2001) Variant 1859G-A (arg620 to gln) of the 'hairless' gene: absence of association with papular atrichia or androgenetic alopecia. (Letter). Am J Hum Genet 69: 235–237

Imperato-McGinley J, Guerrero L, Gautier T, Peterson RE (1974) Steroid 5α-reductase deficiency in man: an inherited form of male pseudohermaphroditism. Science 186:1213–1215

Li L, Hoffman RM (1995) The feasibility of targeted selective gene therapy of the hair follicle. Nat Med 1:705–706

Li M, Marubayashi A, Nakaya Y et al (2001) Minoxidil-induced hair growth is mediated by adenosine in cultured dermal papilla cells: possible involvement of sulfonylurea receptor 2B as a target of minoxidil. J Invest Dermatol 117:1594–1600

Reynolds AJ, Lawrence C, Cserhalmi-Friedman PB, Christiano AM, Jahoda CA (1999) Trans-gender induction of hair follicles. Nature 402:33–34

Trüeb RM (2009) Twenty years of European hair research society. Int J Trichology 1:2

Trüeb RM (2012) Hair India 2012: a letter of appreciation. Int J Trichology 4:235

Examining Hair Loss in Men

2

Observe, record, tabulate, communicate. Use your five senses.
Learn to see, learn to hear, learn to feel, learn to smell,
and know that by practice alone you can become expert.

Sir William Osler (1849–1919)

As with any medical problem, the male patient complaining of hair loss requires a comprehensive medical and drug history, physical examination of the hair and scalp, and, as indicated, appropriate laboratory evaluation to identify the cause. The clinician also has a host of diagnostic techniques that enable classification of the patient's disorder as a shedding disorder or a decreased density disease and documentation of true pathology or only perceived pathology.

Prerequisite for delivering appropriate patient care is an understanding of the underlying pathologic dynamics of hair loss and a potential multitude of cause relationships. By approaching the hair loss patient in a methodical way, and commencing with objects the simplest and easiest to recognize, and ascending step by step, to the knowledge of the more complex, an individualized treatment plan can be designed.

It must be borne in mind that hair loss may result from a combination of factors rather than from a single cause effect. In that case, all factors need to be addressed simultaneously for success. Therefore, it is wise to divide each of the difficulties under examination into as many parts as possible, and as might be necessary for its adequate solution, and finally to make enumerations so complete, and reviews so general, so that nothing is omitted, that might compromise success. For this purpose it is advisable to design a hair database sheet that enables a complete record of collected data.

2.1 Patient History

History taking is of paramount importance in assessing hair loss. By careful and systematic questioning, it is possible to assess the factors pertinent to differential diagnosis and particular lines of further investigation.

In the course of history taking, it is advisable never to accept anything as true, neither from the patient nor from the referring physician, which is not clearly recognizable as such; that is to say, carefully avoid precipitancy and prejudice and comprise nothing more in one's judgement than what is presented to the mind so clearly and distinctly as to exclude all grounds of doubt.

2.1.1 Family History

A detailed family history relating to hair loss is pertinent to the diagnosis of genetic disorders.

While monogenic disorders are usually determined by one gene that has a strong influence on the phenotype, polygenic traits are likely to be determined by a large number of genes that confer variable levels of risk. Moreover, complex polygenic traits usually are not binary in nature, that is, the trait does not exist as one state or the other, such as affected or not affected. More so, the trait presents as a continuous variable that shows a normal distribution across a population. Ultimately, genetic sequence variation is not the only contributing factor that determines the trait.

R.M. Trüeb, W.-S. Lee, *Male Alopecia*,
DOI 10.1007/978-3-319-03233-7_2, © Springer International Publishing Switzerland 2014

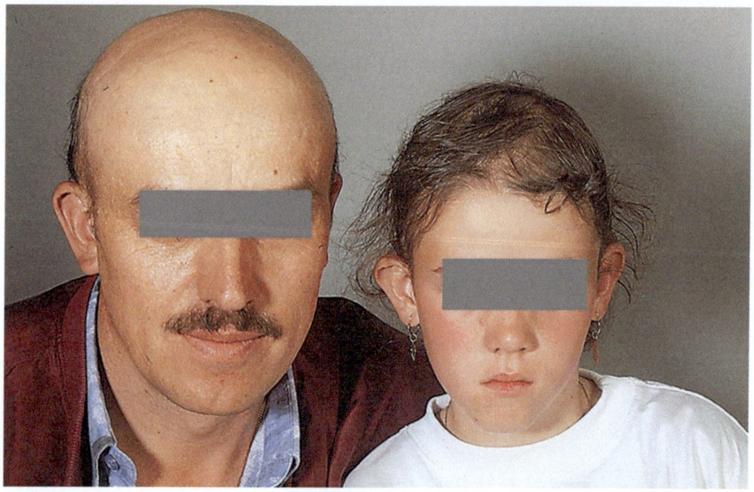

Fig. 2.1 Monogenic trait: hereditary hypotrichosis simplex in father and daughter

Environmental influences also play a role. It is this synergistic interplay between genes and environment that determines a complex phenotype.

Examples for a monogenic disorders leading to hair loss are hereditary hypotrichosis simplex and Marie Unna hereditary hypotrichosis:

Hereditary hypotrichosis simplex is a rare form hereditary hypotrichosis with no associated abnormality or hair shaft anomaly. Affected individuals typically show normal hair at birth, but diffuse hair loss and thinning of the hair shaft start during early childhood and progress with age (Fig. 2.1). In 2000, Baumer et al. reported on a three-generation Italian family with dominant transmission of a form of hereditary hypotrichosis simplex. The nine affected adults presented with sparse, thin, and short hair. Somewhat less sparse and longer hair was observed in the two affected young children in the third generation. The gene locus was mapped to 18p11.32–p11.23. The locus represented the first chromosome region shown to be associated with hereditary hypotrichosis simplex.

Marie Unna hereditary hypotrichosis is distinguished from hereditary hypotrichosis simplex by the presence of a peculiar twisting hair dystrophy. Characteristically coarse, wiry, twisted hairs develop in early childhood and are followed by the development of alopecia beginning in the crown area (Fig. 2.2a–d). The gene locus has been mapped to 8p21.3.

Monilethrix represents yet another monogenic disorder presenting with hair loss. As opposed to hereditary hypotrichosis, loss of hair is due to a hair shaft abnormality with fragility and breakage. It is due to a disorder of hair cortex keratin resulting in brittle hair that tends to fracture and produce varying degrees of alopecia. Individuals with monilethrix have normal hair at birth, but within the first few months of life, sometimes later, develop alopecia. In the mildest forms, only the occipital regions of the scalp are involved, due to friction; however, in severe forms the eyebrows, eyelashes, and secondary sexual hair may also be involved. Follicular hyperkeratosis with predilection for the nape of neck is a consistent feature that is particularly helpful for initially suspecting the diagnosis (Fig. 2.3a). Light microscopic examination is diagnostic and reveals elliptical nodes of normal thickness and intermittent constrictions at which the hair easily breaks (Fig. 2.3b). There may be spontaneous improvement with time, especially during puberty, but the condition never resolves completely. The gene locus has been mapped to 12q.13.13. An autosomal recessive form of *monilethrix-like congenital hypotrichosis* is caused by mutation in the desmoglein 4 gene. The clinical presentation is more severe than in the autosomal dominant form of monilethrix, with more extensive alopecia of the scalp, and body, and a papular

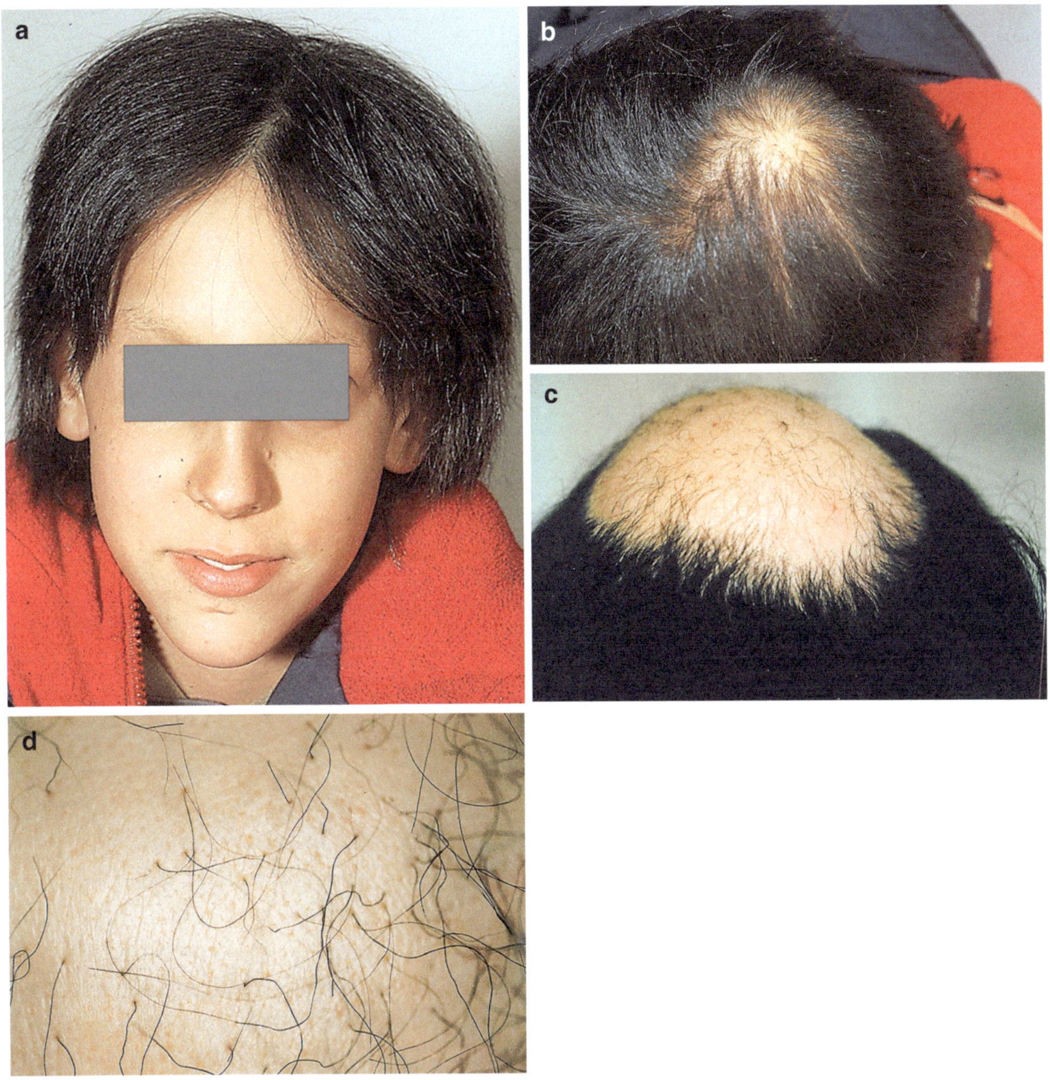

Fig. 2.2 Monogenic trait: Marie Unna hereditary hypotrichosis. (**a**) Coarse hair in child. (**b**) Initial vertex alopecia in child. (**c**) Established vertex alopecia in mother (With courtesy of M. Wyss, M.D.). (**d**) Twisting dystrophy of hair (With courtesy of M. Wyss, M.D.)

rash involving the extremities and periumbilical region.

In everyday clinical practice, we are usually dealing with *androgenetic alopecia* that represents a complex polygenic trait (Fig. 2.4a). The genetic involvement is pronounced, and the importance of genes concurs with marked racial differences in prevalence of androgenetic alopecia, with non-Caucasians exhibiting significantly less balding. The high frequency of androgenetic alopecia has complicated attempts to establish a mode of inheritance. The genes for type 1 and type 2 5α-reductase have been shown not to be associated with the inheritance of androgenetic alopecia. Polymorphism of the androgen receptor (AR) gene is associated with male pattern baldness; however, the AR gene is located on the X chromosome and does not explain the relatively strong concordance of the degree of baldness in fathers and sons. No specific gene has

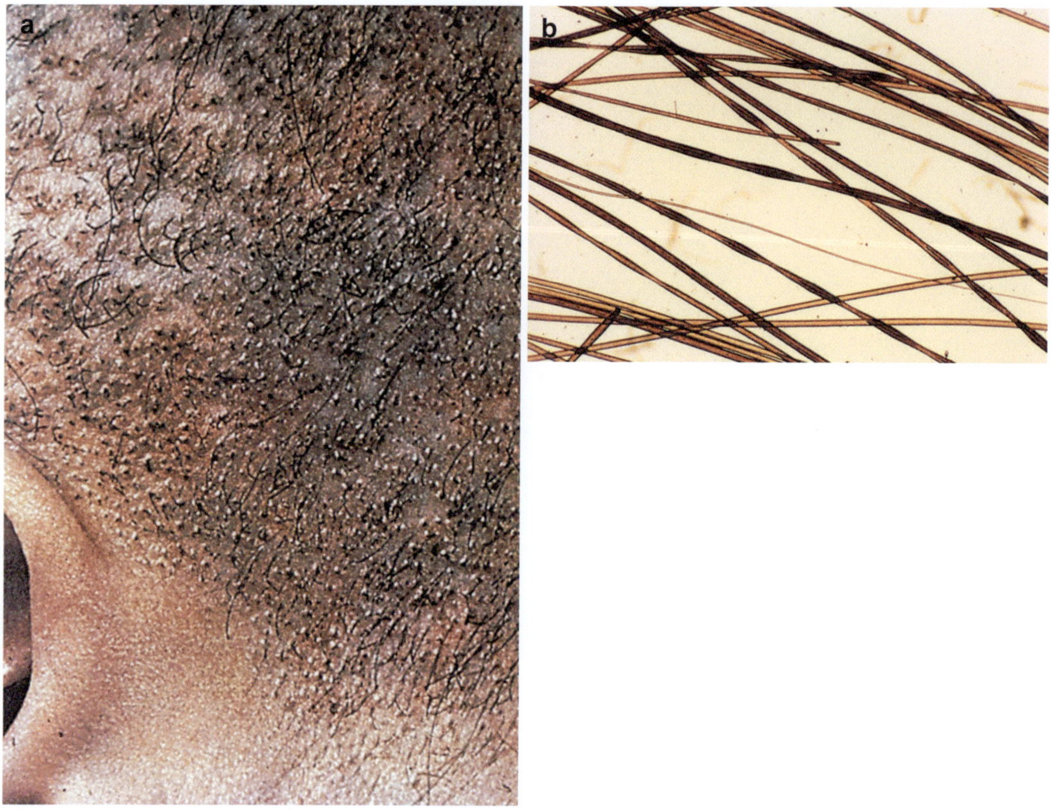

Fig. 2.3 Monogenic trait: monilethrix. (**a**) Follicular hyperkeratosis in the nape of neck. (**b**) Light microscopy: elliptical nodes of normal thickness and intermittent constrictions

been identified so far, though single gene mutations, such as abnormality of the AR, might be necessary, but not sufficient for the phenotype. Other genes relevant to androgens, including those on the Y chromosome, might also be examined. Since the enzyme steroid sulfatase (STS) converts dehydroepiandrosterone sulfate (DHEA-S) to dehydroepiandrosterone (DHEA) that is eventually metabolized to more potent androgens in the periphery, and elevated plasma levels of DHEA-S and DHEA have been reported to correlate with balding in young men, the hypothesis was advanced that men with genetic STS deficiency (X-linked recessive ichthyosis, XRI) do not or only develop minor forms of androgenetic alopecia. Trüeb and Meyer conducted a survey of patients with XRI and demonstrated that this is not the case, since these men also showed advanced androgenetic alopecia. Finally, epigenetic variations that are modifiable by the environment may contribute to striking phenotypic variations between individuals who have a similar genetic makeup. Trüeb reported a 52-year-old monozygotic male twin pair with striking dissimilarity with respect to the extent of vertex alopecia and speculated on the role of lifestyle factors. In summary, predisposition to male pattern balding is a polygenic trait, in which clinical expression represents a threshold effect.

> The risk of premature hair loss usually rises with the frequency and extent of the balding trait within first-degree relatives, while a negative family history does not exclude the diagnosis in a particular individual.

There is circumstantial evidence that *alopecia areata* represents yet another complex polygenic trait. Epidemiological studies provide

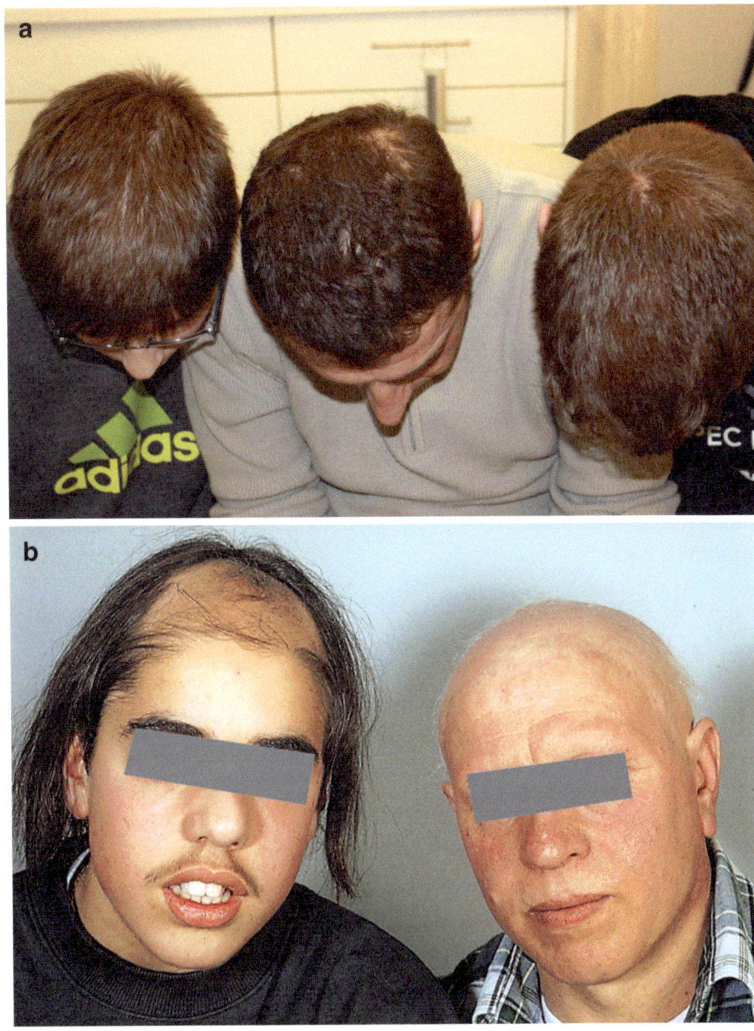

Fig. 2.4 Complex polygenic traits. (**a**) Androgenetic alopecia in father (*middle*) and sons. (**b**) Alopecia areata in son and father

evidence for involvement of alopecia areata susceptibility and severity genes. Alopecia areata with similar times of onset or similar hair loss patterns has been reported in monozygotic twins, and families with several generations of alopecia areata-affected individuals suggest the condition may be a genetically determined disease. Typically 10–20 % of patients with alopecia areata indicate at least one other affected family member (Fig. 2.4b). The triggers for the onset of alopecia areata may be environmental, but the resistance of the alopecia areata lesion to treatment, its persistence and regression, and its extent over the body may be influenced by the presence and interaction of multiple genes.

2.1.2 Personal History

The personal history encompasses on:

- Date of onset of the hair loss problem
- Periodicity of hair loss
- Rate of progression
- Previous investigations and treatments
- Present and past medical history
- Medications, incl. hormone active treatments (anabolics, replacement therapy)
- Associated symptoms relating to the general health status
- Associated symptoms relating to the condition of the scalp

Associated symptoms relating to the condition of the scalp are:

- Greasiness (seborrhoea)
- Dryness (sebostasis)
- Itchiness (pruritus)
- Dandruff
- Burning sensations or hair pain (trichodynia)
- Scratching habit (15 min of scratching will lead to breakage of hair)

In addition, a history of the following lifestyle factors that may impact the condition of hair should be taken:

- Dietary habits and alcohol abuse
- Stressful life events
- Sexual risk behavior and drug abuse (syphilis, HIV infection)
- Cigarette smoking
- UV exposure
- Hair care habits

Dietary Habits. The quantity and quality of hair are closely related to the nutritional state of an individual. Normal supply, uptake, and transport of proteins, calories, trace elements, and vitamins are of fundamental importance in tissues with a high biosynthetic activity such as the hair follicle. Because hair shaft is composed almost entirely of protein, protein component of diet is critical for production of normal healthy hair. The rate of mitosis is sensitive to the calorific value of diet, provided mainly by carbohydrates stored as glycogen in the outer hair root sheath of the follicle. Finally, a sufficient supply of vitamins and trace metals is essential for the biosynthetic and energetic metabolism of the follicle.

In instances of protein and calorie malnutrition, deficiency of essential amino acids, of trace elements, and of vitamins, hair growth and pigmentation may be impaired. In general, malnutrition is due to one or more of following factors: inadequate food intake, food choices that lead to dietary deficiencies, and illness that causes increased nutrient requirements, increased nutrient loss, poor nutrient absorption, or a combination of these factors.

It appears that on a typical Western diet, the hair follicle should have no problem in producing an appropriate hair shaft.

Nevertheless, vitamin and nutritional deficiencies are not uncommonly observed in adolescents feeding on "junk food," people on fad diets, alcoholics, the chronically ill, and especially common in the elderly population.

Iron deficiency is one of the most common of the nutritional deficiencies. Iron is present in all cells in the human body and has several vital functions. Examples include carrier of oxygen to the tissues in the form of hemoglobin, transport medium for electrons within the cells in the form of cytochromes, and integral part of enzyme reactions in various tissues. Total body iron is distributed among storage iron, transport iron, and functional iron. Storage iron is the body's iron reserves that are tissue bound and measured by serum ferritin concentration, transport iron is transported to the tissues and measured by transferrin concentration and saturation, and functional iron consists of iron that is bound to hemoglobin, myoglobin, and diverse enzymes. It is measured by hemoglobin concentration.

Iron deficiency is viewed as a continuum ranging from iron depletion to iron deficiency anemia. In the former, body iron stores are reduced, but functional and transport iron remain normal, leaving little reserves if the body requires more iron; in the latter, storage, transport, and functional iron are severely decreased and can lead to impaired function of multiple organ sites. The ultimate effect of iron deficiency is iron deficiency anemia when the body's stores of iron have been depleted and the body is unable to maintain levels of hemoglobin in the blood. Total body iron averages approximately 3.8 g in men.

Table 2.1 Symptoms of iron deficiency

Symptoms
Fatigue
Decreased exercise tolerance
Dizziness
Skin and conjunctival pallor
Tachycardia
Hair loss
Irritability
Weakness
Pica (appetite for largely nonnutritive substances, such as clay, chalk, dirt, or sand)
Pagophagia (form of pica involving the compulsive consumption of ice or iced drinks)
Brittle or grooved nails (koilonychia)
Plummer–Vinson syndrome (painful atrophy of the mucous membrane covering the tongue, pharynx, and esophagus)
Impaired immune function
Restless legs syndrome

Note: Some patients with iron deficiency and even anemia may remain completely asymptomatic

The recommended daily allowance for men is 8–10 mg iron per day.

Symptoms of iron deficiency may occur before the condition has progressed to iron deficiency anemia. With respect to the relationship between decreased serum ferritin levels and hair loss, the literature has remained controversial, and the respective studies have been performed in females. Moreover, symptoms are not unique to iron deficiency, since iron is needed for many enzymes to function normally, and a wide range of unspecific symptoms may therefore eventually arise. Moreover, some patients with iron deficiency and even anemia may remain completely asymptomatic (Table 2.1).

Before starting treatment, there should be definitive diagnosis of iron deficiency and of the underlying cause. This is particularly the case in older patients, who are most susceptible to gastrointestinal bleeding due to cancer.

> In adults, 60 % of patients with iron deficiency anemia may have underlying gastrointestinal disorders leading to chronic blood loss.

Other causes of iron deficiency are inadequate intake, substances (in diet or drugs) interfering with iron absorption, malabsorption syndromes, and blood donation.

Protein–Calorie Malnutrition. Protein–calorie malnutrition is probably the best studied of possible forms of undernutrition in man. It occurs commonly in developing countries. Kwashiorkor (Ghanian for "copperhead") is due to a deficit of protein in an otherwise calorically adequate diet. Alterations in hair color and texture are short and dry hair, with increased cuticular weathering, reddish-brown to rusty hair color, and a raised telogen count and atrophy of anagen bulbs. Other symptoms include anemia, (hypoproteinemic) edema, and hypopigmentation of skin with dry, fissured areas and cracked appearance ("flaky paint"). Marasmus is due to a deficit of calories exceeding the deficit of protein. The amino acids are utilized to maintain body function. The result is an atrophy of most organs; the hair is thin, sparse, and easily plucked.

> In developed countries, protein–calorie malnutrition predominantly affects chronically ill and hospitalized patients.

It is observed in children on protein restricted diets for management of urea-cycle disorders, such as argininosuccinic aciduria; infants on milk-restricted diets because of suspected lactose intolerance or milk protein allergy; children and adolescents with gastrointestinal disease, cystic fibrosis, and anorexia nervosa; and patients with chronic renal failure, severe neurologic impairment, or malignancy.

Zinc Deficiency. In children, zinc deficiency is a rare autosomal recessive genetic disorder in absorption of zinc resulting in a condition called acrodermatitis enteropathica. It manifests the time of weaning and is associated with reduced absorption of unsaturated fatty acids and impaired desaturation of linoleic and alpha-linoleic acids, which in part explains some of the cutaneous manifestations. These are a characteristic psoriasiform acral and periorificial dermatitis with

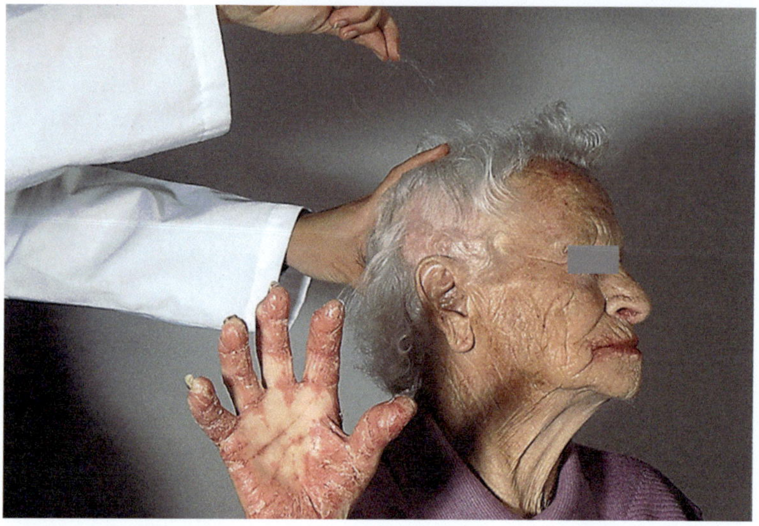

Fig. 2.5 Cutaneous manifestations of zinc deficiency: alopecia and peculiar acrodermatitis

typical histology, susceptibility to infection, superinfection of skin lesions with *Candida albicans* and *Staphylococcus aureus*, stomatitis, angular cheilitis, blepharoconjunctivitis, nail dystrophy, alopecia, and sparse, white, thin, and brittle hair.

In adults and the elderly, the manifestations of acquired zinc deficiency are similar (Fig. 2.5). Intake of 8–10 mg of zinc per day is adequate and obtained in a normal diet.

> Zinc deficiency is seen in chronic alcoholism, anorexia nervosa, kidney disease, or with impaired absorption of zinc due to diet with high phytate content, drugs that chelate zinc (ACE inhibitors), pancreatitis, or gastrointestinal bypass surgery.

Deficiency of Essential Fatty Acids. Deficiency of the long-chain polyunsaturated fatty acids, linoleic acid and alpha-linoleic acid, may be due to impaired fat absorption in children with biliary atresia, cystic fibrosis, or intestinal lymphangiectasia; dietary supplements consisting primarily of medium-chain triglycerides in short-bowel syndrome; and inadequately supplemented parenteral alimentation. Cutaneous manifestations of deficiency of essential fatty acids are: severe dryness and scaling of skin, redness and scaling of scalp and eyebrows, weeping intertriginous lesions, the hair is dry, unruly, lighter in color, and there is a significant telogen hair shedding.

Biotin deficiency is rare, since biotin is synthesized by intestinal bacteria. It is seen in association with parenteral nutrition without biotin supplementation in patients with short-gut syndrome, prolonged antibiotic, anticonvulsant (phenytoin, primidone, carbamazepine) or isotretinoin therapy, and excessive ingestion of raw egg white.

Two forms of rare hereditary biotin deficiency are known: early onset (neonatal) holocarboxylase deficiency and late-onset (3 months) biotinidase deficiency with a characteristic organic aminoaciduria, neurologic symptoms (seizures, ataxia, optic atrophy, neurosensory hearing loss), recurrent infections, periorificial dermatitis, blepharoconjunctivitis, and alopecia.

Symptoms of biotin deficiency are alopecia in combination with periorificial dermatitis, blepharoconjunctivitis, and recurrent infections.

For recommended supplementation dosages of biotin, see Table 2.2.

> Deficiency in zinc, essential fatty acids, and biotin are the three nutritional deficiencies that combine the symptoms of hair loss and scaly skin.

There is evidence that with age, the needs for types and quantities of nutrients may change, and

Table 2.2 Recommended supplementation dosages of biotin

Indication	Daily dosage of biotin
Biotinidase deficiency	10–40 mg daily
Holocarboxylase deficiency in pregnancy	10 mg daily
Holocarboxylase deficiency	Intravenous, solution: 18.4 μmol daily
Parenteral alimentation-induced deficiency	Oral, solution or tablet: 0.1–1 mg daily
Brittle nail disorders	2.5 mg two to three times daily
Nutritional supplementation	30–300 μg daily

it has been found that as many as 50 % of older adults have a vitamin and mineral intake less than the recommended dietary allowance and as many as 30 % of the elderly population have subnormal levels of vitamins and minerals. In the elderly population, socioeconomic status and functional ability have an important influence on nutritional status. When financial concerns are present, meals are skipped and food that is purchased may not provide a nutritionally adequate diet. Declines in both physical and cognitive functional status affect an individual's ability to shop for food and to prepare meals. Nutritional problems are further compromised by social isolation, which commonly leads to apathy about food and decreased intake. Ultimately, the older person has experienced change and loss through retirement, disability, and death of friends and family, as well as change in financial, social, and physical health status. These changes may lead to depression.

Depression is often unrecognized in older persons. Malnutrition may be a presenting symptom of depression in the elderly.

Stressful Life Events. The literature on the subject of hair loss due to stressful life events (psychogenic effluvium) has been more confounding than helpful. The presence of emotional stress is not indisputable proof of its having incited the patient's hair loss. The relationship may also be the inverse. Nevertheless, it has long been recognized that psychosomatic factors play a role in dermatologic conditions. According to the psychosomatic theory, an organ system is vulnerable to psychosomatic ailments when several etiologic factors are operable. These include:

- Emotional factors mediated by the central nervous system
- Intrapsychic processes such as self-concept, identity, or eroticism
- Specific correlations between the emotional drive and the target organ, i.e., social values and standards linked with the organ system
- Constitutional vulnerability of the target organ

Ultimately, the issue of overvalued ideas in relation to the condition of the hair (psychogenic pseudo effluvium) is not always easy to resolve; however, it is important to control stress as a complication of hair loss or fear of hair loss. For this purpose, strong psychological support is essential to help limit patient anxiety, and patients need to be educated about the basics of the hair cycle. Information about the hair cycle can be useful to explain why considerable patience is required for effective cosmetic recovery.

Sexual Risk Behavior and Drug Abuse. A history of sexual risk behavior and drug abuse is relevant with respect to hair loss due to syphilis or HIV infection.

Syphilis (*Alopecia Syphilitica*). Syphilis is a sexually transmitted infection caused by the spirochete bacterium *Treponema pallidum*.

After decreasing drastically with the availability of penicillin for treatment in the 1940s, rates of syphilis infection have increased since the turn of the millennium, often in combination with human immunodeficiency virus. This has been attributed partly to unsafe sexual practices among men who have sex with men, increased promiscuity, prostitution, and decreasing use of condoms.

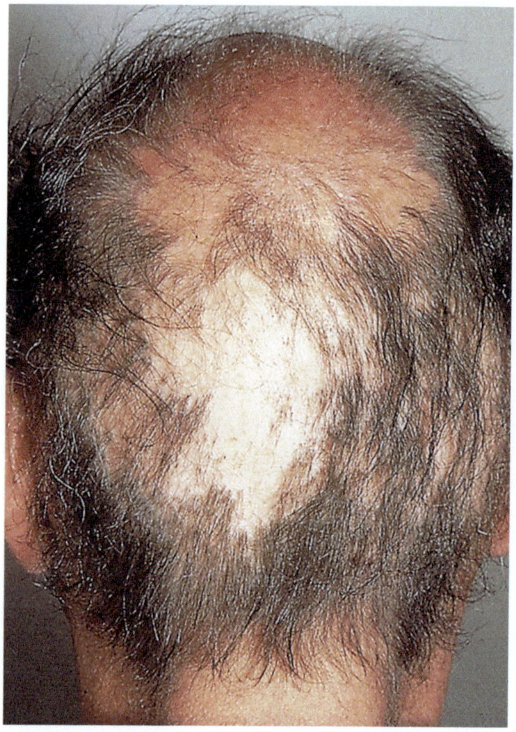

Fig. 2.6 Alopecia syphilitica: moth-eaten pattern of hair loss in a patient with preexisting androgenetic alopecia

The symptoms of syphilis vary depending on the disease stage. The primary stage presents with a firm, painless, non-itchy skin ulceration (chancre); secondary syphilis with a diffuse rash which frequently involves the palms of the hands and soles of the feet; latent syphilis with little to no symptoms; and tertiary syphilis with gummas, neurologic symptoms, or cardiac symptoms. Alopecia syphilitica is an uncommon manifestation of secondary syphilis, occurring in 4 % of affected individuals. It is noninflammatory and non-cicatricial hair loss that can present in a diffuse pattern, a moth-eaten pattern (Fig. 2.6), or a combination of both. The distinguishing clinical and laboratory features of alopecia syphilitica from other forms of diffuse hair loss or hair loss with a moth-eaten pattern include other mucocutaneous changes associated with secondary syphilis, when present, and a positive serology for syphilis.

Human Immunodeficiency Virus (HIV) Infection (HIV Trichopathy). HIV is a slowly replicating retrovirus (lentivirus) that causes acquired immunodeficiency syndrome (AIDS), a condition in which progressive failure of the immune system predisposes to life-threatening opportunistic infections and cancers. HIV infects vital cells in the human immune system such as helper T cells, specifically CD4+ T cells, macrophages, and dendritic cells. HIV infection leads to low levels of CD4+ T cells through a number of mechanisms including apoptosis of uninfected bystander cells, direct viral killing of infected cells, and killing of infected CD4+ T cells by CD8+ cytotoxic lymphocytes that recognize infected cells. When CD4+ T cell numbers decline below a critical level, cell-mediated immunity is lost, and the body becomes progressively more susceptible to opportunistic infections.

A study of 500 patients infected with HIV in a large university-based setting performed by Sadick in 1993 demonstrated that the majority of hair disorders in the study population occurred with helper T cell numbers of less than 150/mm^3.

Papulosquamous problems including seborrheic dermatitis were most commonly noted, followed by disorders of cell growth cycle regulation (telogen effluvium) and trichokeratinization (acquired loose anagen syndrome). In another study, histopathologic studies were performed, and numerous apoptotic or necrotic keratinocytes were seen in the upper external root sheath follicular epithelium in addition to a mild to moderate perifollicular mononuclear cell infiltrate often containing eosinophils. The authors concluded that although telogen effluvium is a common response to a wide spectrum of biological stresses, the presence of apoptotic or necrotic keratinocytes within the upper end of the external root sheath epithelium and dystrophy of hairs may be markers of hair loss in patients with HIV-1 infection.

Another peculiar disorder seen in HIV-infected patient is acquired eyelash trichomegaly, defined

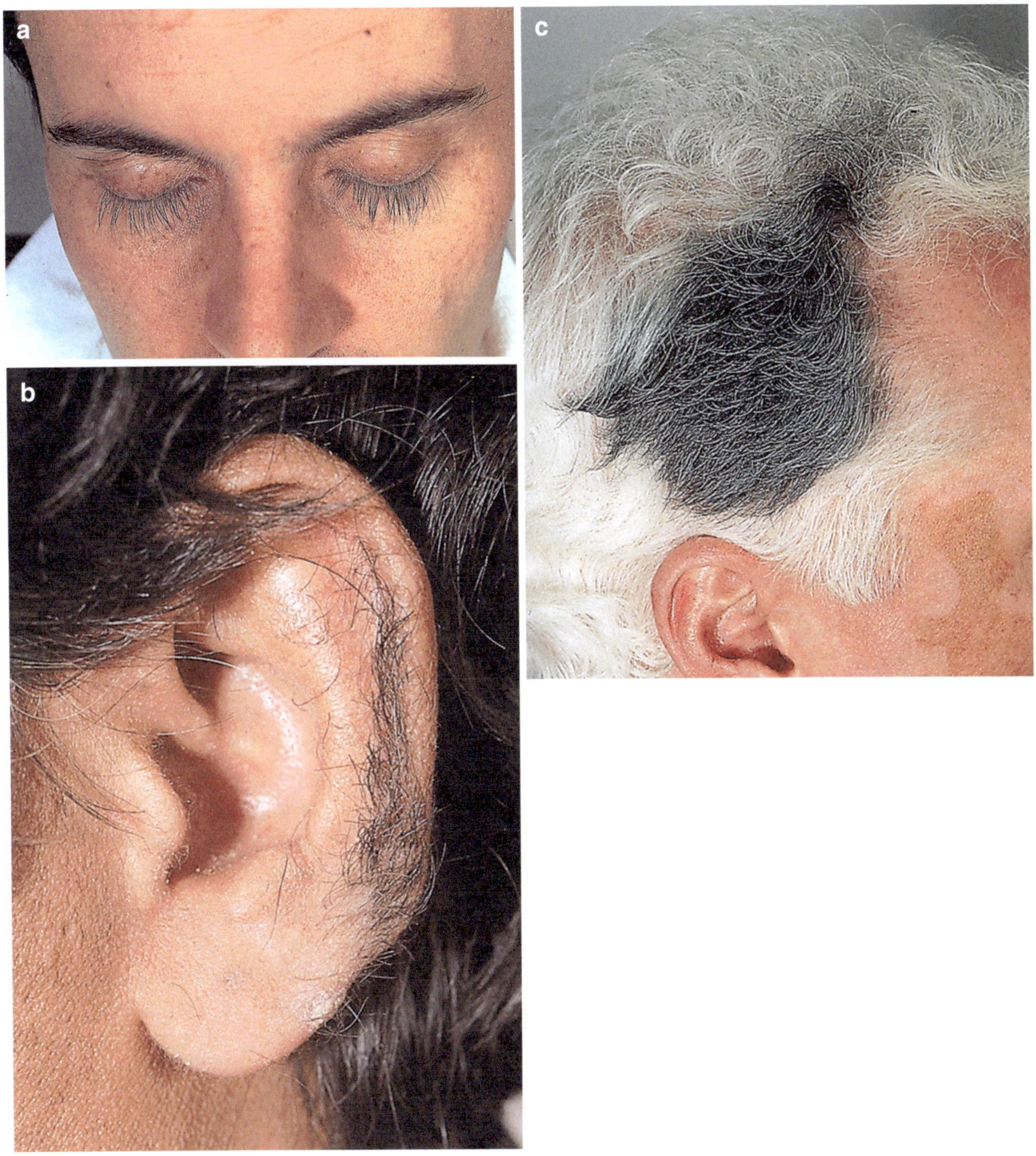

Fig. 2.7 HIV-associated hair changes. (**a**) Acquired eyelash trichomegaly. (**b**) Acquired hairy pinnae. (**c**) Poliosis in recovery phase from alopecia areata in patient with AIDS

as eyelashes which are found to be of increased length, thickness, and pigmentation (Fig. 2.7a). Also, acquired hair pinnae have been reported in association with HIV infection, a finding otherwise frequently encountered as a presumably Y-linked genetic condition in men of southern Indian origin (Fig. 2.7b).

Finally, alopecia areata (and vitiligo) has been reported in association with HIV infection (Fig. 2.7c), as well as in the setting of immune restoration after highly active antiretroviral therapy (HAART).

For the effects of UV exposure and cigarette smoking on the condition of the hair and scalp, see Sect. 3.2.

2.1.3 Drug History

There is a long list of drugs that on occasion have been cited as causing hair loss: all anticoagulant and antithyroid drugs can produce hair loss; some psychotropic drugs are likely to induce a drug-related alopecia; it has been reported that some patients taking lithium developed hair thinning; case reports with tricyclic antidepressants rarely appear in the literature; hair loss is reported secondary to some anticonvulsant agents, mainly valproic acid; among antihypertensive drugs, ACE inhibitors and systemic or topic beta-adrenoceptor antagonists (for treatment of glaucoma) should be considered as possible causes of hair loss; hair loss from nonsteroidal analgesics occurs in a very small percentage of patients; and a few isolated cases have been reported with some hypocholesterolemic or anti-infectious agents.

Diagnosis of drug-induced alopecia remains a challenge. The clinical identification of adverse drug reactions has been based largely on subjective criteria.

> However, the possible culprit of an adverse drug reaction can systematically be assessed based on the following six variables: previous experience with the drug in the general population, alternative etiological causes (usually androgenetic alopecia or may be caused by the disease that is treated with the drug in question), timing of events, drug levels or evidence of overdose, patient reaction to removal of the suspected drug, and patient reaction to rechallenge.

2.1.4 History of Hair Cosmetic Procedures and Trauma

Some patients blame wearing hats, frequent hair washing and blow drying, and hair styling products for their hair loss.

Unless a headdress is worn tight enough to cause long-standing pressure to the scalp or traction to the hair, wearing a hat does not cause hair to fall. In the contrary, coverage of the scalp may contribute positively by blocking UV radiation from the sun to cause damage to the scalp and hair.

> The perception of hair loss in association with the wearing of hats or helmets derives from the fact that male pattern baldness typically starts at an age in which young men become active in the military or in professions with headgears. It represents nothing more than a temporal coincidence.

Neither washing nor blow drying affects the condition of the hair follicle and therefore has no impact on hair growth. Nevertheless, overaggressive shampooing, towelling, and excessive heat from blow dryers may cause physical damage to the hair shaft resulting in brittle hair.

Frequently, patients claim of hair loss in association with the use of a particular shampoo, typically an antidandruff shampoo. This observation is easily explained either through the more intense scrubbing of the head with a special care shampoo causing more telogen hairs to be shed or the shedding of telogen hairs trapped in scales, once these are effectively removed from the scalp. Diffuse hair loss due to an inhibition of mitosis associated with long-term use of shampoos containing keratostatic antidandruff agents, such as selenium sulfide, has been discussed in the older literature and remains controversial. However, absence of effects of dimethicone- and non-dimethicone-containing shampoos on hair loss rates has systematically been demonstrated.

With respect to hairstyling, it is rather the particular hairstyle than the styling product, such as gels, pomades, hair sprays, perm solutions, or coloring, that may result in hair loss.

Again, anything causing long-standing traction to the hair, such as tight ponytails, corn-rows, or chignons will lead to focal hair loss, particularly in association with androgenetic alopecia.

Finally, acute telogen effluvium may be induced by allergic contact dermatitis to hair dyes, particularly to paraphenylenediamine. In these cases, patch testing will reveal the culprit.

For a proper appreciation of the condition of the hair shaft and hair breakage, inquiries therefore should be made on:

- Frequency and type of shampooing
- Use of hair care products
- Hair styling products
- Hair coloring agents
- Hair curling or hair straightening
- Hair grooming habits

2.2 Clinical Examination

The skin and hair are gratifying for diagnosis. One has but to look, and recognize, since everything to be named is in full view. Looking would seem to be the simplest of diagnostic skills, and yet its simplicity lures one into neglect. To reach the level of artistry, looking must be a skillful active undertaking. The skill comes in making sense out of what is seen, and it comes in the quest for the underlying cause, once the disorder has been named. The first look is best made without prejudices of former diagnoses and without bias of laboratory data. In many instances a specific diagnosis is made in a fraction of a second if it is a simple matter of recognition. The informed look is the one most practiced by dermatologists; it comes from knowledge, experience, and visual memory. Where the diagnosis does not come from a glance, the diagnostic tests come in, i.e., the dermatological techniques of examination and the laboratory evaluation.

By definition, *alopecia* is the acquired condition of recognizable hair loss. The term derives from Greek with reference to the loss of hair in patches in foxes afflicted with sarcoptic mange.

In case of congenital absence and lack of hair, the correct terms are *atrichia* and *hypotrichosis*, respectively.

While congenital atrichia is characterized by a total and permanent absence of hair, in congenital hypotrichosis the hair is diffusely thinned, but present.

Hereditary and congenital hypotrichosis and atrichia are among the most complex areas of disorders of hair growth with several distinctive entities occurring either as an isolated defect or as a feature of a complex hereditary syndrome in association with other ectodermal defects (ectodermal dysplasia).

Associated abnormal features include dysplastic or brittle fingernails, skin and tooth defects, or other abnormalities that have to be sought for systematically (for an extensive list, see Online Mendelian Inheritance in Man).

Typical examples include X-linked recessive anhidrotic ectodermal dysplasia of Christ–Siemens–Touraine (Fig. 2.8a) and hidrotic ectodermal dysplasia of Clouston (Fig. 2.8b, c). Also, trichorhinophalangeal syndrome shows characteristic features of fine and sparse scalp hair, a pear-shaped broad nose, and cone-shaped epiphyses of the middle phalanges (Fig. 2.9a, b), while the Rapp–Hodgkin/Hay–Wells syndrome shows coarse and sparse scalp hair, chronic inflammatory dermatitis of the scalp, midfacial hypoplasia, and cleft lip/palate (Fig. 2.10)

In daily clinical practice, we are usually dealing with the alopecias. When examining the scalp, the distribution of hair loss, presence and characteristics of associated skin lesions, and the presence of scarring should be noted. Part widths should be measured and all abnormalities noted.

2.2.1 Pattern Recognition

Male pattern androgenetic alopecia is characterized by its typical bitemporal recession of hair and balding vertex, while *female pattern androgenetic alopecia* is set apart by its rather diffuse thinning of the crown and a usually intact frontal hairline. Ninety-six percent of men affected with androgenetic alopecia have the male pattern and 4 % the female pattern (Fig. 2.11a).

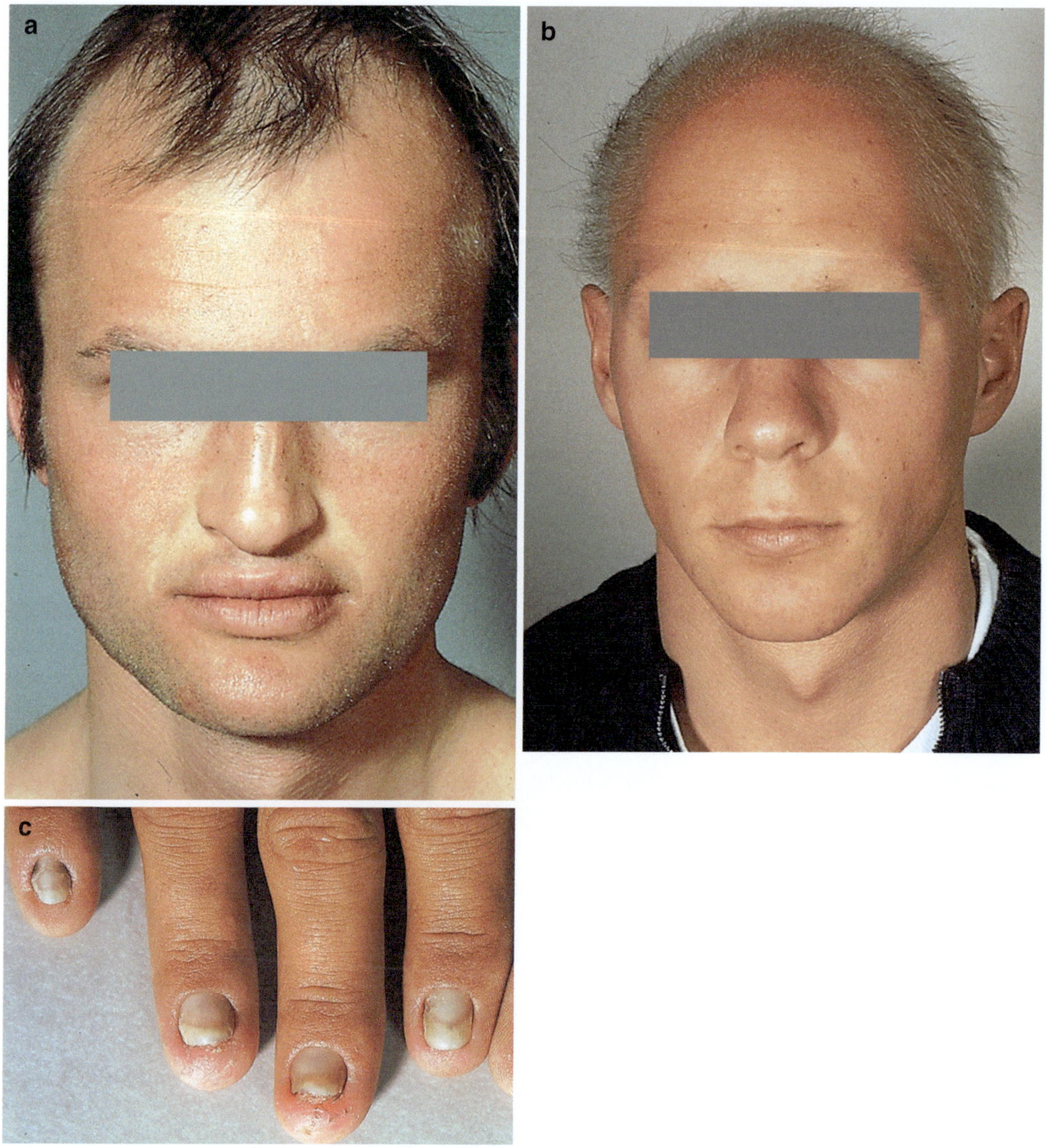

Fig. 2.8 Ectodermal dysplasia. (**a**) Christ–Siemens–Touraine type (anhidrotic) with typical facies (frontal bossing, midfacial hypoplasia, saddle nose, large chin, and thick lips). (**b**) Clouston type (hidrotic) with (**c**) associated nail abnormalities (the nails may be milky white in early childhood and gradually become dystrophic, thick, and distally separated from the nail bed)

When androgenetic alopecia develops early before onset of puberty, it shows exclusively the female pattern (Fig. 2.11b).

> Hair loss in patches signifies either alopecia areata, trichotillomania, or the scarring alopecias.

Alopecia areata typically presents with sudden hair loss causing patches to appear on the scalp (Fig. 2.12a) or other areas of the body (Fig. 2.12b). Some patients show a reticular pattern of alopecia resulting from confluence of multiple small patches of alopecia (Fig. 2.12c). Ophiasis is a form of alopecia areata characterized by the loss of hair in the shape of a wave at the circumference of the head (Fig. 2.12d).

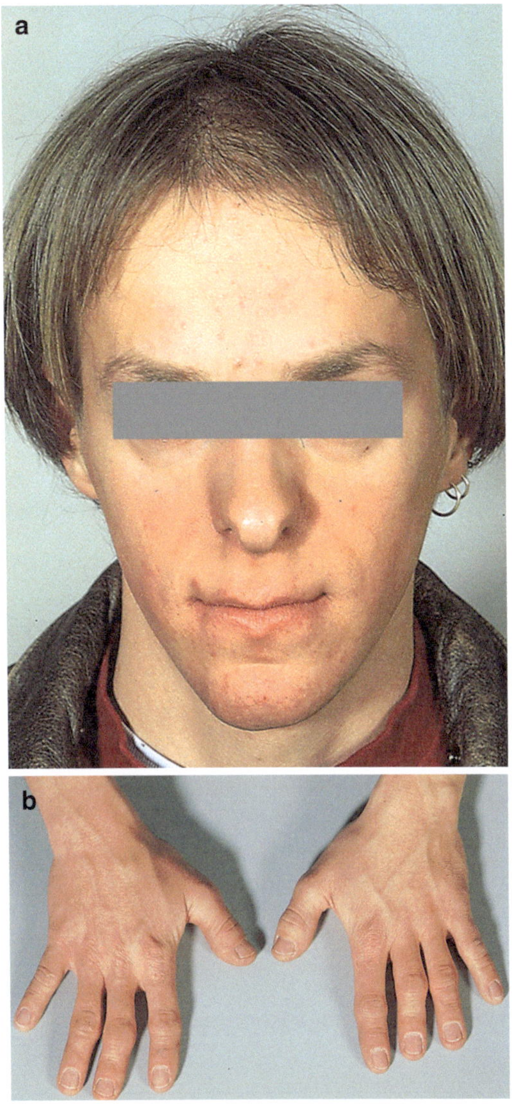

Fig. 2.9 Trichorhinophalangeal syndrome. (**a**) Fine and sparse scalp hair, pear-shaped broad nose. (**b**) Cone-shaped epiphyses of the middle phalanges

The name derives from the Greek word "ophis" for snake, because of the apparent similarity to a snake shape and the pattern of hair loss. Occasionally, alopecia areata may progress to complete baldness, which is referred to as alopecia totalis (Fig. 2.12e), and when the entire body suffers from complete hair loss, it is referred to as alopecia universalis. It is similar to the hair loss that occurs with chemotherapy. The skin within the patches is inconspicuous, and hair follicles are intact.

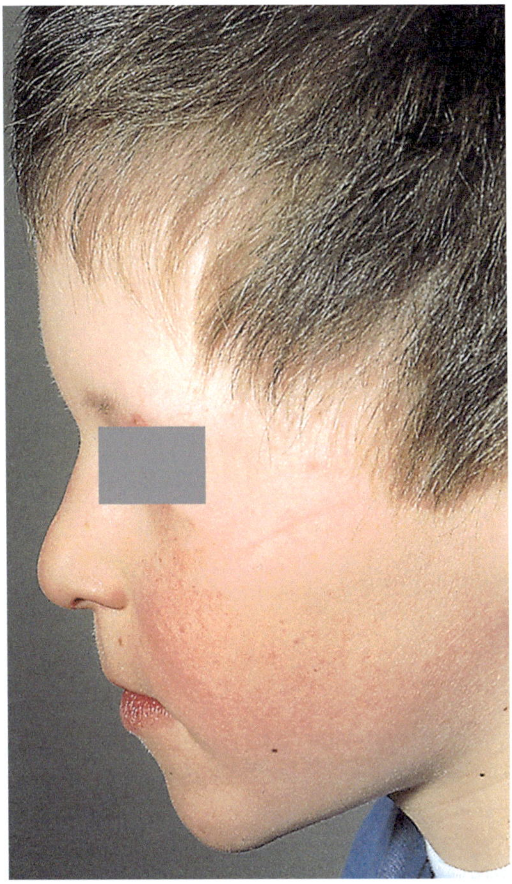

Fig. 2.10 Rapp–Hodgkin syndrome: coarse scalp hair and midfacial hypoplasia

> Ophiasis, alopecia totalis, and alopecia universalis have a poor prognostic significance.

A close mimicker of alopecia areata is *congenital triangular alopecia* (of Sabouraud) that is congenital, but usually appears in childhood as a focal patch of fine vellus hairs with a triangular configuration in the temporal region of the scalp (Fig. 2.13). The suggested frequency for this condition in the general population has been estimated around 0.11 %. The majority of cases are detected in childhood between the ages of 2 and 9 years. The condition presents usually as an isolated finding; rare cases have been associated with Setleis syndrome that is characterized by scar-like, circular depressions

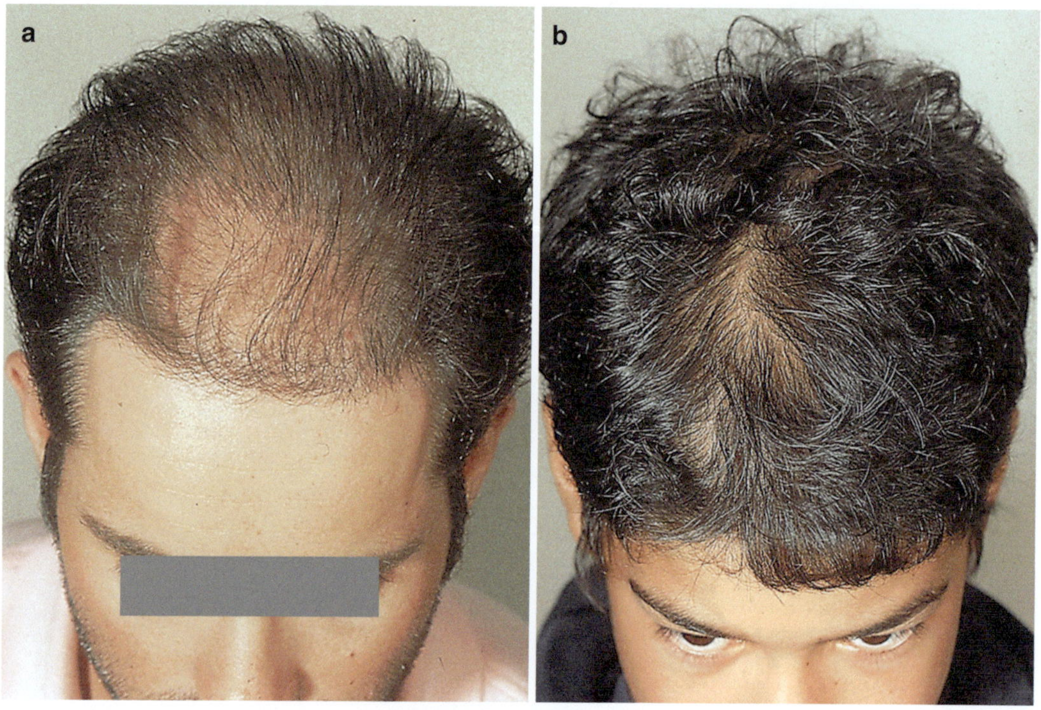

Fig. 2.11 Pattern recognition: female pattern androgenetic alopecia with diffuse thinning of crown area and intact frontal hairline. (**a**) In an adult male. (**b**) In a prepubertal male

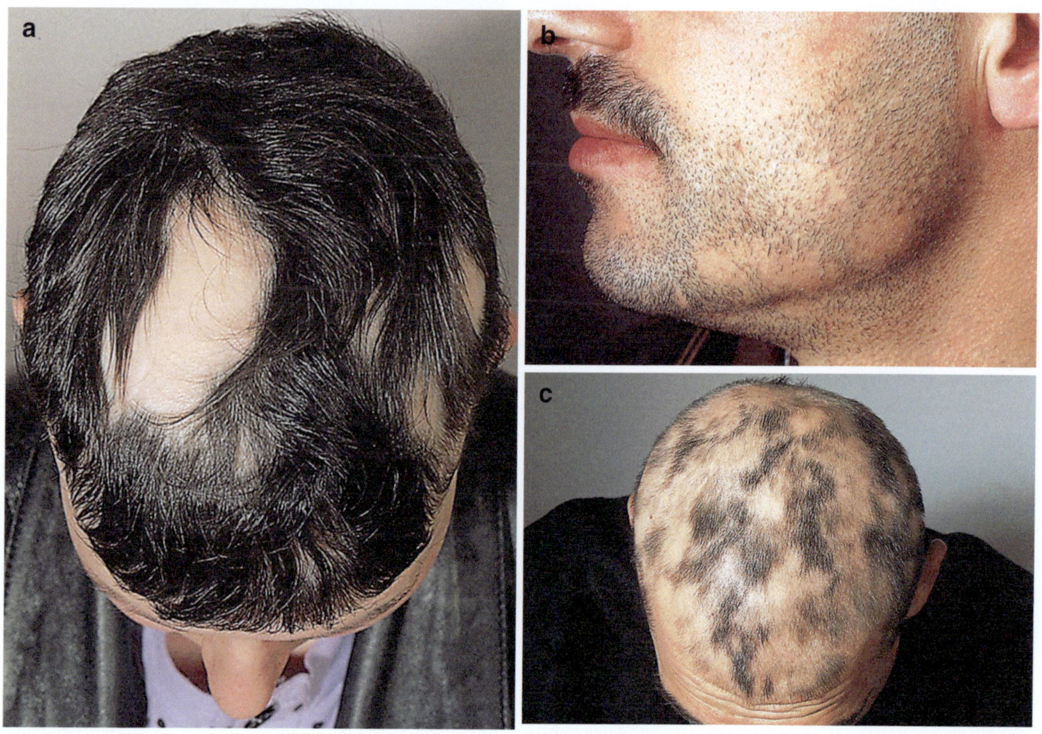

Fig. 2.12 Pattern recognition: alopecia areata. (**a**) Patches of hair loss on the scalp. (**b**) Alopecia areata of the beard. (**c**) Reticular pattern. (**d**) Ophiasis. (**e**) Alopecia totalis. (**f**) Associated nail pitting

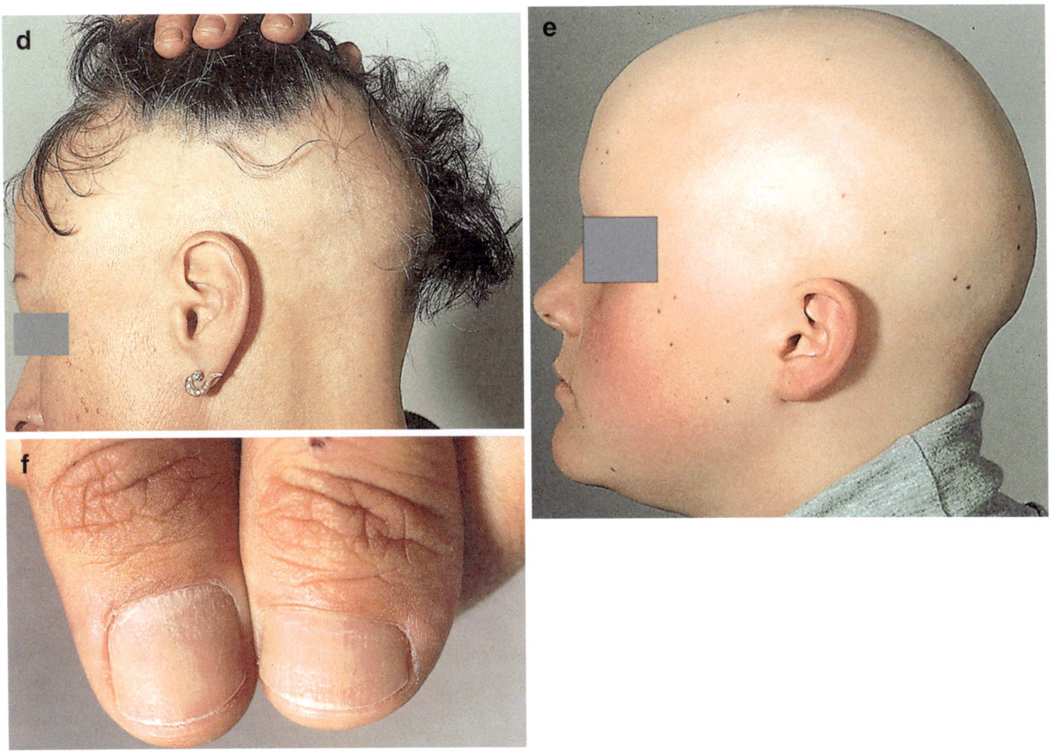

Fig. 2.12 (continued)

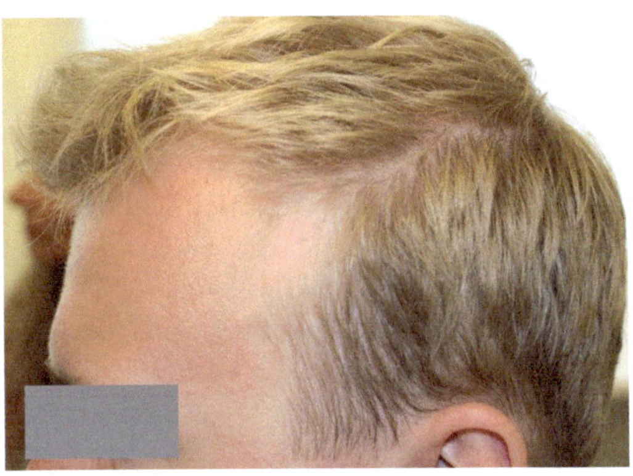

Fig. 2.13 Alopecia triangularis congenita (of Sabouraud): focal patch of alopecia with triangular configuration in the temporal region of the scalp

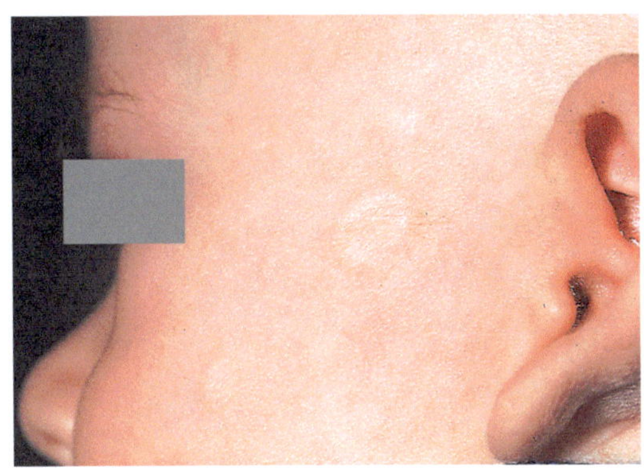

Fig. 2.14 Setleis syndrome: scar-like, circular depressions on the temple

on the temples (Fig. 2.14), which may resemble forceps marks. Also, *aplasia cutis congenita*, a rare, heterogeneous, and polyetiological condition of congenital scalp defect resulting in scarring alopecia (Fig. 2.15a, b), may give rise to litigations with respect to alleged obstetric injury.

In *trichotillomania*, the hair loss is incomplete and usually confined to one or two sites. The disorder represents a disorder of impulse control and usually begins between early childhood and adolescence. It occurs six to seven times more frequently in children than in adults; before the age of six, males predominate and thereafter females. The scalp is the most common pulling site,

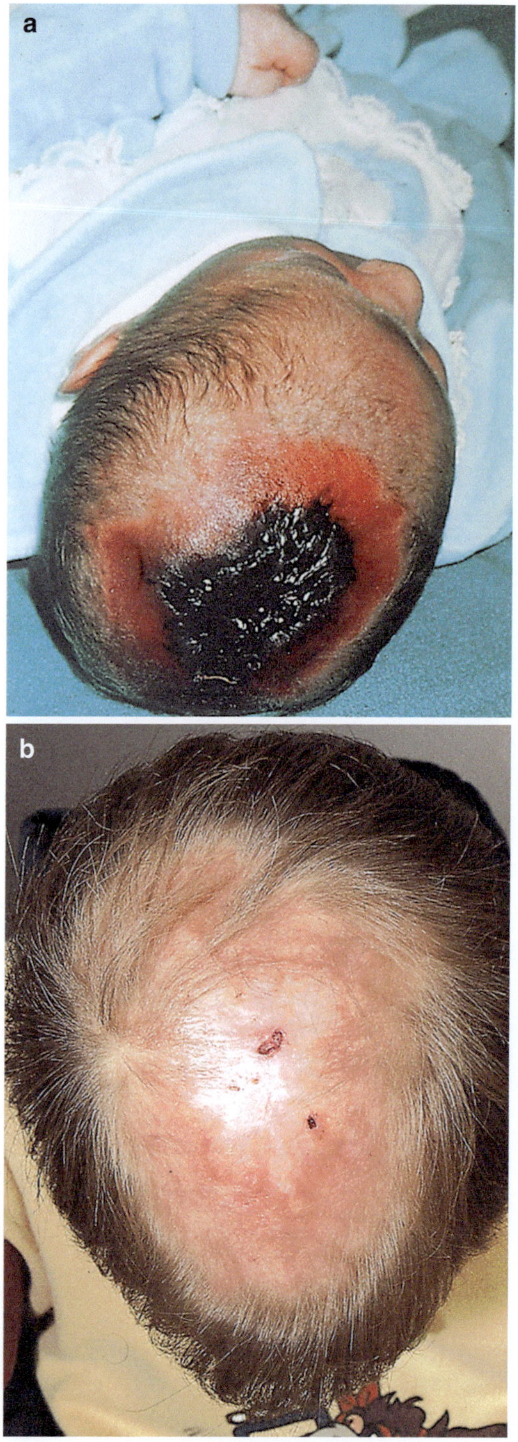

Fig. 2.15 Aplasia cutis congenita: (**a**) congenital scalp defect (**b**) resulting in scarring alopecia

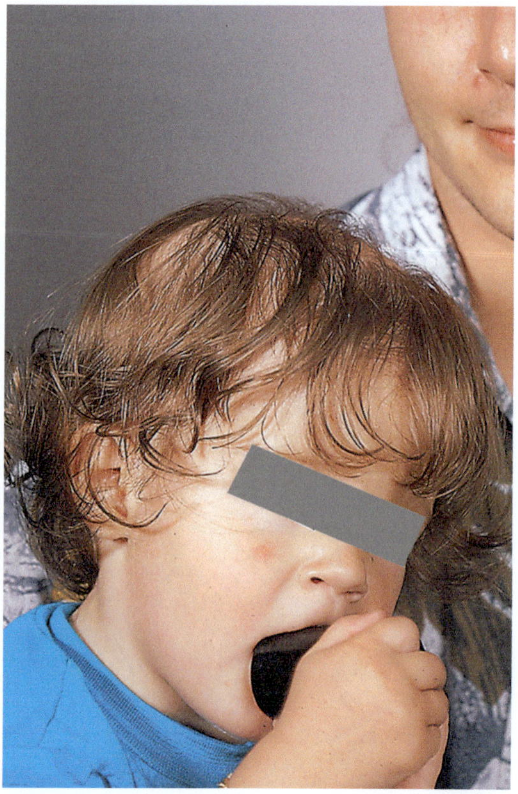

Fig. 2.16 Traumatic alopecia due to child abuse (battered child). Note hematoma on face

followed by the eyebrows and eyelashes, and only rarely face, arms, or legs. Hair is often pulled out, leaving an unusual shape. Within the area of hair loss, the hair exhibits differing lengths; some are broken hairs with blunt ends, some show new growth with tapered ends, and some are broken at mid-shaft or present with an uneven stubble. Scaling on the scalp is not present, overall hair density is normal, and a hair pull test is negative.

Though uncommon, *traumatic alopecia due to child abuse* (*battered child*) is an important differential diagnosis to take into consideration in a child with unexplained hair loss and other signs of physical trauma (Fig. 2.16).

Scarring alopecias usually present with usually irregular patches of alopecia in which the hair follicle ostia are absent. The scarring alopecias encompass a diverse group of disorders

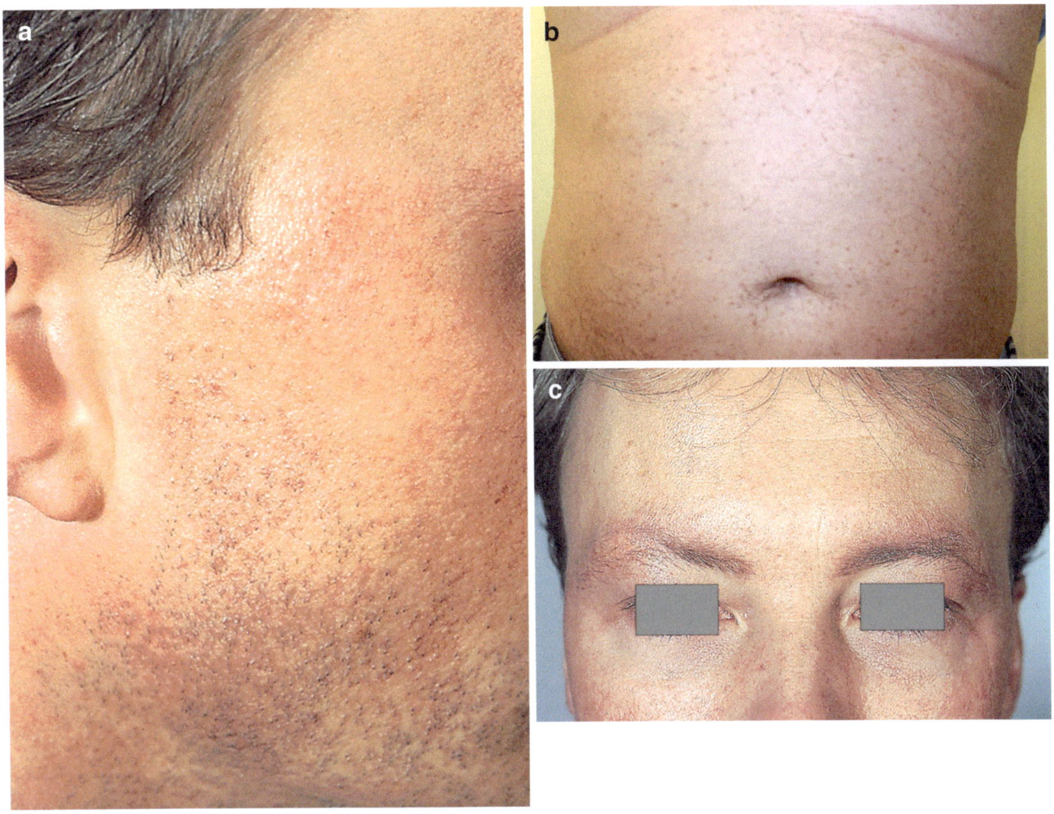

Fig. 2.17 Keratosis follicularis spinulosa decalvans. (**a**) Keratosis pilaris rubra atrophicans of the face. (**b**) Widespread involvement (abdomen). (**c**) Ulerythema ophryogenes (involvement of eyebrows)

characterized by permanent destruction of the hair follicle and irreversible hair loss. The color of the affected scalp, presence of erythema and scaling, its localization and distribution, and presence of pustules, crusting, telangiectasia, atrophy, hypopigmentation, or hyperpigmentation may all be helpful in making a presumptive diagnosis. Usually, a diagnostic scalp biopsy is indicated.

A peculiar form of hereditary scarring alopecia is X-linked *keratosis follicularis spinulosa decalvans* of Siemens that begins with keratosis pilaris (rubra atrophicans) localized on the face (Fig. 2.17a), then evolves to more diffuse involvement (Fig. 2.17b). The condition is accompanied by the loss of eyebrows (ulerythema ophryogenes, Fig. 2.17c), eyelashes, and hair on the face and head. Atopy, photophobia, and keratitis may also occur.

Ultimately, *pseudopeladic state of Degos* represents the nonspecific end stage of a variety of at least 60 types of cicatricial alopecias and is characterized by coalescent patches of ivory-colored alopecia in the absence of clinical signs of inflammation.

By definition, *pseudopelade of Brocq* presents from the beginning with small irregular patches of scarring alopecia in the absence of clinical inflammation (Fig. 2.18) and therefore may be mistaken for alopecia areata (pelade in French).

Alopecia parvimaculata (of Dreuw) is a disease in which hair is lost in very small, irregularly

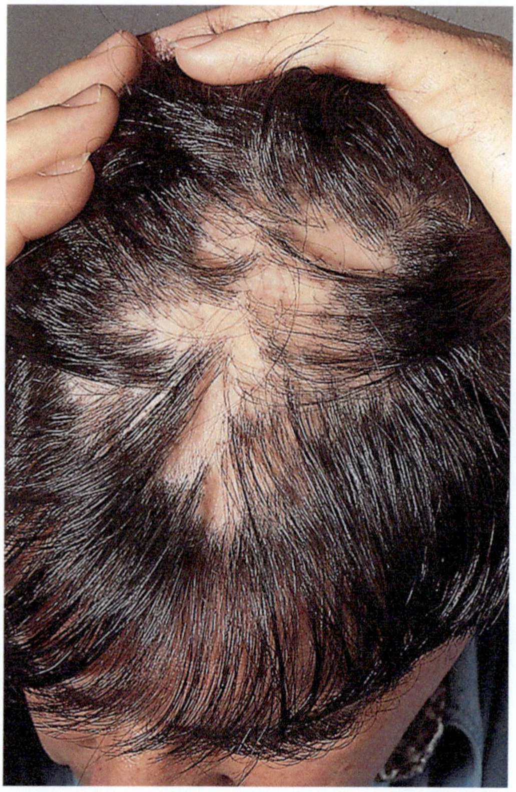

Fig. 2.18 Pseudopelade (Brocq): numerous small irregular patches of scarring alopecia in the absence of clinical inflammation

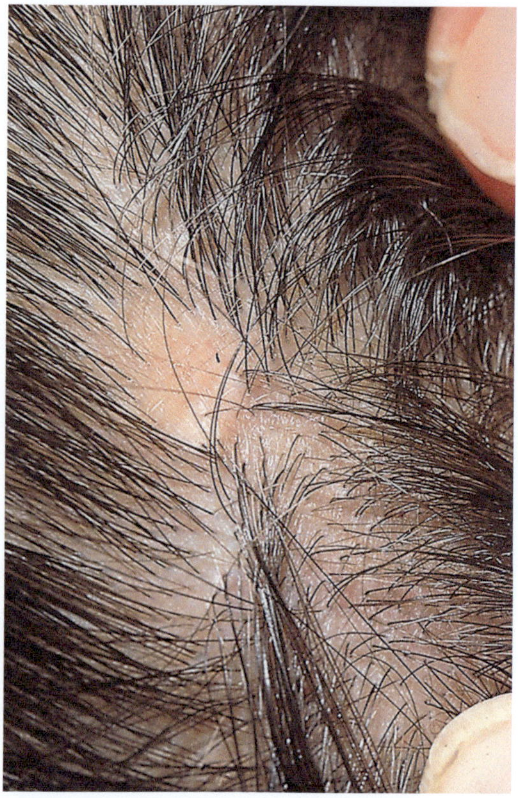

Fig. 2.19 Alopecia parvimaculata (Dreuw): very small patch of alopecia in a child

shaped patches, usually in children (Fig. 2.19). The etiology has remained obscure, but in its original description may have been related to small epidemic outbreaks of parasitic infection.

One of the most distinctive clinical presentations of a scarring alopecia is the more recently described *frontal fibrosing alopecia* that is characterized by a band-like pattern of recession along the frontotemporal and (less commonly) occipital hairline frequently associated with a characteristic loss of eyebrows. The condition was originally described in postmenopausal women, but may also be observed, though less frequently, in men (Fig. 2.20).

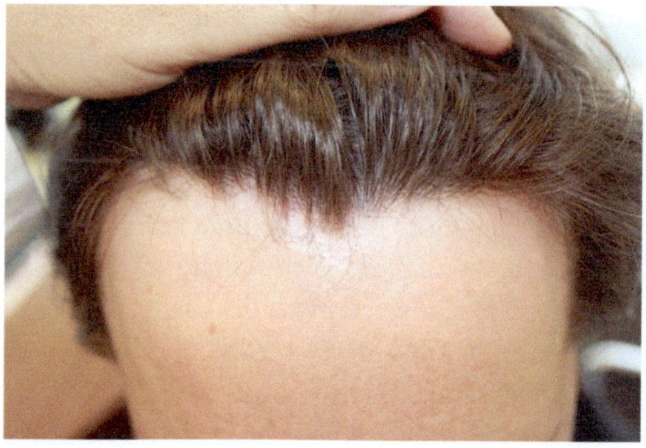

Fig. 2.20 Initial male frontal fibrosing alopecia with lonely hair sign

Diffuse alopecia is characterized by hair loss over the entire scalp including the sides and back of the head (Fig. 2.21). The condition may be due to a variety of causes that have to be sought out systematically. Treating this type of hair loss depends on recognizing and eliminating the actual hair loss cause. In most cases, the hair regrows.

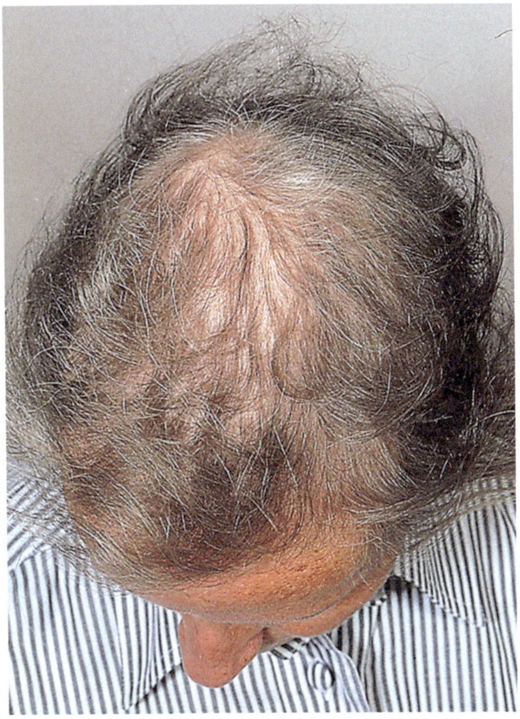

Fig. 2.21 Diffuse alopecia

2.2.2 Black and White Felt Examination

Short, miniaturized hairs in androgenetic alopecia are easily recognized when a contrasting felt background is used. An index card with a piece of black felt glued to one side for identification of light hairs and white felt glued onto the opposite side for identification of dark hairs is used as a contrast material. Fine short hairs with tapered distal ends will project up along the edge of the felt (Fig. 2.22a).

2.2.3 Assessment of Hair Part Width

Assessment of scalp hair density is relevant to patients with active hair shedding or thinned hair. Hair density is frequently relative to the patient's prior assessment of his hair. The assessment of hair part width is one attempt to compare the hair densities in different areas of the scalp or in the course of time. When hair is dense, a very fine, thin-lined part can be seen (Fig. 2.22b), while in areas of decreased density, the part line is very irregular in diameter with small clear areas on both sides of the part line.

Using a comb, a series of coronal parts can be made over the vertex and the part width compared to that in the occipital area. In general, scalp hair is less dense on the vertex, and the thinning increases with age. Widened parts over the vertex are particularly conspicuous in androgenetic alopecia and may tighten in the course of successful treatment.

2.2.4 Hair Pull

The hair pull should be done on every patient who complains of hair loss to assess quickly the amount of hair shed. A cluster of approximately 50 hairs is grasped and held at the ends of the thumb and index finger exerting a slow and constant traction sufficient to tend the scalp slightly while moving toward the distal end of the hair (Fig. 2.22c). At least two different scalp sites are "pulled": in diffuse telogen effluvium or androgenetic alopecia frontal (2 cm behind the forehead and 2 cm lateral) and occipital (2 cm lateral from the occipital protuberance); in circumscribed alopecias, such as alopecia areata or trichotillomania, one sample is taken from the border zone and the control from the normal-appearing contralateral region.

> Normal patients can have up to four hairs epilated per site, but six or more hairs are suggestive of effluvium.

Additional information can be obtained by examining the bulbs of the epilated hairs. They are usually telogen bulbs, increased frontally in androgenetic alopecia and occipitally in diffuse telogen effluvium. In some instances, they may be dystrophic anagen hairs, as seen in dystrophic anagen effluvium, or dysplastic anagen hairs, as seen in loose anagen hair.

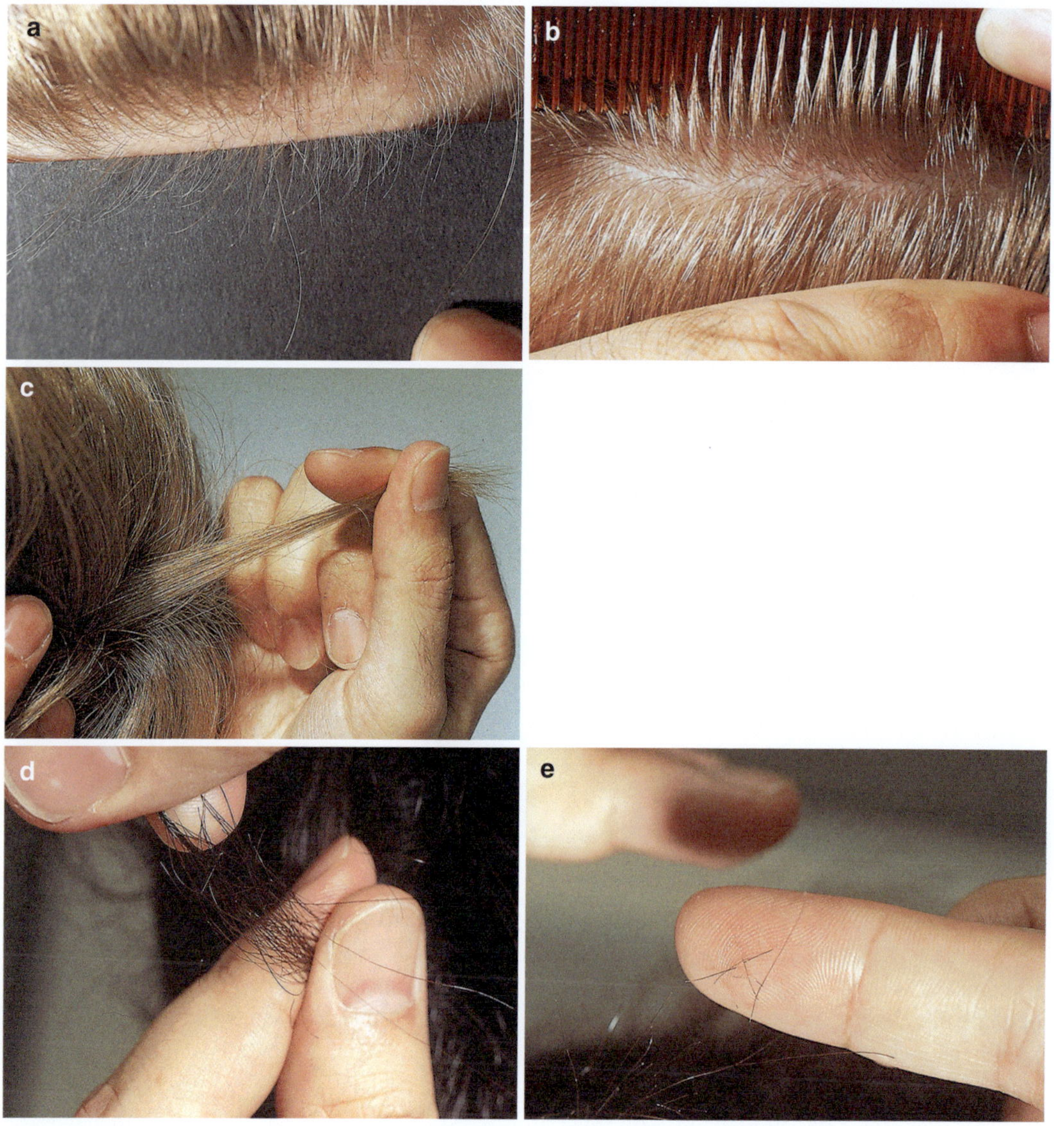

Fig. 2.22 Diagnostic techniques: (**a**) Black felt examination in blond hair. (**b**) Assessment of hair part width. (**c**) Hair pull test. (**d**, **e**) Hair feathering test

2.2.5 Hair Feathering

The hair feathering test is used to determine abnormal hair fragility with hair shaft breakage and should be performed on patients who complain that their hair fails to grow or breaks off. The distal 2–3 cm of the hairs is grasped between the thumb and index finger (Fig. 2.22d). After rubbing the distal hair ends between the thumb and index finger, a brisk pull is made on the ends of the hairs. The thumb and index finger are then checked for short broken hair fragments (Fig. 2.22e).

> In case of increased hair fragility in the hair feathering test, a light microscopic inspection of the hair shaft is warranted to detect the hair shaft defect underlying abnormal breakage.

2.3 Trichoscopy

The naked eye is right for the global look, but for close inspection the additional use of a magnifying glass is practiced. The handheld, single-lens magnifier is the simplest and least expensive, most commonly used by dermatologists, usually at a magnification of 3× to 4×. Although the pathologist lives in a world magnified 100–1,000 times, the clinician does not benefit from a highly magnified view of the patient, lest he performs dermoscopy (10×) and is knowledgeable of the clinicopathologic correlations.

Dermoscopy is a noninvasive diagnostic tool that permits recognition of morphologic structures not visible to the naked eye. Dermatologists involved in the management of scalp disorders have discovered dermoscopy to be also useful in their daily clinical practice. Scalp dermoscopy or trichoscopy is not only helpful for the diagnosis of hair and scalp disorders, but it can also give clues about the disease stage and progression.

> Examination of the scalp by dermoscopy can reassure patients with hair loss that they have received a thorough scalp examination, since patients with hair loss are very distressed and often feel that they are not properly examined.

2.3.1 Using the Dermatoscope for Diagnosing Hair and Scalp Disorders

Studies suggest that the use of dermoscopy in the clinical evaluation of hair and scalp disorders improves diagnostic capability beyond simple clinical inspection and reveals novel features of disease, which may extend our clinical and pathogenetic understanding.

Therefore, dermoscopy of hair and scalp (trichoscopy) is gaining popularity in daily clinic practice as a valuable tool in differential diagnosis of hair and scalp disorders. This method allows viewing of the hair and scalp at high magnifications using a simple handheld dermatoscope (Heine Delta 20®, DermoGenius®, DermLite II PRO HR®, or DermLite DL3®) with alcohol as the interface solution.

2.3.2 Patterns of Scalp Disease Revealed by Dermoscopy

Using dermoscopy, signature patterns are seen in a range of scalp and hair conditions. Some predominate in certain diseases; others can even help making a diagnosis in clinically uncertain cases.

Tosti classified the patterns as either interfollicular or follicular. The interfollicular patterns are further subdivided into vascular and pigment patterns. Scaling can be observed either as epidermal or perifollicular scaling. Finally, the dermatoscope can also be used to visualize hair shaft disorders and exogenous materials on the hair and scalp.

2.3.3 Follicular Patterns

Follicular patterns (Fig. 2.23a–f) encompass distinctive peripilar features that relate to the condition of the hair follicle:

Yellow dots (Fig. 2.23a) are characterized by an array of quite monomorphous, though variably sized, yellow to yellow-pink, round or polycyclic dots that are devoid of hair or contain dystrophic or vellus hair. They correspond to dilated follicular infundibula that contain sebaceous and keratinous material. Yellow dots are a major feature of alopecia areata, where they are found in 95 % of cases. They occasionally (8 %) may also be seen in advanced androgenetic alopecia. In both conditions, they are most apparent in areas of alopecia.

Black dots (Fig. 2.23b) represent pigmented hairs broken off at scalp level. They are seen in acute alopecia areata, tinea capitis (scalp ringworm), and trichotillomania, in which areas of alopecia are studded with follicular black dots. In alopecia areata they represent dystrophic hairs (cadaverized hairs); in tinea capitis, the classical lesion produced by endothrix species (e.g., *Trichophyton tonsurans*, *T. violaceum*) that invade the hair shaft (black-dot ringworm); and in trichotillomania, hairs broken through pathologic hair pulling habit.

Follicular keratosis (Fig. 2.23c) is characterized by follicular plugging with keratotic material. It may produce peripilar (keratin) casts. It is found in keratinization disorders, e.g., monilethrix, but is more commonly seen as an unspecific parakeratotic reaction pattern to follicular inflammation at the level of the isthmus and infundibulum, e.g., lichen planopilaris.

Peripilar signs (*peripilar cupular atrophy*) (Fig. 2.23d) are characterized by the presence of a brown halo, roughly 1 mm in diameter, at the follicular ostium around the emerging hair shaft. This finding has been found to be linked to superficial perifollicular lymphocytic infiltrates in early androgenetic alopecia.

Empty follicles (Fig. 2.23e) are characterized by empty follicular ostia. They represent the physiological interval of the hair cycle in which the hair follicle remains empty after the telogen hair has been extruded and before a new anagen hair

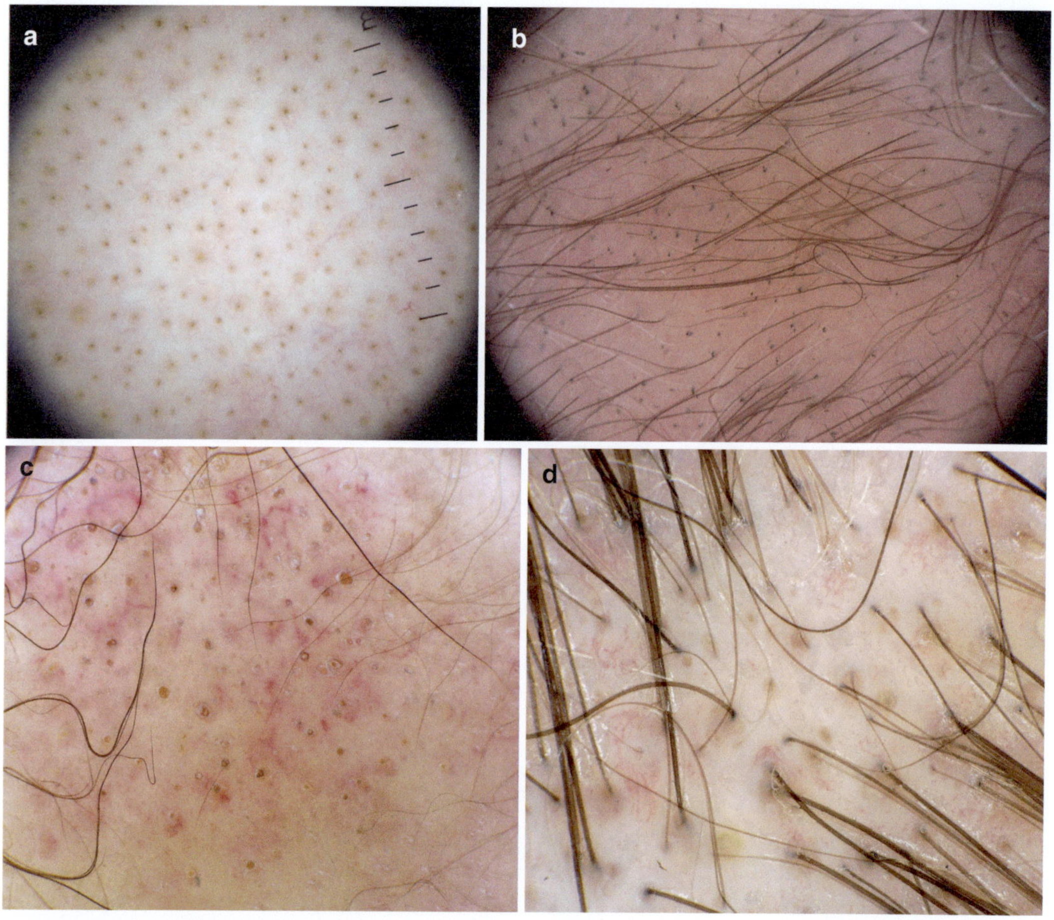

Fig. 2.23 Trichoscopy. (**a–f**) Follicular patterns: (**a**) Yellow dots. (**b**) Black dots. (**c**) Follicular keratosis. (**d**) Peripilar signs. (**e**) Empty follicles. (**f**) Loss of follicular ostia. (**g–l**) Interfollicular patterns (vascular, pigment): (**g**) Simple red loops. (**h**) Arborizing red lines. (**i**) Absent vascular loops. (**j**) Twisted red loops. (**k**) Hair needle vascular loops. (**l**) Honeycomb pigment pattern. (**m**) Scaling. (**n–s**) Hair shaft patterns: (**n**) Hair diameter diversity (anisotrichosis). (**o**) Dystrophic hairs (exclamation mark hair). (**p**) Hair tufting. (**q**) Monilethrix. (**r**) Pili torti. (**s**) Trichorrhexis nodosa. (**t–w**) Exogenous materials: (**t**) Hair dye. (**u**) Camouflage product (hair building fibers). (**v**) Hair spray residues. (**w**) Ectoparasite (head louse). (**x**) Ectoparasite (nit)

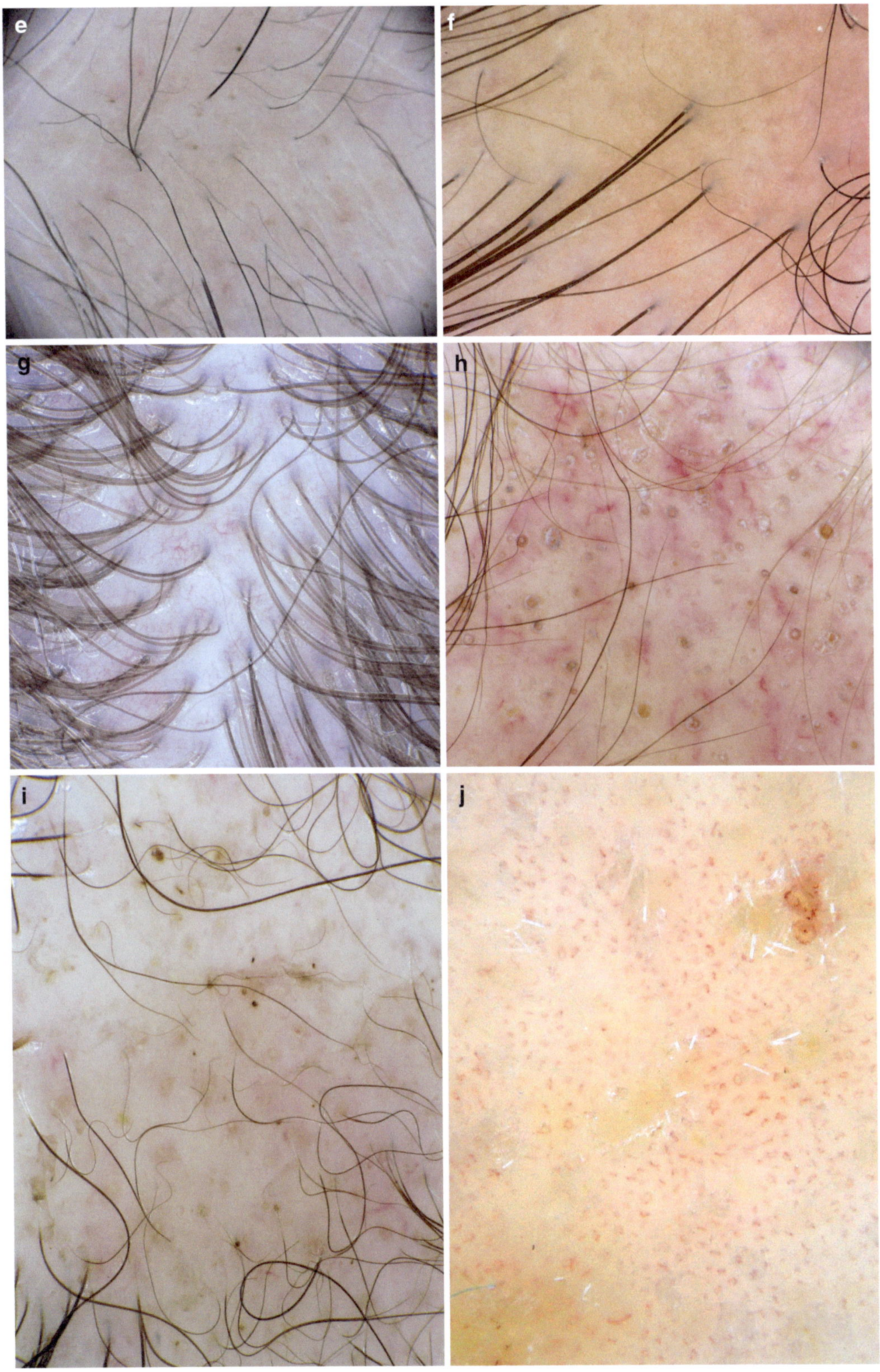

Fig. 2.23 (continued)

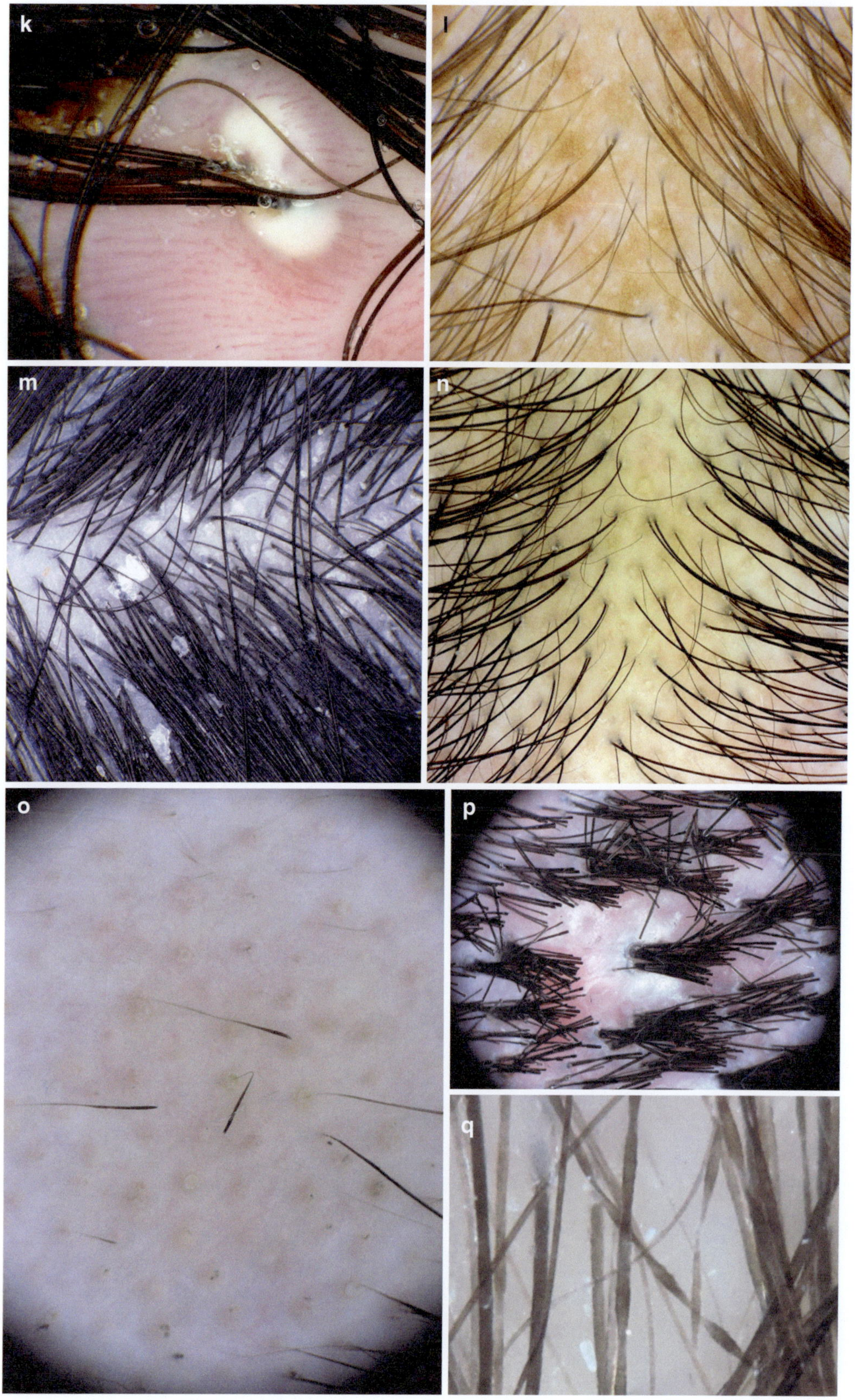

Fig. 2.23 (continued)

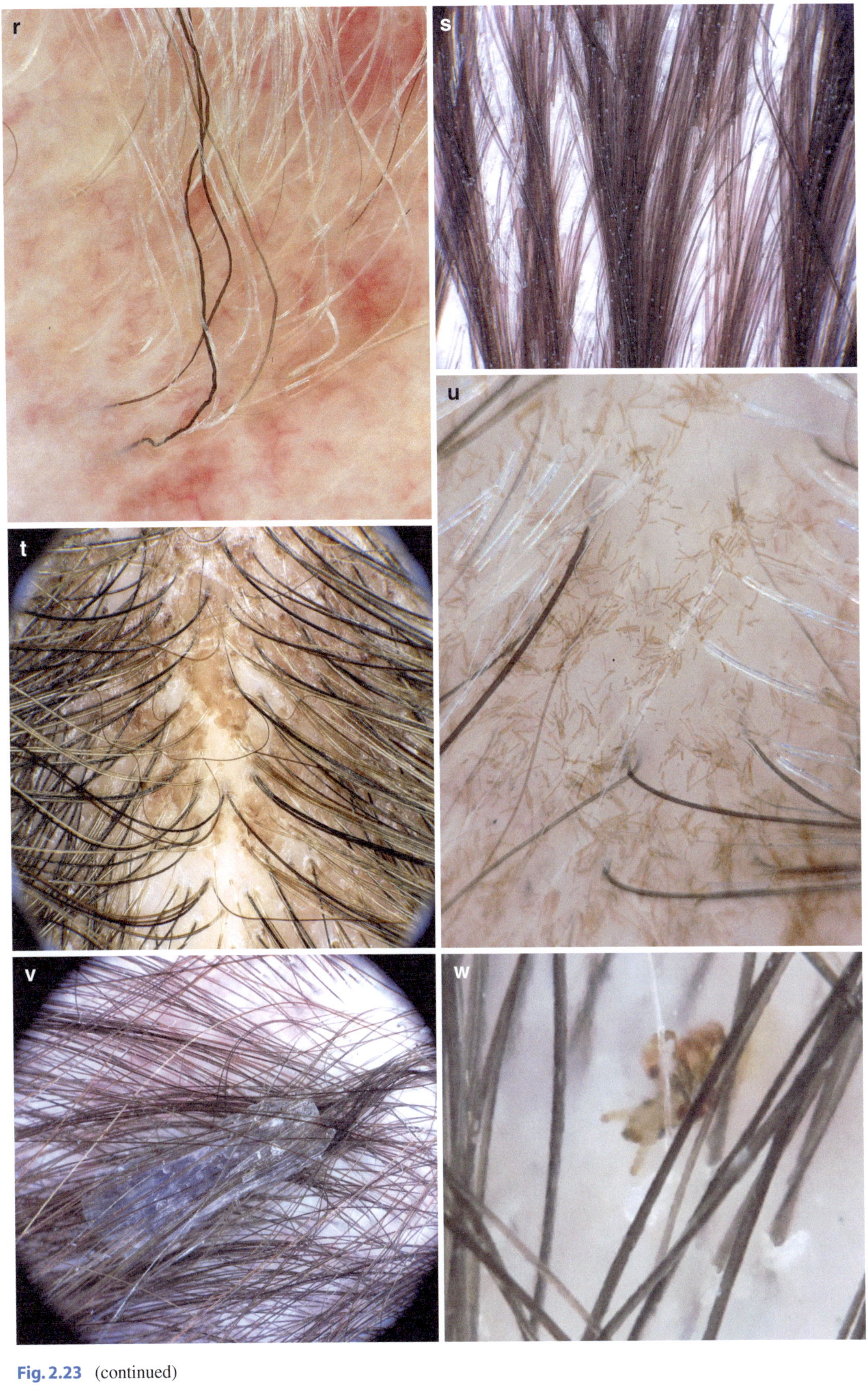

Fig. 2.23 (continued)

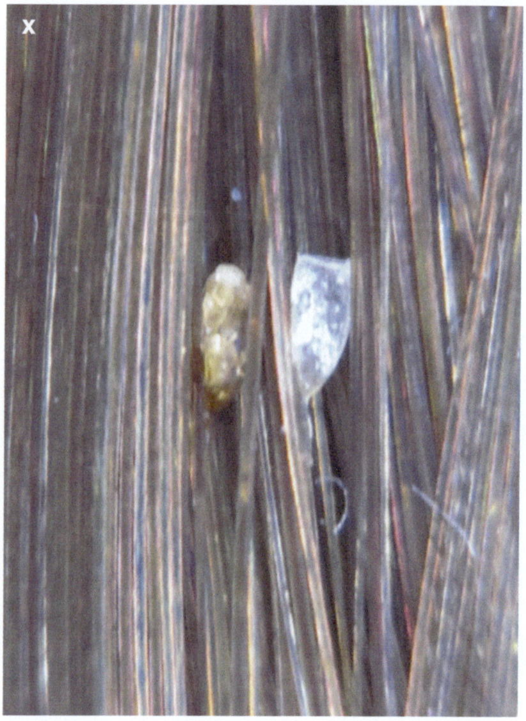

Fig. 2.23 (continued)

emerges (lag phase or kenogen). During kenogen, the hair follicle rests physiologically, but duration and frequency are greater in androgenetic alopecia, possibly accounting for baldness.

Loss of follicular ostia (Fig. 2.23f) is the hallmark of scarring alopecia. By definition, scarring alopecia represents visible loss of follicular ostia with destruction of the hair follicle on histopathologic examination. Classification of the scarring alopecias on the basis of pathology provides the diagnostic framework. Out of this reason, loss of follicular ostia usually represents an indication for diagnostic scalp biopsy.

2.3.4 Interfollicular Patterns (Vascular, Pigment)

Vascular features reflect differences in the skin capillary loop network in relation to the condition of the scalp:

Simple red loops (Fig. 2.23g) are seen in a normal epidermis. The pattern is characterized by multiple, fine, red lasso- or hairpin-shaped structures that are regularly spaced.

Arborizing red lines (Fig. 2.23h) have a wider caliber than the loops and are usually found in a focal pattern. They are seen to underlie and be associated with loops to a variable degree in normal scalp and in diseased scalp of different etiologies.

Effaced or absent loops (Fig. 2.23i) are seen in conditions with epidermal atrophy, for example, in established chronic cutaneous lupus erythematosus, when the epidermis has atrophied.

Twisted red loops occur in states of epidermal hypertrophy proportionate to its degree. Multiple, again relatively evenly spaced, twisted loops are a feature of psoriasis. They are also observed in about 20 % of seborrheic dermatitis and in folliculitis decalvans. Their distribution is diffuse in psoriasis (Fig. 2.23j) and concentrated around actively affected follicles in folliculitis decalvans (Fig. 2.23k). Their number and visibility correlate with disease activity.

Honeycomb pigment pattern is characterized by a relatively homogenous network of adjoining brown rings observed in normal individuals with darker skin colors and in the sun-exposed scalp of light-skinned individuals with thinned hair. Its distribution is diffuse in bald scalp and multifocal when some hair remains in the area (Fig. 2.23l). Usually, the degree correlates with the degree of hair loss and sun exposure.

2.3.5 Scaling

Scaling is an unspecific feature of reactive epidermal hyperproliferation with parakeratosis. The epidermis continuously regenerates itself, and epidermal keratinocytes are pushed outward where they undergo terminal differentiation to corneocytes that eventually flake off. Normally, these flakes of skin are too small to be visible. However, inflammatory conditions of the scalp accelerate cell turnover, especially in the scalp, with abnormal keratinization. The result is that the corneocytes are shed in large clumps, which appear as white or grayish patches on the scalp (Fig. 2.23m). Depending on the cause, the scales differ in localization, size, and greasiness (pityriasis simplex, pityriasis steatoides, pityriasis amiantacea). Scaling severity can be graded on a photographic scale and utilized to evaluate the effect of treatment.

2.3.6 Hair Shaft Patterns

Hair shaft patterns (Fig. 2.23n–s) reflect features that relate to the production and maintenance of the hair shaft:

Hair diameter diversity or *anisotrichosis* (Fig. 2.23n) relates to the presence of hairs with different caliber. This finding is typical of androgenetic alopecia and reflects progressive hair follicle miniaturization due to this condition.

Dystrophic hairs represent hairs that have fractured tips due to any process inhibiting cell division in the hair matrix. Severe inhibition leads to fracture if the narrowing of the hair shaft is marked. The hair shaft may be fractured before emergence from the scalp and then appears as cadaverized hair (also see black dots) or then appears as short exclamation mark hair (Fig. 2.23o).

Hair tufting refers to the emergence of several hair shafts together from the scalp and tufted folliculitis to an inflammatory condition of the scalp that resolves with patches of scarring alopecia within which multiple hair tufts emerge from dilated follicular ostia (Fig. 2.23p). Histologically, a single tuft consists of clustering of adjacent follicular units opening at the bottom of an epidermal depression. While hair tufting to a lesser degree (usually <5 hairs per ostium) may be found on the occipital scalp of healthy young men or represent an unspecific finding in other inflammatory scarring alopecias, i.e., lichen planopilaris and dissecting folliculitis of the scalp, tufted folliculitis of the scalp is considered a distinctive clinicohistological variant of folliculitis decalvans.

Hair shaft abnormalities result from genetic conditions and/or exogenous factors affecting the integrity of the hair shaft. Hair shaft abnormalities may occur as localized or generalized disorders and may lead to unruly hair and brittleness. Diagnosis is based on microscopic examination of the hair shaft. Dermoscopy is an effective tool for quick diagnosis of both congenital and acquired hair shaft disorders. Hair shaft abnormalities that can be visualized by dermoscopy include the following:

Monilethrix (Fig. 2.23q) is characterized by a beaded appearance of the hair due to periodic thinning of the shaft. The uncommon hereditary condition results in hair fragility and patchy dystrophic alopecia. The alopecia is more severe in the occipital region that is more exposed to friction. Typically the occipital scalp also presents follicular keratosis.

Pili torti (Fig. 2.23r) is characterized by hair that is flattened and twisted through 180° on its axis at varying intervals; the hair can additionally be grooved and has then also been termed pili torti et canaliculi. The hair shaft anomaly can be seen as an isolated hereditary trait, in a number of genetic syndromes, including Menkes kinky hair syndrome, Björnstad syndrome (with sensorineural deafness), and the ectodermal dysplasias. More commonly, it is found as acquired pili torti around the edges of patches of cicatricial alopecia, particularly lichen planopilaris, where local inflammatory and fibrosing processes distort the hair follicle.

Pili trianguli et canaliculi refers to the triangular hair shafts with longitudinal grooving underlying the uncombable hair syndrome.

Pili annulati is defined by characteristic alternating light and dark banding in the hair shaft, due to air-filled spaces between the macrofibrillar units of the hair cortex. Their significance lies in that affected hair is more susceptible to weathering, particularly in combination with androgenetic alopecia. With onset of hair thinning due to androgenetic alopecia, progressive reduction of hair shaft diameter may cause increased fragility and trichorrhexis nodosa-like hair shaft fracturing.

Trichorrhexis invaginata or bamboo hair is the marker for Netherton's syndrome, a rare autosomal recessive condition with bamboo hair, ichthyosis, and atopic dermatitis. The hair shaft shows multiple nodes along its length. The nodes consist of a proximal cup-shaped portion and a distal ball-shaped portion, resembling the joint of a bamboo. Hair breakage corresponds to the nodes. Eyebrows are affected as well as scalp hair. Simple examination of eyebrow hairs may increase the likelihood of early diagnosis of Netherton's syndrome in the newborn with congenital erythrodermic ichthyosis.

Trichorrhexis nodosa refers to white knots with transverse fractures along the hair shaft. Dermoscopy reveals brushlike hair fracturing (Fig. 2.23s). In general, trichorrhexis nodosa is an unspecific finding related to excess stress of hair in relation to its fragility. It can be observed in hair shaft abnormalities with increased fragility or more frequently as a consequence of hair weathering.

2.3.7 Exogenous Materials

A variety of exogenous materials of very different origin can be visualized by dermoscopy. These include hair dyes (Fig. 2.23t), camouflage products (Fig. 2.23u), residues from hair styling aids (Fig. 2.23v), and ectoparasites (Fig. 2.23w, x).

2.3.8 Summary and Algorithm of Dermoscopic Features in Common Conditions

A summary and algorithm of dermoscopic features in common conditions of the hair and scalp are given in Table 2.3 and Fig. 2.24, respectively.

Table 2.3 Summary of dermoscopic features in common conditions

Androgenetic alopecia
Hair diameter diversity (anisotrichosis)
Peripilar signs
Empty follicles
Honeycomb pigment pattern
Arborizing red lines
Alopecia areata
Yellow dots
Dystrophic hairs (cadaverized hairs, exclamation mark hairs)
Short regrowing miniaturized hairs
Trichotillomania
Coiled fractured hairs
Longitudinally split short hairs
Black dots
Dermoscopic features of scarring alopecias:
All
Loss of follicular ostia
Lichen planopilaris
Follicular keratosis
Hair casts
Acquired pili torti
Chronic cutaneous lupus erythematosus
Arborizing telangiectasia
Follicular keratotic plugs
Scalp atrophy with effaced or absent vascular loops
Folliculitis decalvans
Severe scaling and crusting
Pronounced hair tufting
Follicular pustules
Numerous coiled capillary loops
Classic pseudopelade of Brocq
No other changes (selective loss of follicular ostia)

2.4 Trichogram

The trichogram or hair pluck test is a semi-invasive technique for hair analysis on the basis of the hair growth cycle. It involves the forceful plucking of 50–100 hairs with a forceps from specific sites of the scalp. A major objective of trichogram measurements is to evaluate and count the status of individual hair roots and to establish the ratio of anagen to telogen roots.

Following the original description of the hair growth cycle by anatomist Mildred Trotter (1899–1991), studies on the dynamics of the follicular cycle have largely depended on the microscopic evaluation of plucked hairs with quantitative measuring of the number of individual hair roots. The method was introduced in 1957 by van Scott et al. as an indicator of hair growth in toxicologic studies with cytotoxic agents. In 1964, the term trichogram was initially used by Pecoraro to describe several hair growth parameters, such as the growth rate, shaft diameter, and telogen rate. Subsequently, the trichogram technique was developed and standardized to serve as a diagnostic tool for evaluation of hair loss in daily clinical practice. For this purpose it is simple to perform, repeatable, and reasonably reliable under standardized conditions.

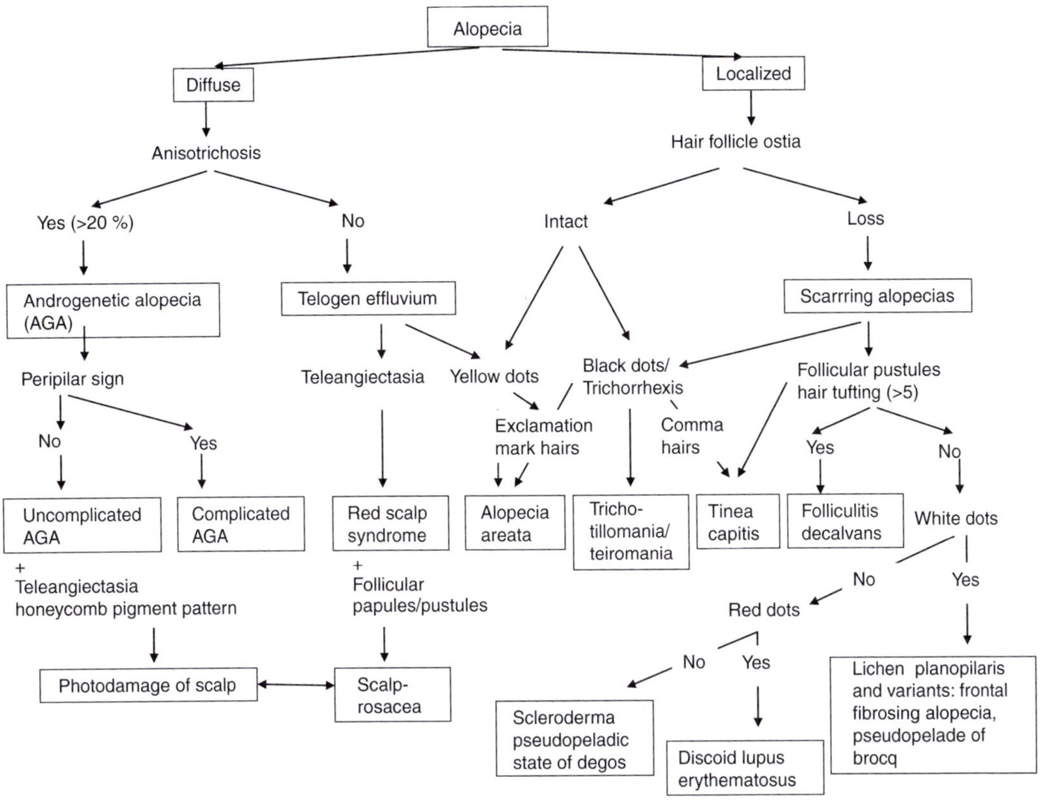

Fig. 2.24 Algorithm of trichoscopy

Since in 95 % of cases hair loss is due to a disorder of hair cycling, trichogram measurements serve as a standard method for quantifying the hair in its different growth cycle phases as it relates to the pathologic dynamics underlying the loss of hair. The percentage of hair roots in anagen, catagen, or telogen reflects either synchronization phenomena of the hair cycle or alterations in the duration of the respective growth cycle phases. Finally, the presence of dystrophic hair roots signalizes a massive damage to anagen hair follicles, either by toxins or drugs in higher concentrations or in severe alopecia areata.

2.4.1 Trichogram Procedure

The trichogram technique provides reliable results under the condition that hair samples are obtained under a standardized procedure.

The materials necessary for performing a trichogram include a tail comb, hair clips, artery forceps covered with rubber tube, a pair of scissors, microslides (76×26 mm), cover glasses (50×24 mm), Eukitt, xylol, a dissecting needle, and a binocular microscope with variable objectives (2.5 and 4.0) (Fig. 2.25a).

> The reproducibility of trichogram measurements relies on the adherence to strict standards in obtaining the hair samples.

Epilation of hair samples for the trichogram should always be performed at least 5 days after the last hair wash to avoid an artificial reduction of the telogen count. To avoid additional loss of telogen hairs, the hairs should also not be cut, curled, waved, or backcombed during that period.

Usually, epilations are carried out from two specified sites at the same time: in diffuse effluvium or androgenetic alopecia frontal (2 cm behind the forehead and 2 cm lateral) and occipital (2 cm lateral from the occipital protuberance); in

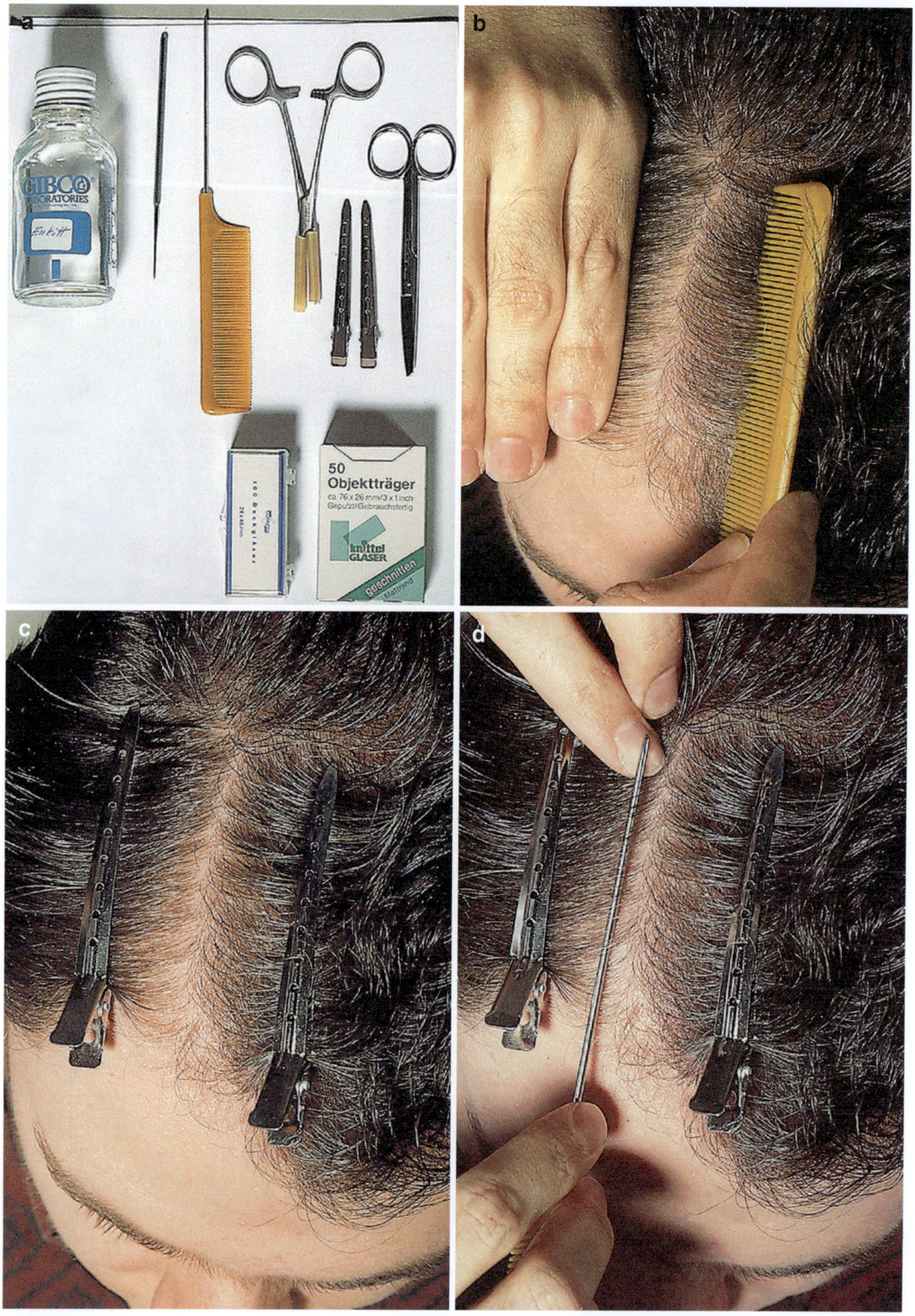

Fig. 2.25 (**a–u**) Trichogram. (**a**) Materials. (**b–o**) Procedure. (**p–t**) Hair root forms. (**p**) Telogen. (**q**) Anagen with root sheaths. (**r**) Anagen without root sheaths. (**s**) Catagen. (**t**) Dystrophic anagen. (**u**) *Demodex folliculorum*

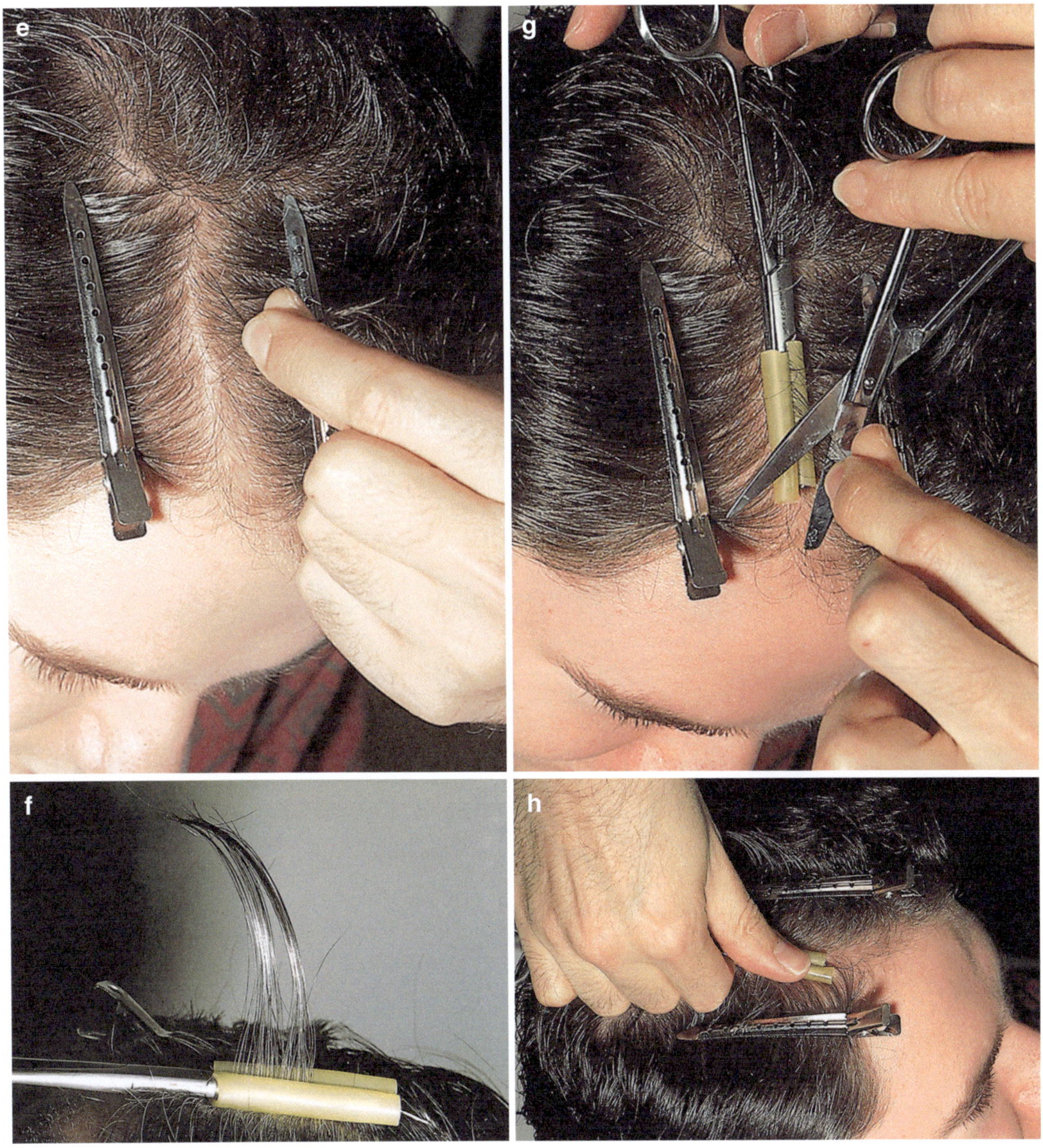

Fig. 2.25 (continued)

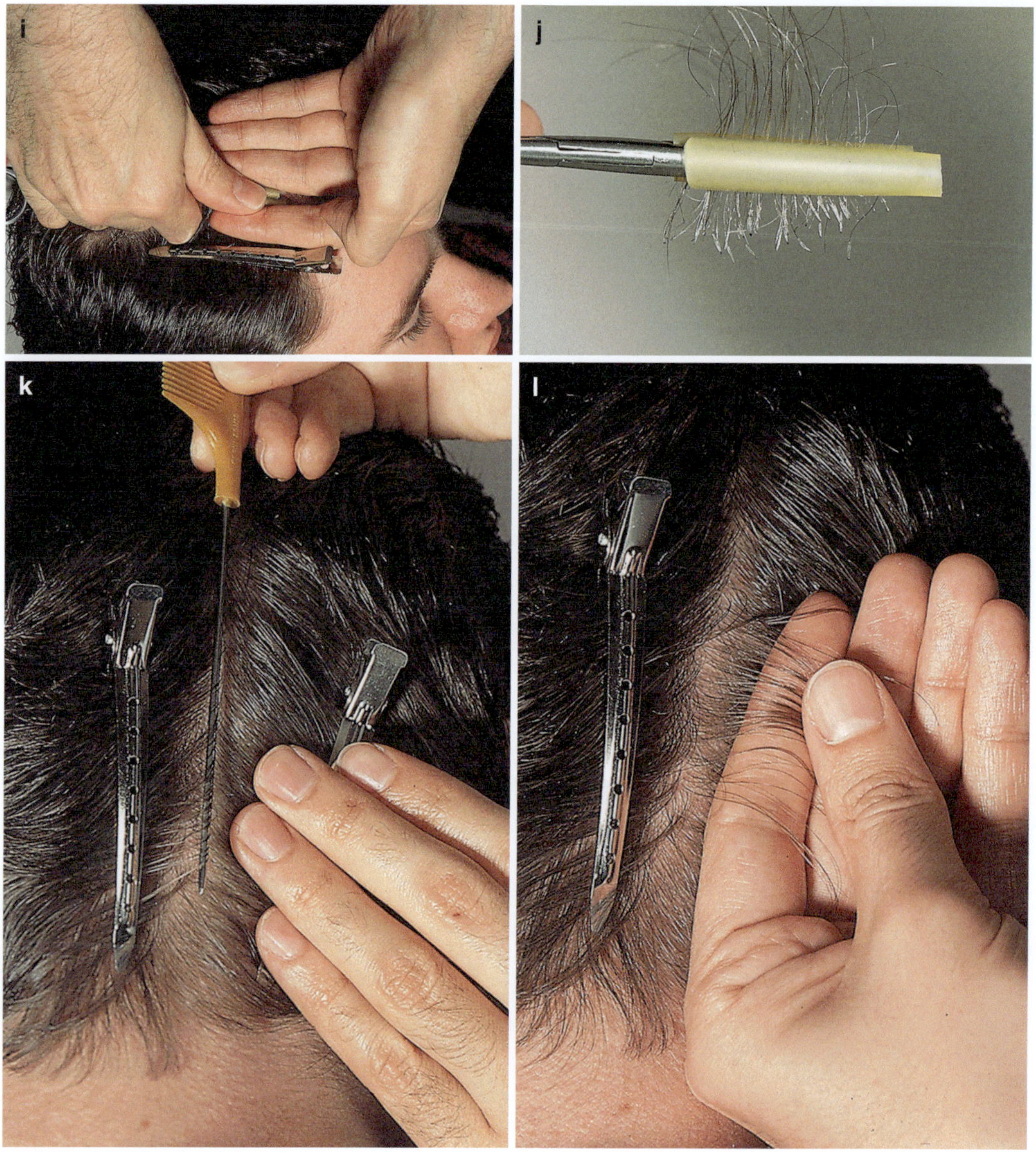

Fig. 2.25 (continued)

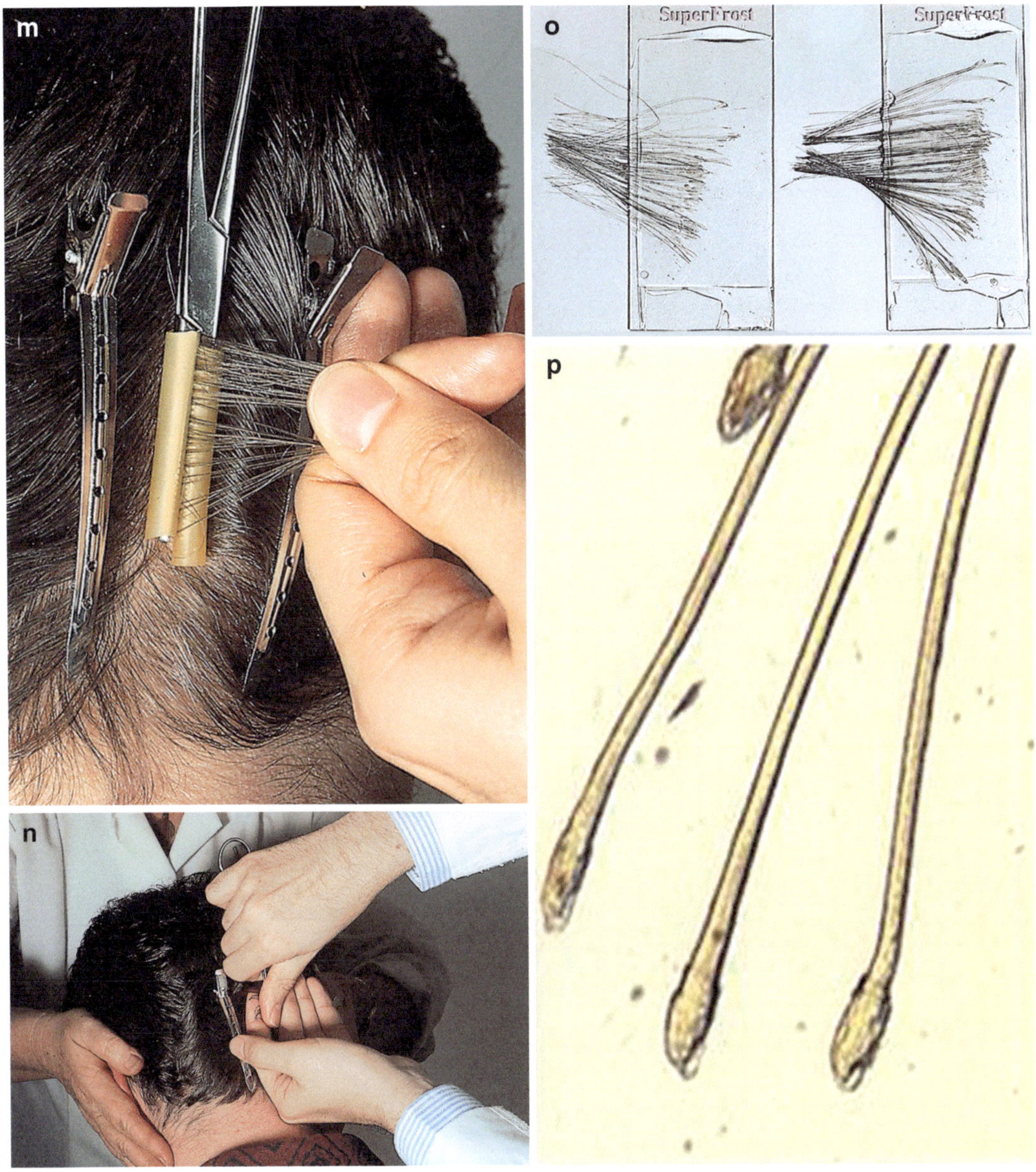

Fig. 2.25 (continued)

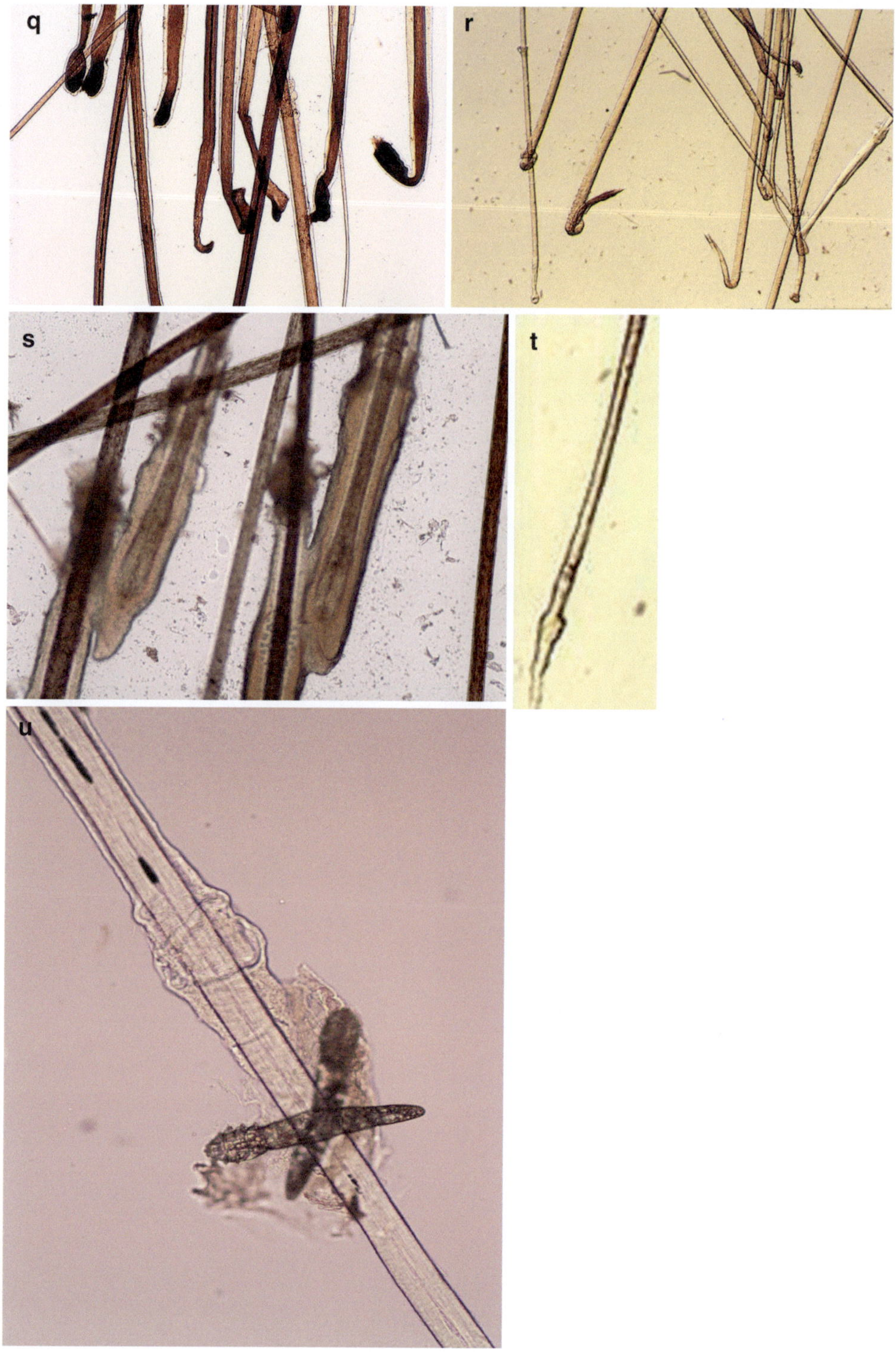

Fig. 2.25 (continued)

circumscribed alopecias, such as alopecia areata or trichotillomania, one sample is taken from the border zone and the control from the normal-appearing contralateral region (Fig. 2.25b–o).

The same standardized scalp regions should always be chosen to permit an optimal comparison of trichogram results in case of a follow-up examination.

Within the chosen area for epilation, the hair is parted and fixed with clips. Along the parting line, a bundle of approximately 50–100 hairs is lifted parallel along the course of the hair and grasped close to the scalp with the forceps whose jaws are covered with the rubber tubes. The forceps jaws are pressed together to the maximum and the tuft of hair is then epilated.

A sharp quick pull and exact plucking in the direction of the emergence angle of the hairs from the scalp are important to obtain a reliable hair root pattern. Slow or hesitant traction or the wrong pulling direction may induce distortions or alterations of the plucked hairs, complicating interpretation.

Embedding of epilated hairs occurs immediately to prevent dehydration of the hair roots. A few drops of Eukitt (after condensation, dilute with xylol) is given on two marked microslides. The tuft of hairs is taken with thumb and pointing finger; the roots are dipped in the embedding material (Eukitt), cut off 2 cm above the roots, and arranged in a fast manner with the dissecting needle in a parallel position before being covered. The evaluation can be done when the embedding material no longer runs, usually after 10 min. Correctly embedded hair roots are suitable for unlimited storage.

The act of plucking scalp hair may cause slight discomfort to the patient and may leave a small linear bald patch, which is why the frontal epilation site is better chosen contralateral to the natural hair part of the patient. The patient should be reassured that plucked hairs grow back after 3–6 weeks.

2.4.2 Trichogram Evaluation

The trichogram is a simple and reliable technique, but it needs critical interpretation. It provides information about the hair growth capacity, it detects disturbances of hair growth, and it detects toxic effects to the hair structure, induced by chemicals or drugs. In addition, the appearance and the size of the hair bulb are also important as atrophy and shrinkage reflect reduced growth activity. Finally, simultaneous microscopic examination of the hair shaft morphology may also help identify abnormalities of the hair shaft.

In every stage of the hair cycle, the hair root is characterized by a typical morphologic structure that is easy to recognize:

Telogen. Telogen hairs are those hairs shed with daily combing. Telogen bulbs are normally epilated with a simple hair pull. When increased numbers of telogen hairs are shed, this suggests the diagnosis of telogen effluvium. The telogen hair root is characteristically club shaped and unpigmented, with smooth contours, and has no attached root sheath structure (Fig. 2.25p).

Anagen with Root Sheaths. Anagen hairs are not normally seen in daily hair collections or epilated with a simple hair pull, with the exception of loose anagen hair that presents with anagen hairs devoid of hair root sheaths. Since anagen hairs are normal-growing hairs, they must be forcibly plucked from the scalp. The normal anagen hair root has a large base with an equally large diameter throughout. The bulb tip is usually pigmented and the adjacent hair shaft has a white coating composed of both the inner and outer root sheath (Fig. 2.25q)

Anagen Without Root Sheaths (Dysplastic Anagen Hair). These represent an epilation artifact in thin but obviously growing anagen hairs, with a diminished matrix diameter and devoid of hair root sheaths. The lower end of the hair shaft is usually wavy or bent like the handle of a bishop's crozier (Fig. 2.25r).

Catagen. The hair root in catagen generally has an equal diameter throughout or can become narrower toward the base. The hair roots look like club hair in the telogen phase, but still shows root sheaths, which increasingly become shorter (Fig. 2.25s).

Dystrophic Anagen. Under normal circumstances, dystrophic roots appear very seldom. Basically, they represent thin, nongrowing anagen hairs. Any pathologic condition that causes rapid cessation of mitosis in the hair matrix results in tapering of the diameter of the hair shaft that breaks off at the narrowest level with a pencil-like broken end tip (Fig. 2.25t).

Broken-off Hairs. They represent normally growing anagen hairs that have broken off on plucking. They can be easily recognized, since the broken ends appear smooth with a remaining diameter equal to that of the hair shaft.

Miniature Hairs. In addition to hairs of normal diameter, patients with androgenetic alopecia have a second population of hairs in the androgen-dependent area resulting from progressive narrowing and shortening of the hair shaft. These hairs represent terminal-to-vellus hair transformation. They are approximately 1 cm long and often have finely tapered tips. By definition vellus hairs have a shaft diameter of <40 μm.

In cases of androgenetic alopecia with seborrhea, occasionally *Demodex folliculorum* may be found, at times in considerable numbers, and nested within the outer hair root sheath (Fig. 2.25u). Their significance has remained elusive, though *Demodex* spp. are well recognized as the cause of demodectic mange in canines (remember, the term "alopecia" derives from Greek with reference to the loss of hair in patches in foxes afflicted with sarcoptic mange).

2.4.3 Trichogram Interpretation

Normally a maximum of 15 % of scalp hair bulbs are in telogen and 85 % are in anagen.

Normally a maximum of 20 % of scalp hair bulbs are anagen hairs devoid of hair root sheaths (dysplastic anagen hairs).

Trichograms with >10 % broken-off hairs cannot be evaluated correctly. Unless they are due to fragile hair, plucking should be repeated (Table 2.4).

The trichogram is diagnostic for telogen effluvium if more than 20 % of bulbs are in telogen. An increase of the frontal telogen rate together with a normal occipital telogen rate is diagnostic for androgenetic alopecia, while an increase of the occipital telogen rate is diagnostic for diffuse telogen effluvium (Table 2.5).

Greater than 10 % of dystrophic hairs are indicative of dystrophic anagen effluvium. If the cause is not obvious from the patient's history, toxicologic studies may be indicated. In a completed anagen effluvium in which only a few hairs remain on the scalp, all the epilated hairs are telogen bulbs (Table 2.6).

In children and in persons with thin hair, the rate of dysplastic anagen can occasionally reach >50 % (Table 2.7).

In trichotillomania, 100 % of the hair bulbs are in anagen, since the patient epilates the telogen hair.

Broken-off hair may amount up to a maximum of 10 % of the total number; their prevalence is higher either when the hair is fragile or

Table 2.4 Normal distribution pattern of hair roots in the trichogram of the scalp

Hair roots	Percentage (%)
Anagen with root sheaths	60–80
Anagen without root sheaths (dysplastic anagen)	5–20
Catagen	1–3
Telogen	12–15
Dystrophic anagen	<2
Broken-off hairs	5–6

From: Blume-Peytavi U, Orfanos CE (1995) Microscopy of the hair – the trichogram. In: Derup J, Jemec GBE (eds) Handbook of non-invasive methods and the skin. CRC Press, London, pp 549–554

Table 2.5 Causes for telogen effluvium

Postpartal effluvium
Postfebrile effluvium
Postinfectious effluvium
Effluvium from chronic diseases and malignancies
Effluvium from iron deficiency
Effluvium from endocrinologic diseases
Effluvium from cytostatic, anticoagulant, or chemical substances or ionizing radiation in low doses
Alopecia areata with slow progression
Androgenetic alopecia
Psychogenic effluvium

Modified from Braun-Falco O, Heilgemeir GP (1985) The trichogram. Structural and functional basis, performance, and interpretation. Semin Dermatol 4:40–52

Table 2.6 Causes for dystrophic anagen effluvium

Effluvium from cytostatic, anticoagulant, or chemical substances, toxins (heavy metals, plant toxins), or ionizing radiation in high doses
Alopecia areata with rapid progression

Modified from Braun-Falco O, Heilgemeir GP (1985) The trichogram. Structural and functional basis, performance, and interpretation. Semin Dermatol 4:40–52

Table 2.7 Causes for increase in anagen hairs devoid of hair root sheaths

Children
Loose anagen hair (>80 %, usually 90–100 % anagen hairs without hair root sheaths)
Thin hair
Androgenetic alopecia (frontal increase in % anagen hairs without hair root sheaths)
Inadequate epilation technique

Table 2.8 Trichogram characteristics of androgenetic alopecia

Increase in frontal telogen rate (telogen effluvium) >20 %
Increase in frontal anagen roots without root sheaths (thinning of hairs) >20 %
Increase in frontal catagen rate >2 %
Increase in percentage miniature hairs (terminal-to-vellus hair transformation) >13 %

when the plucking technique was not adequate. A light microscopic hair shaft examination is indicated to exclude a hair fragility disorder.

Presence of >13 % miniature hairs is indicative of androgenetic alopecia (Table 2.8).

2.4.4 Light Microscopic Hair Shaft Examination

In case of complaint of hair breakage, a pathologic hair feathering test, or if there is a high percentage of broken-off hairs in the trichogram, light microscopic examination of hair shaft is indicated. In general the patient with a hair shaft disorder presents with an abnormality or change in hair texture, appearance, manageability (so called unruly hair), or ability to grow long hair. Paramount to the clinical evaluation is to determine whether there is increased fragility or not by performing a hair feathering test. An algorithmic approach to narrow the differential diagnosis is to classify hair shaft disorders into congenital or acquired conditions, and in those with (which consequently give rise to alopecia) and those without increased hair fragility (Table 2.9). Finally, a systematic patient history and total clinical examination of the patient with emphasis on the teeth, nails, and sweat glands are needed, especially in the congenital disorders.

Table 2.9 Classification of hair shaft abnormalities (with corresponding SEM)

Congenital
With increased fragility
Classical pili torti (Fig. 2.26a)
Menkes kinky hair syndrome
Pili torti-like (pili torti et canaliculi) and corkscrew hairs (Fig. 2.26b) in the ectodermal dysplasias
Trichorrhexis invaginata (in Netherton's syndrome) (Fig. 2.26c)
Monilethrix (Fig. 2.26d)
Pseudomonilethrix (Fig. 2.26e)
Trichothiodystrophies (trichoschisis)
Congenital trichorrhexis nodosa (in argininosuccinase deficiency)
Without increased fragility
Twisting dystrophy in Marie Unna hereditary hypotrichosis
Woolly hair and woolly hair syndromes
Uncombable hair (pili trianguli et canaliculi) (Fig. 2.26f, g)
Pili annulati (may acquire increased fragility with weathering)
Pili pseudoanulati
Acquired
With increased fragility
Trichorrhexis nodosa (Fig. 2.26h)
Trichoclasia (Fig. 2.26i)
Without increased fragility
Whisker hair (allotrichia circumscripta symmetrica)
Acquired progressive kinking of the hair
Drug-induced acquired curly hair
Knotting of scalp hair (trichonodosis) (Fig. 2.26j)
Bird's nest hair (matting of scalp hair)
Twisted and rolled body hairs with multiple, large knots (Fig. 2.26k)
Hair casts (Fig. 2.26l)

Usually, a hair mount and examination of shafts provides important clues to the diagnosis. For this purpose, hair must be cut off, as they break at the point of fragility upon plucking. They are embedded in a similar way as in the trichogram technique. Using the light microscope and polarization, the great majority of congenital or acquired hair shaft disorders can be diagnosed in the office. Many hair shaft abnormalities can be recognized also by dermoscopy (see Sect. 2.3.6). Current knowledge of structural changes has been amplified by scanning electron microscopy (SEM: Fig. 2.26a–l).

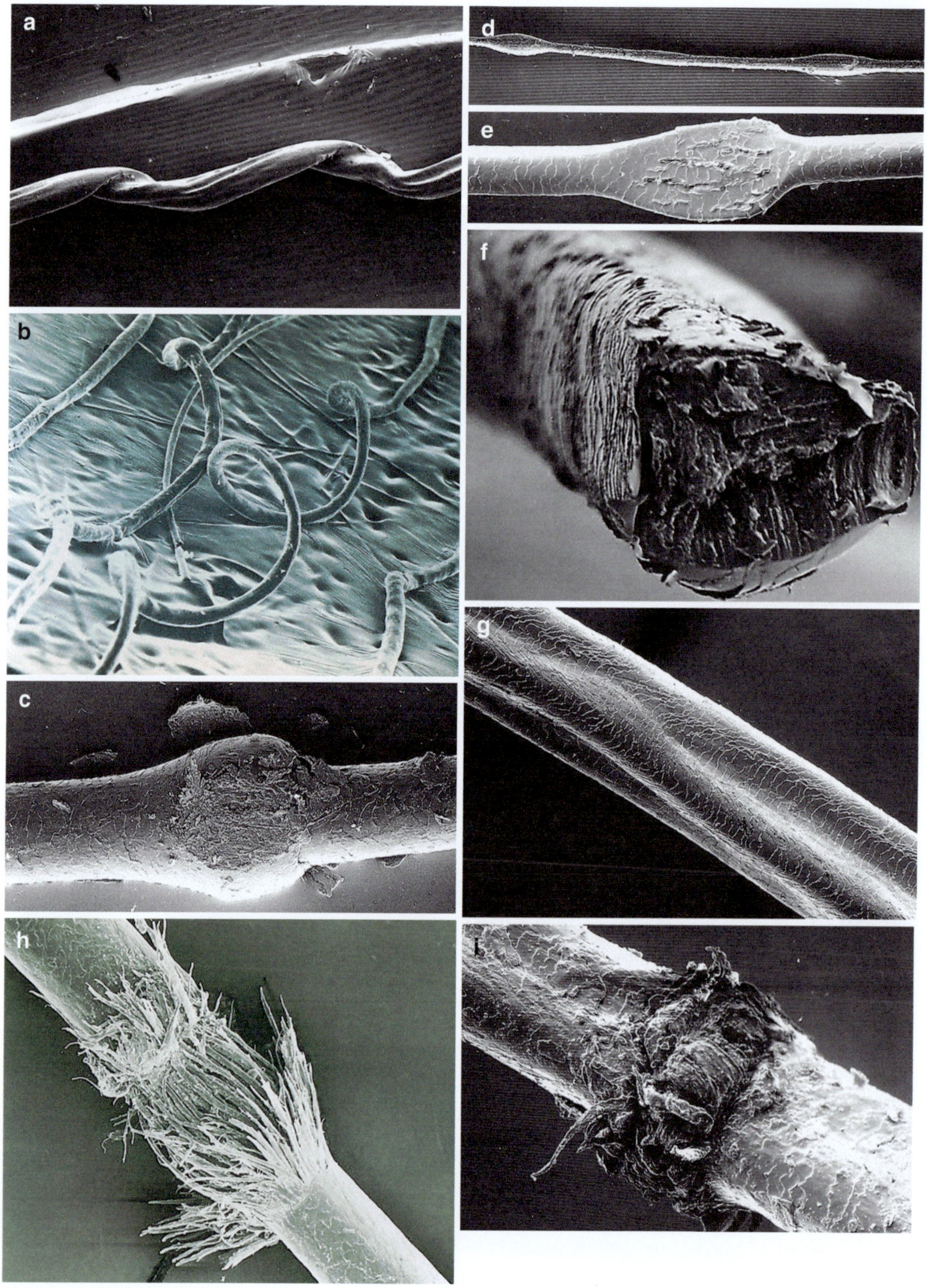

Fig. 2.26 (**a–k**) Scanning electron microscopy. (**a**) Classical pili torti. (**b**) Pili torti-like (pili torti et canaliculi) and corkscrew hairs (ectodermal dysplasia). (**c**) Trichorrhexis invaginata (in Netherton's syndrome). (**d**) Monilethrix. (**e**) Pseudomonilethrix. (**f, g**) Pili trianguli et canaliculi. (**h**) Trichorrhexis nodosa. (**i**) Trichoclasia. (**j**) Knotting of scalp hair (trichonodosis). (**k**) Twisted and rolled body hairs with multiple, large knots (Courtesy of Prof. P. Itin). (**l**) Hair cast

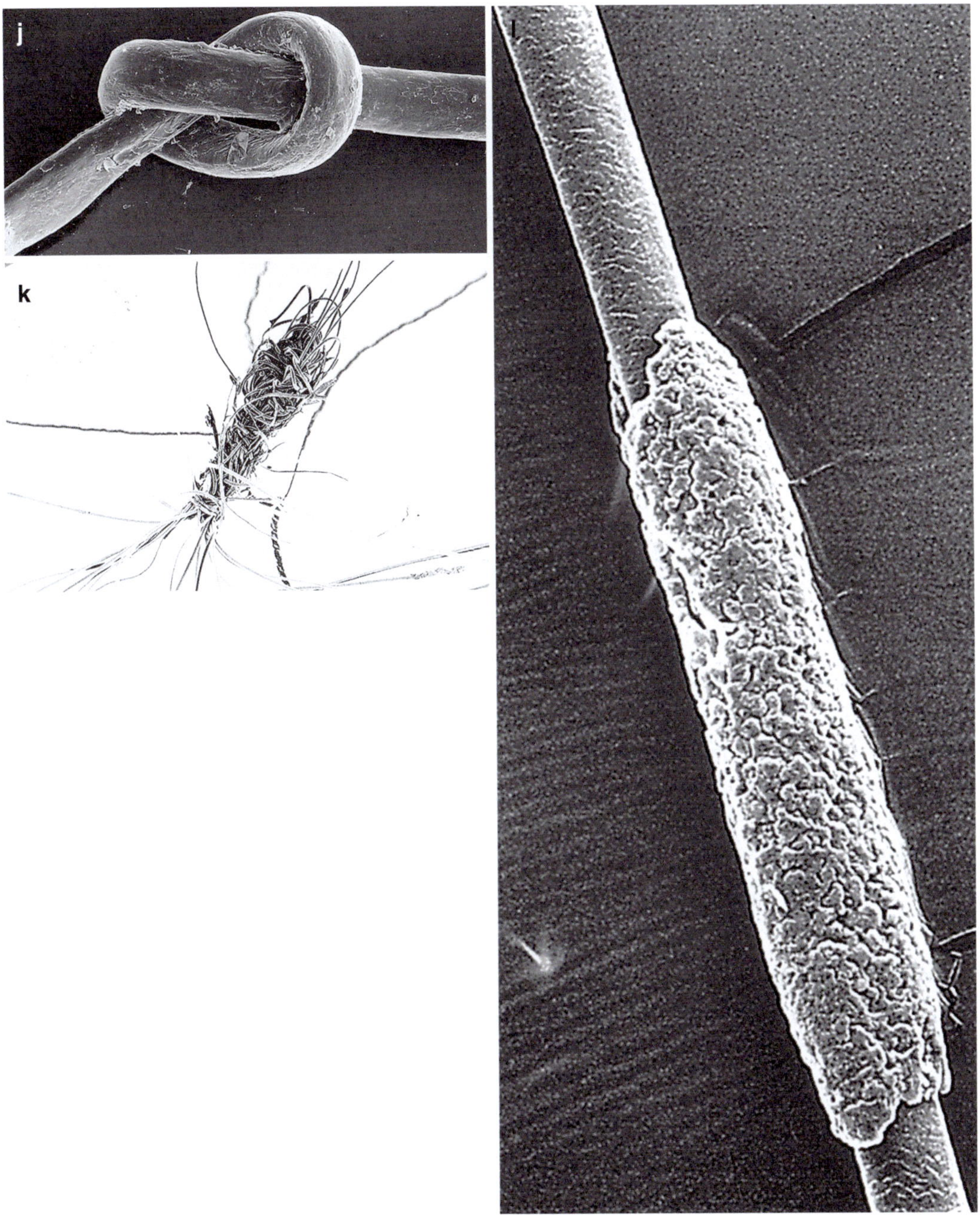

Fig. 2.26 (continued)

2.5 Laboratory Evaluation

Diagnostic tests are useful when the probability of a disease being present is neither high nor low, since high degree of clinical certainty overrides the uncertainty of the laboratory data.

> The greater the number of different tests done, the greater the risk of getting false-positive or irrelevant leads. The possibilities for laboratory errors increase in the automated multiple-screen procedures. Therefore, laboratory testing must be kept sharply focused.

Clinical suspicion is the determinant, and knowledge of clinical dermatology is the prerequisite for combining medical sense with economic sense in requesting laboratory tests.

2.5.1 Biochemical Investigations

In men, laboratory testing for the diagnosis of androgenetic alopecia is unnecessary, unless the patient history or examination provide clues for another underlying disorder or associated disease. Measurement of ferritin level, thyroid-stimulating hormone, and syphilis serology (PRP or VDRL and TPPA) may be considered depending on the individual history and clinical findings, especially in diffuse telogen effluvium.

Serum ferritin levels are measured in medical laboratories as part of the iron studies workup for anemia. Storage iron is the body's iron reserves that are tissue bound and measured by serum ferritin concentration, transport iron is transported to the tissues and measured by transferrin concentration and saturation, and functional iron consists of iron that is bound to hemoglobin, myoglobin, and diverse enzymes. It is measured by hemoglobin concentration. The normal ranges for serum ferritin levels can vary between laboratories but are usually between 30 and 300 ng/mL (=μg/L) for males.

> Ferritin levels may be artificially high in cases of chronic disease where ferritin is elevated in its capacity as an acute phase protein.

In children or adolescents with premature onset of androgenetic alopecia, an interdisciplinary approach with a pediatric endocrinologist may be considered, though androgenetic alopecia without associated signs of premature puberty is usually not associated with endocrinologic abnormalities.

Finally, in men above 45 years considered for oral finasteride treatment of androgenetic alopecia, measuring the prostate-specific antigen (PSA) level is recommended before, after starting therapy, and thereafter on a twice yearly basis.

> Finasteride reduces PSA levels by ca. 50 % and can delay diagnosis or mask detection of prostate cancer. In case of increase >0.4 ng/ml/year, patient must be referred to a urologist.

Since alopecia areata is considered to be an organ-specific autoimmune disease and, at least in localized patchy disease, the clinical appearance would seem sufficient to make a diagnosis, further laboratory investigation could seem unnecessary or even inappropriate. Nevertheless, in recurrent cases or patients presenting with extensive alopecia areata, certain laboratory investigations may be indicated to detect associated autoimmune diseases and/or comorbidities that may affect the disease course (Table 2.10). An increased incidence of other autoimmune diseases, like Hashimoto's thyroiditis and pernicious anemia, is seen among alopecia areata patients, while low serum ferritin or zinc levels and HIV infection may have an influence on the disease course. Ultimately, the detection of anti-thyroid or anti-parietal cell autoantibodies may represent markers for autoimmunity in favor of the diagnosis of alopecia areata.

Table 2.10 Proposed comorbidities screening in alopecia areata

Test	Purpose
To detect associated autoimmune disorders	
Antithyroid antibodies	To detect associated thyroid autoimmunity
Anti-parietal cell antibodies	To detect associated parietal cell autoimmunity
Thyroid function tests	To detect associated autoimmune thyroid disease
Vitamin B12 level	To detect associated pernicious anemia
To detect potentially disease-modifying comorbidities	
CRP and ferritin level	Iron deficiency
Zinc level	Zinc deficiency
Vitamin D3 level	Vitamin D deficiency
HIV serology	HIV infection/AIDS
To rule out other causes of patchy alopecia	
Antinuclear antibody test	Lupus erythematosus
RPR test (or VDRL and TPPA depending on laboratory)	Syphilis II (alopecia areolaris)

The diagnosis of heavy metal toxicity requires observation of presenting symptoms, obtaining a thorough history of potential exposure (occupational, environmental, accidental), and the results of laboratory tests. Laboratory tests routinely used for seriously exposed persons include blood and urine analysis.

In a study performed by Pierard, toxic metals in abnormal amount in blood and urine were observed only when >10 % of hair bulbs in the trichogram were dystrophic.

2.5.2 Microbiological Studies

Microbiological studies are mandatory in inflammatory conditions of the scalp with scaling, crusting, and/or pustulation.

While in children fungal infections (tinea capitis) predominate, in the adult, bacterial infection with *S. aureus* is the most prominent.

At times, repeated microbiological studies are recommended, since with prolonged antibiotic treatments, typically in folliculitis decalvans, new and resistant pathogens may emerge, e.g., Gram-negative folliculitis.

Diagnosis of fungal and bacterial skin infections requires swabs and test systems for direct visualization of pathogens (KOH preparation, Gram's stain), cultures and special tests for species identification, and the availability of the appropriate laboratory infrastructure.

2.5.3 Misuse of Hair Analysis as a Diagnostic Tool

Hair analysis refers to the chemical analysis of a hair sample. Its most widely accepted use is in the fields of forensic toxicology and, increasingly, environmental toxicology. Hair analysis is also used for the detection of recreational drugs, including cocaine, heroin, benzodiazepines, and amphetamines, and to detect the presence of illegal drugs. Chemical hair analysis may prove particularly useful for retrospective purposes when blood and urine are no longer expected to contain a particular contaminant, typically a year or less.

On the other hand, an increasing number of commercial laboratories are committed to providing multielemental hair analyses in which a single test is used to determine values for many minerals simultaneously. This type of analysis is used by several alternative medicine fields with the claim that hair analyses can help diagnose a wide variety of health problems and can be used as the basis for prescribing natural chelation therapy, mineral, trace elements, and/or vitamin supplements. However, these uses remain controversial for a number of reasons:

Most commercial hair analysis laboratories have not validated their analytical techniques by checking them against standard reference materials.

Hair mineral content can be affected by exposure to various substances such as shampoos, bleaches, and hair dyes. No analytic technique enables reliable determination of the source of specific levels of elements in hair as bodily or environmental.

The level of certain minerals can be affected by the color, diameter, and rate of growth of an individual's hair; the season of the year; the geographic location; and the age and gender of the individual.

Normal ranges of hair minerals have not been defined.

For most elements, no correlation has been established between hair level and other known indicators of nutrition status. It is possible for hair concentration of an element to be high even though deficiency exists in the body, and vice versa.

2.6 Scalp Biopsy

In some cases of alopecia, a diagnosis cannot be made based on results of physical examination, diagnostic hair techniques, and laboratory studies. This is particularly the case in the scarring alopecias. In these cases, a scalp biopsy may provide the specific diagnosis. In addition, it must be kept in mind that two types of alopecia may coexist within the same patient.

In all cases of scarring alopecia, a scalp biopsy is mandatory.

2.6.1 Algorithm of Scalp Histopathology

By definition, scarring alopecia is characterized by a visible loss of follicular ostia due to a destruction of the hair follicle on histopathologic examination. The biopsy will help to identify the cause and rule out infiltrating malignant disease.

In the non-cicatricial alopecias where the follicular ostia are intact, a scalp biopsy is optional for morphometric studies on transverse sections (hair follicle density, anagen/telogen ratio, terminal/vellus hair ratio) or to detect specific findings for a particular diagnosis, such as trichomalacia in trichotillomania and the peribulbar lymphocytic infiltrate in alopecia areata.

In the inflammatory scarring alopecias with active inflammation, the type of inflammatory infiltrate (lymphocytic, neutrophilic, mixed, granulomatous), the pattern of inflammation, and its relation to the hair follicle usually enable a specific diagnosis. Where active inflammation is missing, an elastin stain will help to identify the scarring process and its pattern (Fig. 2.27).

Frequent problems related to the scalp biopsy are the reluctance of many dermatologists to perform a scalp biopsy and therefore lack of experience with the proper procedure and the lack of familiarity of many pathologists with scalp histopathology.

Scalp biopsies are often inadequately performed: superficial (without subcutaneous tissue), small, often tangential to the hair follicle, and with crush artifacts. Finally, the hair follicle and its derangements are complex and dynamic, while a biopsy only gives a momentary snapshot of the pathology.

Nevertheless, if done and examined properly, the scalp biopsy should be an easy, relatively painless, and bloodless procedure that represents an invaluable adjunct for confirming or establishing the diagnosis of a specific type of alopecia, whether scarring or non-scarring.

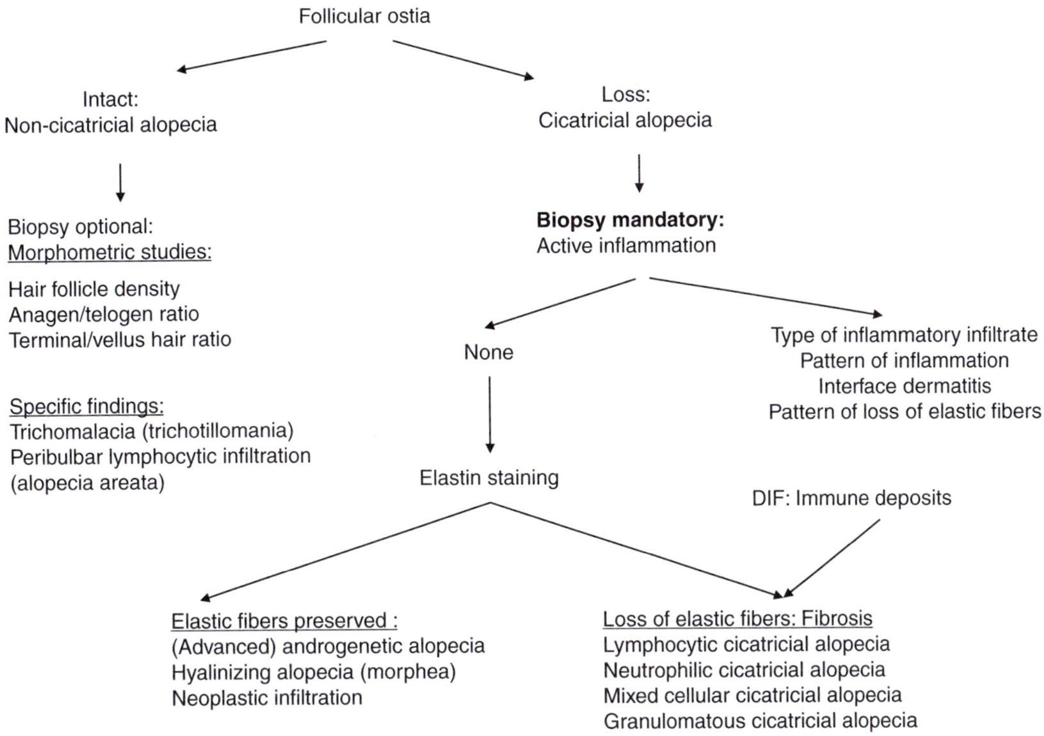

Fig. 2.27 Algorithm of scalp histopathology

2.6.2 Procedure of Scalp Biopsy

The scalp specimen obtained for histopathologic study should be large enough to include multiple hairs, deep enough to contain the hair bulb, and properly angled so that microscopic sectioning shows the entire follicular structure.

For a biopsy an area of the scalp is chosen where the disease is active; frequently the margin of the involved area shows the pathologic changes best, while areas should be avoided where there are no hair follicles present. After choosing the appropriate site, the hairs are clipped in a 1 cm^2 area, leaving a 2-mm stubble (Fig. 2.28a). The area is prepared with 70 % alcohol. For adequate anesthesia and hemostasis, 1.5 ml of 1.0 % lidocaine with epinephrine is injected, raising a large wheal (Fig. 2.28b). To obtain an adequate vasoconstrictor effect, it is advisable to wait 20–30 min before proceeding to the biopsy. Also, areas are to be avoided that lie over the temporal or occipital arteries or in which an arterial palpation can be detected. To avoid tying long hairs in the suture material, paper tape is placed over the uncut hairs surrounding the biopsy site. An adequate biopsy specimen can be obtained by using a 6-mm punch instrument that is placed parallel to the emerging angle of the hair stubbles (Fig. 2.28c). The punch is turned through the dermis and subcutaneous fat to a level including the hair bulbs. The biopsy specimen can be grasped at the edge with a fine-toothed forceps (Fig. 2.28d), while it is cut free of attachment deep in the fat with small, curved scissors. Alternatively, a thin 1-cm ellipse can be made, especially if the scalp is very tight or scarred, and a 6-mm punch site may not be closed with sutures. The biopsy site is sutured with blue 4-0 Prolene (Fig. 2.28e). Three to four stitches are usually adequate for hemostasis. The specimen is then cut in half with a # 15 blade parallel to the longitudinal axis of the hair shafts (Fig. 2.28f). One half of the specimen is submitted for the routine hematoxylin and eosin examination, while the other half for immunofluorescence studies as indicated (Fig. 2.28g). In some instances, transverse sectioning of a second, entire punch according to the Headington technique may be done for quantitative morphometric analyses of the follicles and hair.

For a discussion of the specific histopathologic conditions, the reader should consult a standard dermatopathology textbook.

2.6.3 Value of Direct Immunofluorescence Studies

In a study of 136 scalp biopsies obtained for histopathology and direct immunofluorescence (DIF) studies at the Department of Dermatology, University Hospital of Zurich, Trachsler and Trüeb

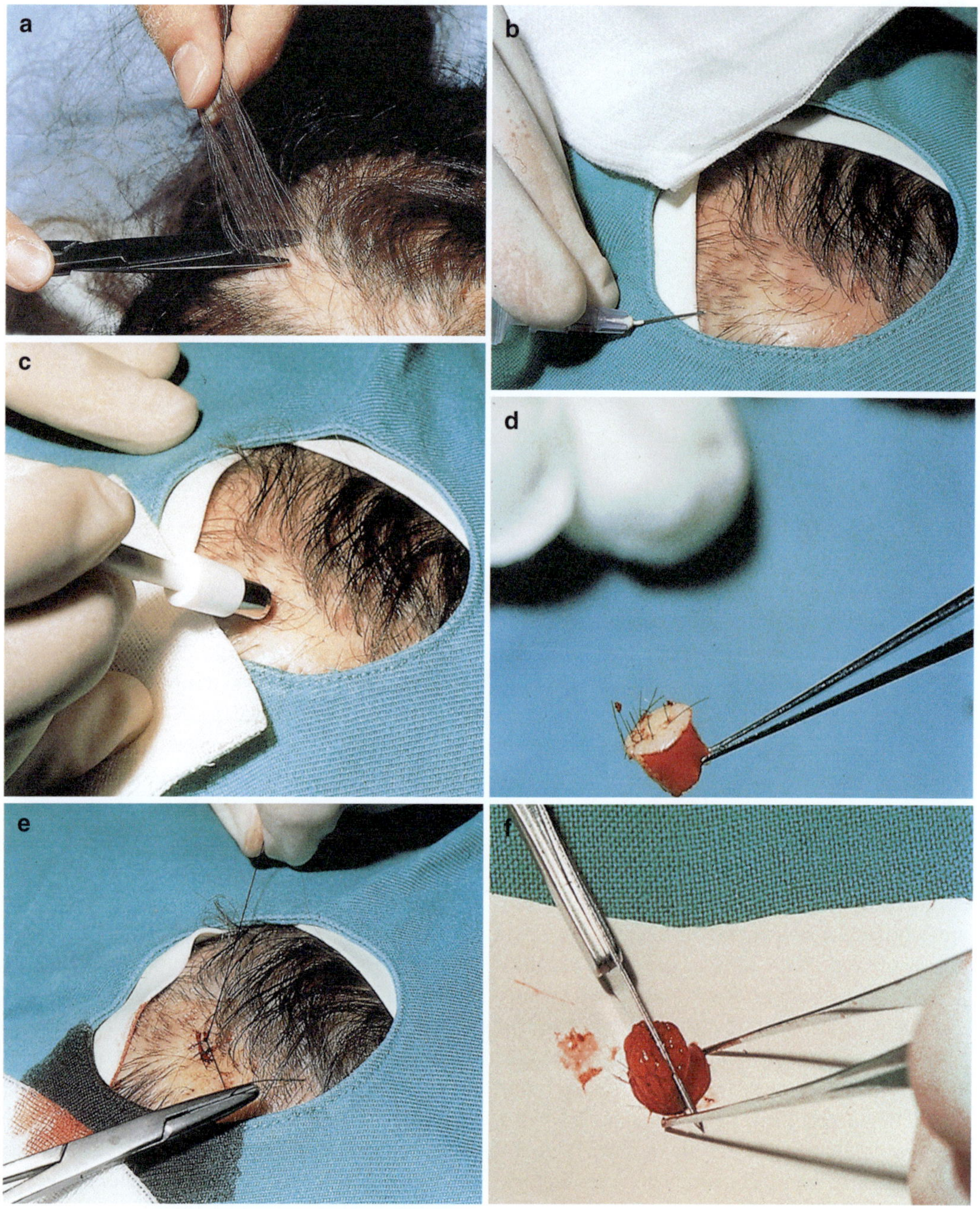

Fig. 2.28 (**a**–**g**) Scalp biopsy

g

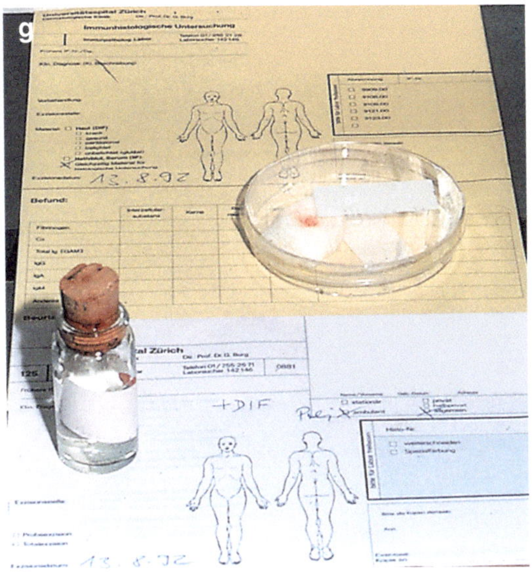

Fig. 2.28 (continued)

made a definitive diagnosis in 126 of 136 biopsies. In 97 % the definitive diagnosis was made on the basis of histopathology alone. Characteristic DIF patterns showed high specificity (98 %) but low sensitivity (34 %) for lichen planopilaris (Fig. 2.29a) and high specificity (96 %) and sensitivity (76 %) for lupus erythematosus (Fig. 2.29b).

> The diagnostic yield of DIF studies performed on scalp biopsies is highest when the diagnosis of cutaneous lupus erythematosus is in question.

Schaerer and Trüeb were the first to propose DIF studies on plucked hairs for diagnosis of autoimmune pemphigus. Hair is plucked in the same manner as for the trichogram and snap frozen and processed much the same way as scalp biopsies for DIF studies. Our observation of positive immunofluorescence within the outer hair root sheath of plucked anagen hairs (Fig. 2.29c) in patients with pemphigus vulgaris and foliaceus has stimulated subsequent authors to further elaborate on the method. Positive DIF findings are seen in scalp hair, irrespective of the presence of scalp lesions. All pemphigus variants (pemphigus vulgaris, foliaceus, erythematosus, and vegetans) have positive DIF findings in the outer hair root sheaths. Currently, utility of the method for evaluation of immunological remission in patients with pemphigus is being studied.

> Regarding the high sensitivity of DIF on plucked hair in autoimmune pemphigus patients, it seems that hair plucking is a suitable alternative to the more invasive techniques of skin or mucosal biopsy for obtaining specimens for DIF.

2.7 Quantifying Hair Loss

Reliably assessing the actual shedding of hair is a crucial diagnostic point in trichological practice. To fulfill office requirements, the test should be easy, noninvasive, and not time-consuming. Many methods have been proposed, but all need standardization. The hair pull represents a poorly sensitive method, while telogen percentage in the trichogram does not correlate with severity of hair loss.

2.7.1 Daily Hair Counts

Daily hair counts are done by the patient at home to provide a *quasi*-quantitative assessment of the number of hairs shed daily. For this purpose, the patient is instructed to collect all hairs that fall out during the morning grooming, including hairs on the pillow, sink, comb, brush, and shoulders as well as all hairs that come out with the morning shampoo. Placing a piece of nylon netting or gauze over the drain will help secure hairs otherwise lost during washing. The entire morning's collection is placed in a clear, smooth, plastic bag. The date and information on whether the hair has been shampooed or not is written on a label placed on the bag. The patient is also asked to count every hair in the bag and to record the total count on the label as well. Typically, hair collection should be done for 14 consecutive days, and all 14 bags are brought to the physician's office (Fig. 2.30).

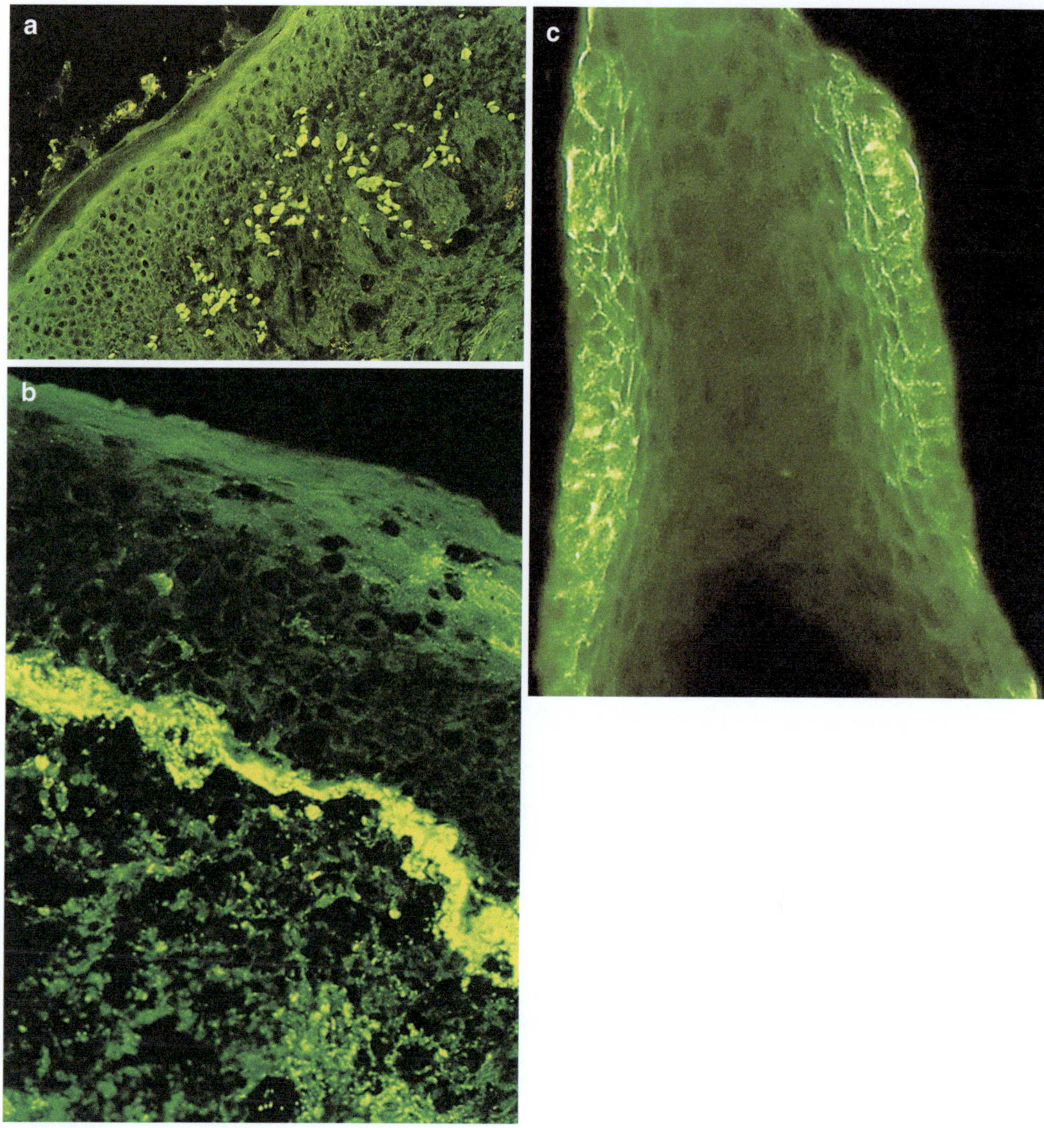

Fig. 2.29 (**a–c**) Direct immunofluorescence studies: (**a**) Pattern for lichen planopilaris: cytoid bodies. (**b**) Pattern for lupus erythematosus: lupus band. (**c**) Chicken wire pattern within outer hair root sheath of plucked anagen hairs in pemphigus

> It is more practical to ask patients to collect and count the hairs on 5–7 days prior to the trichogram (daily hair counts) and after washing the hair following the trichogram (hair wash test).

The amount of normal hair shed may vary from 35 to 180 hairs, depending on the amount of scalp hair and seasonal factors. The number is usually higher on the day of shampoo, especially when the hair is not shampooed daily.

> In diffuse telogen effluvium and anagen effluvium, the number of hairs shed daily is in the 100 s, while in androgenetic alopecia, it may well be less than 100.

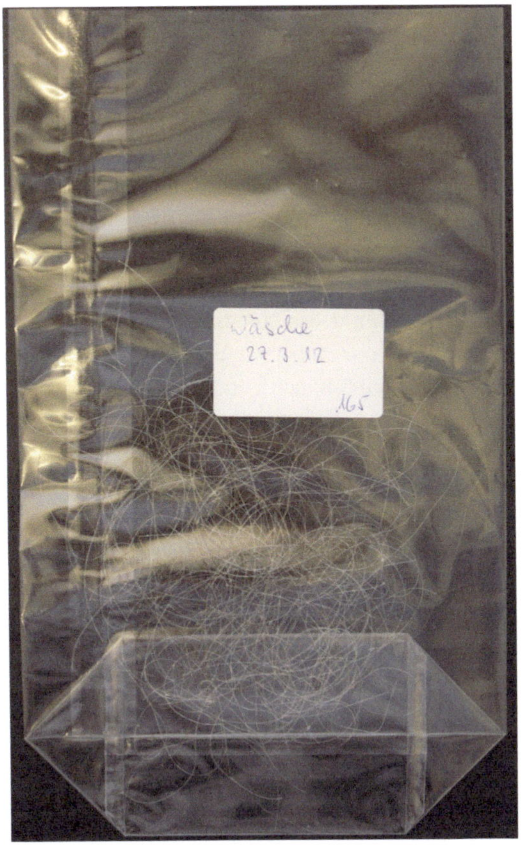

Fig. 2.30 Daily hair count

Therefore, it is not wise to trust in rules of thumb, such as a daily hair count of up to 100 is normal, when evaluating hair loss.

2.7.2 Hair Wash Test and Modified Wash Test

While the daily hair count is a cumbersome procedure, it has been proposed that the wash test is probably the best method to adopt. In the wash test, the patient, 5 days after the last shampoo, washes the hair in the sink with its drain covered by gauze. The hairs entrapped in the gauze are then counted. In one study assessing hair shedding in children, the wash test proved to be reliable, with a cutoff point of normality close to 11. Wash test values increase with age. Age-dependent normal values in adults do not exist.

In an attempt to find a simple method to evaluate reliably the diagnosis and activity of androgenetic alopecia and telogen effluvium, Guarrera et al. adopted the modified wash test, which accomplishes such a task through the assessment of the number of shed hair and the vellus percentage. The collected hairs after washing are counted and divided into ≤ 3 and ≥ 5 cm in length. The technique has originally been adapted to differentiate telogen effluvium from female androgenetic alopecia. The test demonstrated that in female androgenetic alopecia, 58.9 % of hair is vellus, whereas in chronic telogen effluvium, only 3.5 %.

2.7.3 Office-Based Computer-Assisted Image Analysis

Eventually, measurement of the effects of treatment needs to be quantified reliably. The method should be more sensitive than the wash test and capable of analyzing relevant parameters of hair growth, which are hair density, hair diameter, hair growth rate, and anagen/telogen ratio.

For this purpose, computer-assisted image analysis has been proposed: Some patents have been filed and publications followed since the 1980s. However, it soon became clear that hair is a tricky material for automated computer-assisted image analysis and that numbers might not all be considered as reflecting hair measurements. Physical properties of hair, that is, the object and the variability of the skin, and their background are very complex. The multilayered fiber is composed of a nonpigmented cuticle, a cortex with presence or absence of pigment granules, and a medulla filled with proteinaceous material or air cavities. On top, its organization and orientation at the exit point from the skin must also be taken into account. A follicular unit comprising a number of hair follicles (occasionally up to five) may exit from a single orifice at the skin surface and it may be difficult to count individual hair fibers. Some attempts have suggested that use of fully automatic systems may be an option, but this has not been made available to the public.

A software named TrichoScan combining epiluminescence microscopy with digital image analysis has been proposed and marketed for automated image analysis of scalp hair. This method requires the use of hair dyes for improved detection of less pigmented and thinner hair.

Advocates for the method declare that a system must be able to analyze the biological parameters that constitute hair growth, which are (1) hair density (n/cm^2), (2) hair diameter (μm), (3) hair growth rate (mm/day), and (4) anagen/telogen ratio. Intra-class correlation of approximately 91 % within the same operator and an interclass correlation of approximately 97 % for different operators suggested that the method was very precise and reproducible.

Using standardized photographic equipment and calibrated processing for contrast-enhanced phototrichogram (CEPTG) analysis, van Neste established a protocol that was equally sensitive as scalp biopsies for hair detection and growth staging. Taking this as a reference method, van Neste and Trüeb performed a study to evaluate the advantages and limits of TrichoScan for human hair growth analysis. The study was prompted by a number of variations that were unexpected after considering the original claims for accuracy promoting the TrichoScan method for hair growth measurement. The investigation did not corroborate these claims. With the available software, numbers were displayed for hair counts (all fibers detected by the software in the target area and those that touched the border of the target area). This number is also split into resting hair (telogen) and those considered growing, that is, in anagen phase of the hair growth cycle. The commercially available software provided to dermatologists and hair clinics for office-based use originally did not display the thickness of hair fibers and the hair growth rate. Although cumulative thickness may be an indirect way to approach the hair thickness measurement, it provides a global measure that depends on hair cycle duration. Also, that TrichoScan measures growth accurately was challenged. First, there are no growth rates on the data display. Second, the precision of anagen hair detection is not optimal. Indeed, the anagen percentage was underestimated (difference >5 %) in two out of four scalp sites as well as in the beard area, but it was overestimated when thinning was more important (overestimation of 32 % anagen hair proportion in the vertex). A number of these errors (especially with thin hair detection) have been described by others using the TrichoScan method in normal scalp sites, especially a density that was underestimated by 22 % and the lack of detection of thinner hair. As thinning is a phenomenon associated with androgenetic alopecia, published documents and our experimental study clearly documented that especially thin hair counts as well as growth staging generated by the TrichoScan method may not be considered as reliable. Therefore, it was concluded that TrichoScan in the present form would not qualify as a test method for quantification of hair loss according to our internal and other standards particularly in patients with androgenetic alopecia.

Computerized methods require further optimization. Ease of use and fast image processing, as pointed out by others, are certainly appreciated.

> Albeit speed is considered smart in our culture, customers, that is, clinicians, patients, and pharmaceutical or cosmetic companies, deserve the highest standard and a better service than merely a fast one. All should be given the best possible and clinically most relevant information about hair measurements – both qualitatively and quantitatively – that have diagnostic, prognostic, and therapeutic relevance.

Ultimately, Guarrera et al. assessed the reliability of TrichoScan in comparison with the modified wash test. They studied 41 female subjects complaining of hair loss due to androgenetic alopecia or telogen effluvium and compared the results obtained with TrichoScan versus the modified wash test. The concordance between the clinical diagnosis and that of the modified wash test was found to be fair and that between clinical diagnosis and TrichoScan fair enough, though less satisfactory. TrichoScan and the modified wash test were concordant in only 17/41 patients (41 %). The modified wash test proved better in general and especially at detecting telogen effluvium. The authors concluded that clinical observation should be assisted by the modified wash test and dermoscopy, leaving the scalp biopsy for very difficult cases. TrichoScan proved less useful and may be even misleading in telogen effluvium.

2.8 Hair Database Sheet

The patient and family history, history of hair cosmetic procedures, clinical examination findings (of hair loss pattern and scalp condition), diagnostic techniques, laboratory data, and results from microbiological studies and scalp biopsy, as indicated in the individual case, enable a definitive diagnosis to be made. For documentation purposes and facilitation of interpretation, findings are recorded on a hair database sheet (Fig. 2.31)

HAIR DATA BASE SHEET

Patient History

Family History — negative ☐ androgenetic alopecia ☐ other: ______

Personal History ______

Drug History ______

Hair Cosmetic Procedures — negative ☐ positive: ______

Clinica l Examination

Hair Loss Pattern — androgenetic ☐ diffuse ☐ localized ☐

Scalp Examination ______

Felt Examination ______

Part Width Assessment ______

Hair Pull — frontal ____/50 occipital____/50 lesional____/50

Hair Feathering — normal ☐ pathologic ☐

Trichoscopy

Follicular Patterns — peripilar sign ☐ yellow dots ☐ loss of follicular ostia ☐; empty follicles ☐ black dots ☐ follicular keratosis ☐

Vascular/Pigment Patterns — vascular ☐ ______ pigment ☐ ______

Hair Shaft Patterns — anisotrichosis ☐ Other ______

Exogenous Materials ______

Trichogramm	Frontal	Occipital	Contralateral
Anagen with outer root sheath	___%	___%	___%
Anagen without outer root sheath	___%	___%	___%
Catagen	___%	___%	___%
Telogen	___%	___%	___%
Dystrophic	___%	___%	___%
Broken - off	___%	___%	___%
Miniaturized	___%		

Laboratory Evaluation

Biochemical Investigations ______

Microbiological Studies ______

Scalp Biopsy Specimen ______

Hair Counts

Daily ______

Hair Wash/Modified Wash ______

Final Diagnosis: ______

Fig. 2.31 Hair database sheet

Further Reading

Patient History

Archer VE, Luell E (1960) Effect of selenium sulfide suspension on hair roots. J Invest Dermatol 35:65–67

Baumer A, Belli S, Trüeb RM, Schinzel A (2000) An autosomal dominant form of hereditary hypotrichosis simplex maps to 18p11.32-p11.23 in an Italian family. Eur J Hum Genet 8:443–448

Bi MY, Cohen PR, Robinson FW, Gray JM (2009) Alopecia syphilitica-report of a patient with secondary syphilis presenting as moth-eaten alopecia and a review of its common mimickers. Dermatol Online J 15:6

Carlini P, Di Cosimo S, Ferretti G et al (2003) Alopecia in a premenopausal breast cancer woman treated with letrozole and triptorelin. Ann Oncol 14:1689–1690

Cho M, Cohen PR, Duvic M (1995) Vitiligo and alopecia areata in patients with human immunodeficiency virus infection. South Med J 88:489–491

Daneschfar A, Davis CP, Trüeb RM (1993) Trichomegaly in HIV infection. Schweiz Med Wochenschr 123:1941–1944

Ellis JA, Stebbing M, Harrap SB (1998) Genetic analysis of male pattern baldness and the 5alpha-reductase genes. J Invest Dermatol 110:849–853

Ellis JA, Stebbing M, Harrap SB (2001) Polymorphism of the androgen receptor gene is associated with male pattern baldness. J Invest Dermatol 116:452–455

Grover RW (1956) Diffuse hair loss associated with selenium (Selsun) sulfide shampoo. J Am Med Assoc 160:1397–1398

Johnson KA, Bernard MA, Funderberg K (2002) Vitamin nutrition in older adults. Clin Geriatr Med 18:773–799

Kullavanijaya P, Gritiyarangsan P, Bisalbutra P (1992) Absence of effects of dimethicone- and non-dimethicone-containing shampoos on daily hair loss rates. J Soc Cos-met Chem 43:195–206

Mirmirani P, Hessol NA, Maurer TA et al (2003) Hair changes in women from the Women's Interagency HIV Study. Arch Dermatol 139:105–106

Nikolic DS, Viero D, Tijé VC, Toutous-Trellu L (2013) Alopecia universalis associated with vitiligo in an 18-year-old HIV-positive patient: highly active antiretroviral therapy as first choice therapy? Acta Derm Venereol. doi:10.2340/00015555-1651, Epub ahead of print

Orentreich N, Berger RA (1964) Selenium disulfide shampoo. It's influence on hair growth and the follicular cycle. Arch Dermatol 90:76–80

Ostlere LS, Langtry JA, Staughton RC, Samrasinghe PL (1992) Alopecia universalis in a patient seropositive for the human immunodeficiency virus. J Am Acad Dermatol 27:630–631

Riedel-Baima B, Riedel A (2008) Female pattern hair loss may be triggered by low oestrogen to androgen ratio. Endocr Regul 42:13–16

Rockey D, Cello J (1993) Evaluation of the gastrointestinal tract in patients with iron-deficiency anemia. N Engl J Med 329:1691–1695

Sadick NS (1993) Clinical and laboratory evaluation of AIDS trichopathy. Int J Dermatol 32:33–38

Sawin CT, Geller A, Herschman JE (1979) The aging thyroid: increased prevalence of elevated serum TSH levels in the elderly. JAMA 242:247–250

Schulpkis KH, Georgala S, Papakonstantinou ED, Michas T, Karikas GA (1999) The effect of isotretinoin on biotinidase activity. Skin Pharmacol Appl Skin Physiol 12:28–33

Sereti I, Sarlis NJ, Arioglu E, Turner ML, Mican JM (2001) Alopecia universalis and Graves' disease in the setting of immune restoration after highly active antiretroviral therapy. AIDS 15:138–140

Smith KJ, Skelton HG, DeRusso D, Sperling L, Yeager J, Wagner KF, Angritt P (1996) Clinical and histopathologic features of hair loss in patients with HIV-1 infection. J Am Acad Dermatol 34:63–68

Stewart MI, Smoller BR (1993) Alopecia universalis in an HIV-positive patient: possible insight into pathogenesis. J Cutan Pathol 20:180–183

Tosti A, Gaddoni G, Peluso AM, Misciali C, Piraccini BM, Menni B (1993) Acquired hairy pinnae in a patient infected with the human immunodeficiency virus. J Am Acad Dermatol 28:513

Tosti A, Piraccini BM, van Neste DJ (2001) Telogen effluvium after allergic contact dermatitis of the scalp. Arch Dermatol 137:187–190

Trüeb RM (2003) Association between smoking and hair loss: another opportunity for health education against smoking? Dermatology 206:189–191

Trüeb RM, Meyer JC (2000) Male-pattern baldness in men with X-linked recessive ichthyosis. Dermatology 200:247–249

York J, Nicholson T, Minors P, Duncan DF (1998) Stressful life events and loss of hair among adult women, a case–control study. Psychol Rep 82:1044–1046

Zlotogorski A, Marek D, Horev L, Abu A, Ben-Amitai D, Gerad L, Ingber A, Frydman M, Reznik-Wolf H, Vardy DA, Pras E (2006) An autosomal recessive form of monilethrix is caused by mutations in DSG4: clinical overlap with localized autosomal recessive hypotrichosis. J Invest Dermatol 126: 1292–1296

Clinical Examination

Caserio RJ (1987) Diagnostic techniques for hair disorders part III: clinical hair manipulations and clinical findings. Cutis 40:442–448

Degos R, Rabut R, Duperrat B, Leclercq R (1954) Pseudopeladic state; comments on one hundred cases of circumscribed cicatricial alopecia, apparently primary, of pseudopelade type. Ann Dermatol Syphiligr (Paris) 81:5–26

Dreuw H (1910) Klinische Beobachtungen bei 101 haarkranken Schulknaben. Monatsh prakt Dermatol 51:103–118
Dunn PM (1992) Litigation over congenital scalp defects. Lancet 339:440
Frieden IJ (1986) Aplasia cutis congenita: a clinical review and proposal for classification. J Am Acad Dermatol 14:646–660
Hamilton JB (1951) Patterned loss of hair in man; types and incidence. Ann N Y Acad Sci 53:708–728
Ludwig E (1977) Classification of the types of androgenetic alopecia (common baldness) occurring in the female sex. Br J Dermatol 97:247–254
Norwood OT (1975) Male pattern baldness: classification and incidence. South Med J 68:1359–1365
Tosti A, Miteva M, Torres F (2011) Lonely hair: a clue to the diagnosis of frontal fibrosing alopecia. Arch Dermatol 147:1240

Trichoscopy

Annessi G (1998) Tufted folliculitis of the scalp: a distinctive clinicohistological variant of folliculitis decalvans. Br J Dermatol 138:799–805
Bakos RM, Bakos L (2007) Dermoscopy for diagnosis of pediculosis capitis. J Am Acad Dermatol 57:727–728
de Lacharrière O, Deloche C, Misciali C et al (2001) Hair diameter diversity: a clinical sign reflecting the follicle miniaturization. Arch Dermatol 137:641–646
Deloche C, de Lacharrière O, Misciali C et al (2004) Histological features of peripilar signs associated with androgenetic alopecia. Arch Dermatol Res 295:422–428
Galliker NA, Trüeb RM (2012) Value of trichoscopy versus trichogram for diagnosis of female androgenetic alopecia. Int J Trichology 4:19–22
Guarrera M, Rebora A (1996) Anagen hairs may fail to replace telogen hairs in early androgenic female alopecia. Dermatology 192:28–31
Guarrera M, Rebora A (2005) Kenogen in female androgenetic alopecia. A longitudinal study. Dermatology 210:18–20
Hidvégi B (2008) Dermoscopy of hair and scalp disorders. Eur J Dermatol 18:607
Hofbauer GF, Tsambaos D, Spycher MA, Trüeb RM (2001) Acquired hair fragility in pili anulati: causal relationship with androgenetic alopecia. Dermatology 203:60–62
Inui S, Nakajima T, Itami S (2007) Dry dermoscopy in clinical treatment of alopecia areata. J Dermatol 34:635–639
Inui S, Nakajima T, Nakagawa K, Itami S (2008a) Clinical significance of dermoscopy in alopecia areata: analysis of 300 cases. Int J Dermatol 47:688–693
Inui S, Nakajima T, Itami S (2008b) Significance of dermoscopy in acute diffuse and total alopecia of the female scalp: review of twenty cases. Dermatology 217:333–336
Inui S, Nakajima T, Shono F, Itami S (2008c) Dermoscopic findings in frontal fibrosing alopecia: report of four cases. Int J Dermatol 47:796–799
Itin PH, Schiller P, Mathys D, Guggenheim R (1997) Cosmetically induced hair beads. J Am Acad Dermatol 36:260–261
Kossard S, Zagarella S (1993) Spotted cicatricial alopecia in dark skin. A dermoscopic clue to fibrous tracts. Australas J Dermatol 34:49–51
Kurwa AR, Abdel-Aziz AH (1973) Pili torti-congenital and acquired. Acta Derm Venereol 53:385–392
Lacarrubba F, Dall'Oglio F, Nasca MR, Micali G (2004) Videodermoscopy enhances diagnostic capability in some forms of hair loss. Am J Clin Dermatol 5:205–208
Loewenthal JA (1947) "Compound" and grouped hairs of the human scalp: their possible connection with follicular infection. J Invest Dermatol 8:263–273
Olszewska M, Rudnicka L, Rakowska A et al (2008) Trichoscopy. Arch Dermatol 144:1007
Powelll J (2000) Increasing the likelihood of early diagnosis of Netherton syndrome by simple examination of eyebrow hairs. Arch Dermatol 136:423–424
Rebora A, Guarrera M (2002) Kenogen. A new phase of the hair cycle? Dermatology 205:108–110
Requena L, Sarasa JL, Ortiz Masllorens F et al (1995) Follicular spicules of the nose: a peculiar cutaneous manifestation of multiple myeloma with cryoglobulinemia. J Am Acad Dermatol 32:834–839
Ross EK, Vincenzi C, Tosti A (2006) Videodermoscopy in the evaluation of hair and scalp disorders. J Am Acad Dermatol 55:799–806
Rudnicka L, Olszewska M, Rakowska A et al (2008) Trichoscopy: a new method for diagnosing hair loss. J Drugs Dermatol 7:651–654
Sewell LD, Elston DM, Dorion RP (2007) "Anisotrichosis": a novel term to describe pattern alopecia. J Am Acad Dermatol 56:856
Tončić RJ, Lipozenčić J, Pastar Z (2007) Videodermoscopy in the evaluation of hair and scalp disorders. Acta Dermatovenerol Croat 15:116–118
Tosti A (2007) Dermoscopy of hair and scalp disorders with clinical and pathological correlations. Informa healthcare, Andover/Hampshire
Tosti A, Whiting D, Iorizzo M et al (2008) The role of scalp dermoscopy in the diagnosis of alopecia areata incognita. J Am Acad Dermatol 59:64–67

Trichogram

Adya KA, Inamadar AC, Palit A, Shivanna R, Deshmukh NS (2011) Light microscopy of the hair: a simple tool to "untangle" hair disorders. Int J Trichology 3:46–56
Argenziano G, Monsurrò MR, Pazienza R, Delfino M (1998) A case of probable autosomal recessive ectodermal dysplasia with corkscrew hairs and mental retardation in a family with tuberous sclerosis. J Am Acad Dermatol 38:344–348

Blume-Peytaivi U, Orfanos CE (1995) Microscopy of the hair – the trichogram. In: Derup J, Jemec GBE (eds) Handbook of non-invasive methods and the skin. CRC Press, London, pp 549–554

Braun-Falco O, Heilgemeir GP (1985) The trichogram. Structural and functional basis, performance, and interpretation. Semin Dermatol 4:40–52

Caserio RJ (1987) Diagnostic techniques for hair disorders part III: clinical hair manipulations and clinical findings. Cutis 40:442–448

Itin PH, Bircher AJ, Lautenschlager S, Zuberbühler E, Guggenheim R (1994) A new clinical disorder of twisted and rolled body hairs with multiple, large knots. J Am Acad Dermatol 30:31–35

Mirmirani P, Huang KP, Price VH (2011) A practical, algorithmic approach to diagnosing hair shaft disorders. Int J Dermatol 50:1–12

Mortimer PS (1985) Unruly hair. Br J Dermatol 113:467–473

Trüeb RM, Spycher MA, Schumacher F, Burg G (1994a) Pili torti et canaliculi in ectodermal dysplasia. Hautarzt 45:372–377

Trüeb R, Burg G, Bottani A, Schinzel A (1994b) Ectodermal dysplasia with corkscrew hairs: observation of probable autosomal dominant tricho-odonto-onychodysplasia with syndactyly. J Am Acad Dermatol 30:289–290

Whiting DA, Dy LC (2006) Office diagnosis of hair shaft defects. Semin Cutan Med Surg 25:24–34

Laboratory Evaluation

Barrett S Commercial hair analysis: a cardinal sign of quackery. http://www.quackwatch.com/01QuackeryRelatedTopics/hair.html

Blume-Peytavi U, Blumeyer A, Tosti A, Finner A, Marmol V, Trakatelli M, Reygagne P, Messenger A, European Consensus Group (2001) S1 guideline for diagnostic evaluation in androgenetic alopecia in men, women and adolescents. Br J Dermatol 164:5–15

Hambidge KM (1982) Hair analyses: worthless for vitamins, limited for minerals. Am J Clin Nutr 36:943–949

Park H, Kim CW, Kim SS, Park CW (2009) The therapeutic effect and the changed serum zinc level after zinc supplementation in alopecia areata patients who had a low serum zinc level. Ann Dermatol 21:142–146

Pierard GE (1979) Toxic effects of metals from the environment on hair growth and structure. J Cutan Pathol 16:237–242

Sherertz E (1985) Misuse of hair analysis as a diagnostic tool. Arch Dermatol 121:1504–1505

Zlotken SH (1985) Hair analysis, A useful tool or a waste of money? Int J Dermatol 24:161–164

Scalp Biopsy

Caserio RJ (1987) Diagnostic techniques for hair disorders part III: clinical hair manipulations and clinical findings. Cutis 40:442–448

Daneshpazhooh M, Asgari M, Naraghi ZS, Barzgar MR, Akhyani M, Balighi K, Chams-Davatchi C (2009) A study on plucked hair as a substrate for direct immunofluorescence in pemphigus vulgaris. J Eur Acad Dermatol Venereol 23:129–131

Daneshpazhooh M, Naraghi ZS, Ramezani A, Ghanadan A, Esmaili N, Chams-Davatchi C (2011) Direct immunofluorescence of plucked hair for evaluation of immunologic remission in pemphigus vulgaris. J Am Acad Dermatol 65:e173–e177

Elston DM, McCollough ML, Angeloni VL (1995) Vertical and transverse sections of alopecia biopsy specimens. Combining the two to maximize diagnostic yield. J Am Acad Dermatol 32:454–457

Harries MJ, Trüeb RM, Tosti A et al (2009) How not to get scar(r)ed: pointers to the correct diagnosis in patients with suspected primary cicatricial alopecia. Br J Dermatol 160:482–501

Headington JT (1996) Cicatricial alopecia. Dermatol Clin 14:773–782

Kumaresan M, Rai R, Sandhya V (2011) Immunofluorescence of the outer root sheath: an aid to diagnosis in pemphigus. Clin Exp Dermatol 36:298–301

Rao R, Dasari K, Shenoi SD, Balachandran C, Dinesh P (2013) Monitoring the disease activity in pemphigus by direct immunofluorescence of plucked hair: a pilot study. Indian J Dermatol 58:164

Ross EK, Tan E, Shapiro J (2005) Update on primary cicatricial alopecias. J Am Acad Dermatol 53:1–37

Schaerer L, Trüeb RM (2003) Direct immunofluorescence of plucked hair in pemphigus. Arch Dermatol 139:228–229

Solomon AR (1994) The transversely sectioned scalp biopsy specimen: the technique and a algorithm for its use in the diagnosis of alopecia. Adv Dermatol 9:127–157

Sperling LC (2001) Scarring alopecia and the dermatopathologist. J Cutan Pathol 28:333–342

Templeton SF, Solomon AR (1994) Scarring alopecia: a classification based on microscopic criteria. J Cutan Pathol 121:97–109

Trachsler S, Trüeb RM (2005) Value of direct immunofluorescence for differential diagnosis of cicatricial alopecia. Dermatology 211:98–102

Quantifying Hair Loss

Guarrera M, Semino MT, Rebora A (1997) Quantitating hair loss in women: a critical approach. Dermatology 194:12–16

Guarrera M, Cardo PP, Rebora A (2011) Assessing the reliability of the Modified Wash Test. G Ital Dermatol Venereol 146:289–294

Guarrera M, Fiorucci MC, Rebora A (2013) Methods of hair loss evaluation: a comparison of TrichoScan(®) with the modified wash test. Exp Dermatol 22:482–484

Hoffmann R (2001) TrichoScan: combining epiluminescence microscopy with digital image analysis for the measurement of hair growth in vivo. Eur J Dermatol 11:362–368

Ihm CW, Lee JY (1991) Evaluation in daily hair counts. Dermatologica 182:67

Lee SH, Kwon OS, Oh JG et al (2004) Phototrichogram: evaluation of modified methods with bleaching and Trichoscan. Seoul, Korea, poster presentation at the European Hair Research Society, Berlin, 2004

Olsen EA (1993) Clinical tools for assessing hair loss. In: Olsen EA (ed) Disorders of hair growth: diagnosis and treatment. McGraw-Hill, New York, pp 59–69

Rampini P, Guarrera M, Rampini E, Rebora A (1999) Assessing hair shedding in children. Dermatology 199:256–257

Rebora A, Guarrera M, Baldari M, Vecchio F (2005) Distinguishing androgenetic alopecia from chronic telogen effluvium when associated in the same patient: a simple noninvasive method. Arch Dermatol 141:1243–1245

Van Neste D, Trüeb RM (2006) Critical study of hair growth analysis with computer-assisted methods. J Eur Acad Dermatol Venereol 20:578–583

Hair Database Sheet

Caserio RJ (1987) Diagnostic techniques for hair disorders part III: clinical hair manipulations and clinical findings. Cutis 40:442–448

Diagnosis and Treatment

3

Diagnosis is not the end, but the beginning of practice.

Martin H. Fischer (1879–1962)

Clinical trichology should represent an integral part of medical training, and the dermatologist participates with the other medical disciplines in the diagnosis and treatment of all types of hair problems relating to systemic disease. On the other hand, hair loss is an important cause of discomfort and disability. The general physician is not always aware of the significance of hair loss and therefore may fail to refer patients with hair disorders to the dermatologist for appropriate management. Too often, the delay of correct diagnosis, and as a result the delay of appropriate therapy, leads to potentially irreversible loss of hair, prolongs the discomfort, and promotes the disfigurement. Knowledge of the main types of hair loss is prerequisite to providing appropriate patient care.

3.1 Male Androgenetic Alopecia

Androgenetic alopecia is the most common type of hair loss that occurs after puberty in both sexes. Patients typically present with progressive thinning and shortening of hair in affected scalp area. It is also referred to as male pattern hair loss, male pattern baldness, or common baldness in men; represents an age-related, heritable, androgen-dependent phenomenon; and occurs in a defined pattern.

It is assumed that the genetically predisposed hair follicles are the target for androgen-stimulated hair follicle miniaturization, leading to gradual conversion of large, thick pigmented hairs (terminal hairs) to barely visible, thin, depigmented hairs (vellus hairs) in the affected scalp area. The result is a progressive decline in visible scalp hair density. It is characterized by its typical bitemporal recession of hair and balding vertex and affects at least 50 % of men by the age of 50 years and up to 70 % of all males in later life.

3.1.1 Pathobiology of Androgenetic Alopecia

Hair follicles are subject to constant turnover in a three-phase cycle, consisting of a period of growth (anagen), involution (catagen), and rest (telogen), after which the hair is shed, before a new anagen phase sets in again. Each phase of the follicular cycle underlies the influence of various hormones, most importantly androgens. The loss of hair in androgenetic alopecia is the result of a gradual reduction in the duration of anagen, a prolongation of the latent period of the hair cycle, and miniaturization of terminal hair follicles.

The loss of hair in androgenetic alopecia is mediated by inhibitory autocrine factors released by dermal papilla cells, likely in response to activation of androgen receptors by androgenic hormones. Many studies have shown that patients with androgenetic alopecia have increased levels of androgen receptor present in the dermal papilla of frontal hairs compared with occipital hairs. It also has been shown that men with androgenetic

R.M. Trüeb, W.-S. Lee, *Male Alopecia*,
DOI 10.1007/978-3-319-03233-7_3,

alopecia have increased activity of 5α-reductase, an enzyme important in converting testosterone to the more potent androgen dihydrotestosterone (DHT), in balding areas compared with non-balding areas of the scalp. These studies support the idea that increased levels of DHT interact with increased expression of androgen receptor (AR) in dermal papilla cells to cause the release of inhibitory factors that result in changes in the hair follicle, ultimately leading to the transformation of terminal to vellus hairs.

The molecular control of the anagen–catagen transformation of the hair cycle has been revealed by a number of studies: catagen has been suggested to begin with a decrease in the expression of anagen-maintaining factors, such as insulin-like growth factor 1 (IGF-1), basic fibroblast growth factor (bFGF), and vascular endothelial growth factor (VEGF), and an increase in the expression of cytokines, such as transforming growth factor beta 1 (TGF-1), interleukin-1 alpha (IL-1α), and tumor necrosis factor alpha (TNF-α) (Table 3.1). Of the several factors, IGF-1 has been recognized to alter with stimulation by androgens in vitro. At the tissue level in humans, testosterone induces IGF-1 in a dose-dependent fashion from cultured dermal papilla cells in both beard and parietal scalp hair.

Table 3.1 Function of various molecules in pathogenesis of androgenetic alopecia

Molecule	Function
Beta-catenin	Facilitates cell–cell communication in adult epithelial cells by binding neighboring cells Essential role for the fate of hair stem cell in embryogenesis through Wnt signaling pathway
Lymphoid enhancer-binding factor-1 (LEF-1)	Reacts with beta-catenin and forms beta-catenin-LEF-1 complex Binds to cellular DNA and activates the genes instructing the cell to become hair follicle
p63	Homologue of tumor suppressor p53 Plays an essential role in the morphogenesis of epidermis and ectodermal differentiation during embryogenesis
Insulin-like growth factor (IGF-1), basic fibroblast growth factor (bFGF), vascular endothelial growth factor (VEGF)	Anagen-maintaining factors Promote to start catagen phase when level of these factors decrease
Transforming growth factor (TGF) β1	The cohesion of androgen and androgen receptor in balding dermal papilla cells facilitates production of the factor Leads to beginning of catagen phase Inhibits the growth of hair follicle
IL-1α, tumor necrosis factor (TNF) α	Leads to beginning of catagen phase
Stem cell factor (SCM)	Production of SCM is achieved to greater extent in androgen-dependent beard cells than in control non-balding scalp tissue cells Ligand for cell surface receptor c-kit on melanocyte Role in hair pigmentation
Nexin-1	Protease located in dermal papilla cells Altered by androgens
Dickkopf-1 (DKK-1)	Located in balding dermal papilla cells Increases the level of 5α dihydrotestosterone

3.1.2 Androgens, Androgen Metabolism, and the Androgen Receptor

Androgens are a mediator for hair growth in all body parts. In the absence of androgens or with the diminution of its action, scalp hair continues to grow, whereas hairs in other parts of the body diminish in growth. This paradoxical effect may be due to differences in the number of androgen receptor in different body sites, in variations in the formation of potent androgens, and in peculiarities of androgen metabolism.

The correlation between androgens and androgenetic alopecia was emphasized by Hamilton in 1942. According to his observations, men deprived of androgens by castration before puberty neither developed baldness nor recession of the frontal hairline. However, men castrated after puberty showed the typical phenotypic expression of male pattern baldness. In these patients, progressive hair loss in a defined pattern was observed with less than physiological levels of testosterone administration. Since patients who retained an intact hairline despite testosterone injection had no family history of androgenetic alopecia, it was strongly suggested that androgenetic alopecia was also dependent on a genetic predisposition.

Since the discovery of the role of androgens in androgenetic alopecia, there have been numerous studies on blood levels of androgens in men with or without baldness. It has been known that there is no difference in plasma testosterone and urinary androgen level in balding and non-balding men. However, a few studies show higher levels of specific androgens in men with alopecia. No definitive relationship has been found between androgenetic alopecia and other androgen-related markers, including sebum secretion, body hair density, and bone, skin, or muscle thickness.

Androgen metabolism, in the broadest sense, includes the secretion, transport, tissue uptake, peripheral transformation, and excretion of C-19 steroids. Androgen metabolism pathway starts with pregnenolone, a 21-carbon steroid substrate. Cholesterol, a precursor of pregnenolone, is synthesized in Leydig cells through de novo pathway or diverted from plasma lipoprotein. Pregnenolone is then converted into testosterone and DHT by the enzymes 3β-hydroxysteroid dehydrogenase-isomerase 2 (3β-HSD2), 17β-hydroxysteroid dehydrogenase 3 (17β-HSD3), and 5α-reductase. Of above phases, the first four phases occur in the adrenal glands, testes, and ovaries (in females), and the rest take place in peripheral target tissue including the scalp. The most important protein involved in androgen transport is sex hormone-binding globulin (SHBG). Normally, 70 % of testosterone is bound to SHBG and 19 % to albumin. The rest exists as free, unbinding form. Some circulating testosterone and androstenedione can be turned into estrogen by the enzyme aromatase (CYP19) in peripheral tissue.

5α-reductase is responsible for androgen metabolism in the scalp. It has two isoforms, type 1 and type 2, that differ in biochemical and pharmacologic characteristics as well as tissue expression patterns. Type 1 isoenzyme is mainly expressed in sebaceous glands and type 2 isoenzyme in the genitourinary system and hair follicle. In the hair follicle, type 1 5α-reductase expression is mainly localized to the sebaceous gland, but also noted in other areas of the hair follicle including dermal papilla. Type 2 5α-reductase expression is seen in the outer root sheath, inner root sheath, and dermal papilla. In dermal papilla cells, 5α-reductase activity is higher in balding vertex scalp versus non-balding occipital scalp. Also in scalp biopsy samples, more DHT production was observed in balding area versus non-balding areas as a result of elevated 5α-reductase activity in balding area.

The role of type 2 5α-reductase on hair growth found attention in 1974 with the report of a peculiar genetic disorder due to type 2 5α-reductase deficiency. The disorder results in considerably diminished DHT formation, but normal testosterone levels. Otherwise normal 46XY patients show ambiguous external genitalia at birth, but at puberty normal virilization sets in with normal testosterone levels, including musculature. However, these men have less facial and body hair and neither develop androgenetic alopecia nor prostate hyperplasia with age. This implicates the role of type 2 5α-reductase for the development of androgenetic alopecia. Up to date, there has been no report of type 1 5α-reductase-deficiency yet, and it is unknown in what phenotype this abnormality would result.

Testosterone is metabolized to DHT by 5α-reductase in target tissue. DHT is five times more potent in affinity to AR than testosterone. The levels of DHT are affected mainly by the activity of 5α-reductase, as well as by the supply of precursors, and the metabolism of DHT. The major precursor of DHT in men is testosterone and in women dehydroepiandrosterone (DHEA). 17β-hydroxysteroid dehydrogenase (17β-HSD) converts 17-ketosteroids (DHEA, androstenedione, estrone) into 17β-hydroxysteroids (androstene-3β, 17β-diol

[5diol], testosterone, 17β-estradiol), respectively. It also plays an important role in androgen metabolism, and it is proven by the fact that 17β-HSD deficiency induces pseudohermaphroditism.

More than five isoforms of 17β-HSD have been discovered so far, and they have different properties and take place in different hormone metabolism pathways. Type 1 17β-HSD reduces testosterone to 17 β-estradiol, and type 2 17β-HSD regulates the reverse oxidative sequence. Type 3 17β-HSD and type 5 17β-HSD reduce androstenedione to testosterone, and type 2 17β-HSD inactivates testosterone to androstenedione. Histochemically, 17β-HSD locates in the outer root sheath of anagen hair follicle and tends to reduce as baldness progresses. Moreover, balding scalp shows lower 17β-HSD than non-balding scalp. Although most studies on androgenetic alopecia have dealt with 5α-reductase rather than 17β-HSD, it seems as well to play a certain role in the development of androgenetic alopecia.

Some of DHT produced by 5α-reductase is converted to weak androgen, androsterone, and androstanediol. However, they can be diverted into strong DHT by oxidative 3α-HSD, which is displayed in dermal papilla, worsening alopecia. Another enzyme in androgen metabolism is 3β-hydroxysteroid dehydrogenase (3β-HSD), which is essential in the production of androgen, estrogen, mineralocorticoids, and glucocorticoids. 3β-HSD converts DHEA to androstenedione and is expressed in many tissues including the scalp. It is higher in activity in balding scalp than non-balding scalp.

Androgens, like other steroid hormones, bind to cytosolic or nuclear receptor protein after crossing plasma membranes. AR complex combines with DNA and induces alteration of DNA transcription and protein formation. The AR binds with various steroid hormones with different levels of affinity, in order of as follows: DHT, testosterone, estrogen, and progesterone. DHT–AR complex has stronger affinity for receptors in the nuclear chromatin than does the testosterone–AR complex, and the former is more stable and persists longer in cells. AR is mostly distributed in dermal papilla. It is also found in dermal sheath cells, and this supports the fact that dermal sheath cells form the part of dermal papilla. AR expression is 30 % higher in frontal scalp follicles than in occipital follicles in male alopecia and is strongly expressed in dermal papilla cells of balding area versus non-balding area.

With reference to the various respective studies, the mechanisms by which androgens regulate hair growth or baldness after binding with the AR mainly located with the dermal papilla can be explained as follows: testosterone is converted to DHT in balding dermal papilla with high 5α-reductase activity and binds to AR which is largely distributed in the balding area. This diminishes the production of growth factors in dermal papilla or induces the production of growth-inhibiting factors. This has been demonstrated in various experiments: for instance, the addition of testosterone to cultured dermal papilla cells or outer hair root sheath cells of beard hair follicles increases mitosis slightly, whereas the addition of testosterone to the coculture of dermal papilla cells and outer hair root sheath cells induces three times more DNA synthesis. Moreover, conditioned medium of balding dermal papilla cells inhibits the growth of keratinocytes in response to testosterone, unlike those of non-balding dermal papilla cells. These studies support that androgens regulate the growth of hair through dermal papilla.

3.1.3 Genetic Involvement

Unlike monogenic disorders that can be determined only by a phenotype of one or few genes, polygenic disorders such as androgenetic alopecia possess complex traits that require their features to be determined by a much larger number of genes. Each gene possesses variable levels of risk, and these diseases are not typically binary (strictly divided into a group of disease or no disease).

> The general consensus on polygenic disorders is that along with variations of genetic sequence, environmental influences also play a role in determining the onset and progression of disease.

Androgenetic alopecia clearly possesses a highly heritable trait, proven by twin studies. Yet the high prevalence of the condition and a wide distribution in age of onset and range of severity suggest that the disease is not controlled by a single gene (single gene traits rarely occur with a frequency >1 in 1,000). Therefore, a polygenic mode of inheritance is highly suggested for the development of androgenetic alopecia.

In the early studies on the genetic involvement in androgenetic alopecia, the focus has been based on the genes involved in androgen metabolism. Therefore, geneticists initially concentrated on chromosomes 2 and 5, the sites of the 5 α-reductase enzyme genes, SRD5A2, and SRD5A1. Yet no difference in young bald men and older non-bald male controls were found, ruling out an association between androgenetic alopecia and genes encoding the two 5 α-reductase isozymes.

The shift then turned to the AR gene located on the X chromosome (Xq11-12). Ellis et al. discovered a polymorphism in the AR gene, and reportedly, there was association between AR and the susceptibility to the development of androgenetic alopecia. It is believed that variations in the AR gene may increase the activity of AR in hair follicles. Of a special note in the variations of the AR gene is a single nucleotide polymorphism (SNP) in exon 1, StuI (rs6152, restriction fragment length polymorphism [RFLP], E211 G>A) that shares a strong association with androgenetic alopecia in Caucasian men. The StuI RFLP in exon 1 is present in 98 % of young bald men and 92 % of old bald men, but the fact that it is also found in 77 % of non-bald older men suggests that androgenetic alopecia indeed is a polygenic condition. It can be inferred that non-balding men with StuI RFLP probably lack additional factors that are necessary for onset of androgenetic alopecia. Moreover, AR's location on the X chromosome cannot explain the father-to-son transmission of androgenetic alopecia.

In conclusion, only a small portion of heritability of androgenetic alopecia can be explained by variations in AR. Also, it is unclear as to how genetic changes in AR increase the risk of hair loss. Studies estimate that genetic variations in AR account for about 40 % of heritability, meaning that 60 % of heritability is not yet known. Combination of sequence variation in undiscovered genes that affect the regulatory elements in the noncoding sequences and changes to genomes not based on DNA sequences, also known as epigenetic variation, might take part in genetic involvement of androgenetic alopecia, and further research on such fields should be conducted in the future.

3.1.4 Gene Polymorphism Diagnostics in Androgenetic Alopecia

Phenotype of inheritance in androgenetic alopecia depends on genotype inherited from parents along with influences of various environmental factors. Although it is difficult to accurately predict the onset of androgenetic alopecia by mere genetic screening, the field of predictive medicine based on diagnostics and treatment of the genetic polymorphisms (SNP) is on the rise.

Currently, a screening test for androgenetic alopecia has been developed by a company, HairDx LLC (Irvine, California, USA), for assessing the risk for development of androgenetic alopecia. The supposed end goal of this test is to allow an early detection of androgenetic that will enable patients to undergo treatment with finasteride as soon as possible. The test is conducted on a cheek swab and evaluates StuI SNP in the AR gene. The test claims that a patient who tests positive for AR variant, together with a positive family history for androgenetic alopecia in the father, will have a >80 % risk of developing androgenetic alopecia. On the other hand, a patient who tests negative and has a father without a history of androgenetic alopecia will have >90 % chance of not developing androgenetic alopecia.

Thus, if a patient has a reasonable risk of balding from the test, the patient can benefit from early initiation of treatment, while the patient with a higher chance of not balding can avoid undergoing an unnecessary and costly treatment. Despite the availability of genetic tests for early diagnosis of androgenetic alopecia, patients must be aware of the screening method's limitations: only a small portion of heritability of androgenetic alopecia can be explained with AR gene variations, and data are limited in explaining the clinical relevance.

> Patients must be aware that current genetic testing relies on AR gene variations, while onset of androgenetic alopecia is actually due to polygenic contributions from other genes or epigenetic mechanisms.

3.1.5 Syndromatic Androgenetic Alopecia

On a rare occasion, early-onset or an unusually severe androgenetic alopecia may be the symptom of a complex genetic disorder.

Examples are trichorhinophalangeal syndrome (see Sect. 2.2), the progerias (see Sect. 3.4.1), Laron syndrome, and Curschmann–Steinert's myotonic dystrophy.

The *Laron syndrome* (primary growth hormone insensitivity) is an autosomal recessive disorder characterized by an insensitivity to growth hormone, caused by a variant of the growth hormone receptor. The principal feature of the syndrome is abnormally short stature (dwarfism). Physical symptoms include prominent forehead with frontal hair recessions, depressed nasal bridge, underdevelopment of mandible, truncal obesity, and a very small penis. Seizures are frequently seen secondary to hypoglycemia. Some genetic variations have an impact upon intellectual capacity. The hair of patients with Laron syndrome is thin and easy to pluck. Young adults have various degrees of alopecia, more pronounced in males. Electron microscopy of hair shows pathologic, though unspecific, features.

Curschmann–Steinert's myotonic dystrophy is an autosomal dominant disorder characterized by wasting of the muscles (muscular dystrophy), cataracts, heart conduction defects, endocrine changes, and myotonia. Myotonia is the designation for a peculiar form of muscle disorder characterized by delayed relaxation (prolonged contraction) of the skeletal muscles after voluntary contraction or electrical stimulation. Although early frontoparietal alopecia is one of the most common symptoms in myotonic dystrophy (Fig. 3.1), it has not received the deserved attention. Another peculiar dermatologic finding in patients with myotonic dystrophy is the development of multiple pilomatrixomata, often before signs of myotonic dystrophy. Since the onset of multiple pilomatrixomata may precede the signs of myotonic dystrophy, they can serve as potential early cutaneous marker for this systemic disorder.

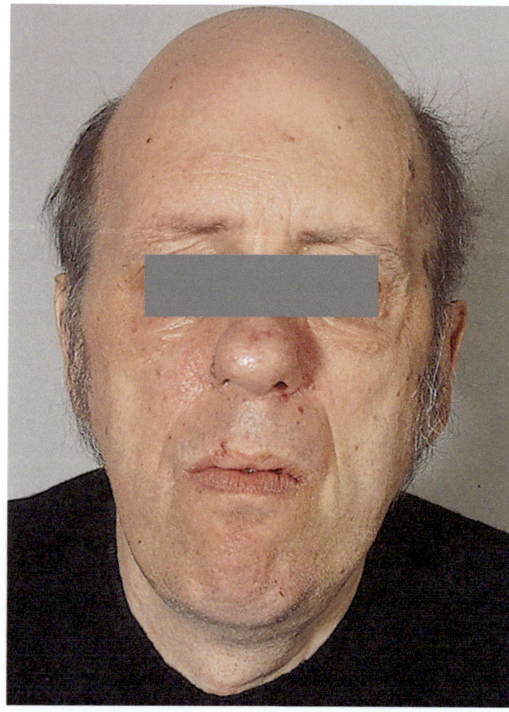

Fig. 3.1 Curschmann–Steinert's myotonic dystrophy. Note pronounced alopecia and myopathic facies

3.1.6 Premature Alopecia

Androgenetic alopecia that is clinically manifest between the ages of 10 and 20 is called premature alopecia or alopecia praecox. In children before puberty it presents in both females and males exclusively with the female pattern (Fig. 3.2).

In 2005, Tosti et al. originally reported the first case series of androgenetic alopecia in children in the age range from 6 to 10 years. All had normal physical development. Clinical examination

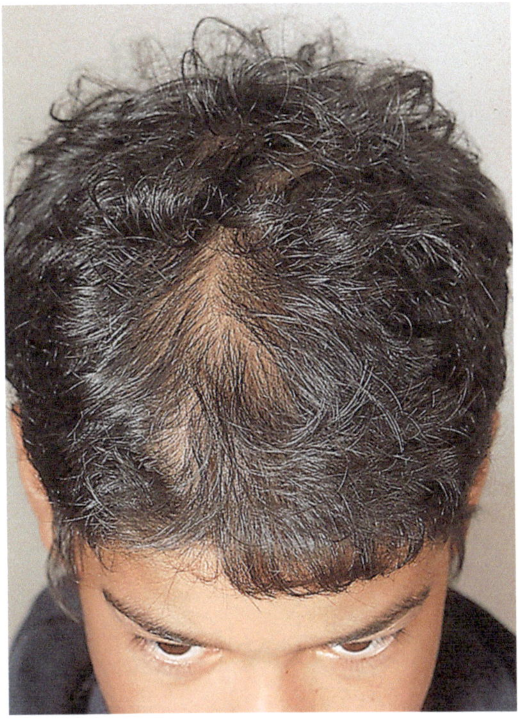

Fig. 3.2 Premature alopecia. Note female pattern

showed hair loss with thinning and widening of the central parting of the scalp, both in boys and girls. There was a strong family history of androgenetic alopecia in all patients.

In children and adolescents with early-onset alopecia, it is first important to differentiate whether hair loss is congenital or acquired. The differential diagnosis of congenital hair loss includes hypotrichosis simplex (without associated abnormalities) and ectodermal dysplasia (with associated delayed physical/psychological development, sweating, dental, or nail abnormalities). Premature androgenetic alopecia is an acquired hair loss with a characteristic pattern distribution and no associated abnormalities. It is important to assess the child's general health status, physical and mental development, and particularly early onset of puberty. Premature androgenetic alopecia without signs of premature puberty is usually not associated with endocrinological abnormalities; nevertheless, referral to a pediatric endocrinologist is recommended.

Treatment with topical 2 % minoxidil solution (before the age of 12 once daily, thereafter twice daily) is usually very effective (Fig. 3.3a–c). Systemic side effects of topical minoxidil (hypertrichosis and cardiovascular) are observed more frequently in children, especially at higher than the recommended dosages.

3.1.7 Clinical Presentations and Classifications

The main characteristics of male androgenetic alopecia are recession of the frontal hairline and balding of the vertex. Finally, alopecia may coalesce resulting in a rim of normal hair growth at the sides and occipital scalp (Fig. 3.4).

Androgenetic alopecia is a continuous sustained process rather than a series of separate phases and has widely different features for individual patients. Nevertheless, hairs within the balding regions may become gradually shorter and thinner, in the end vanishing completely, or demonstrate a more diffuse decrease in hair density with maintenance of normal hair diameter in the remaining hair. There are racial differences in the clinical characteristics of androgenetic alopecia.

> A more diffuse pattern of hair loss over the vertex and frontal hairline, resembling female pattern hair loss, seems to be more common in Asian men, whereas it is less than 5 % of Caucasian men.

It is not easy to evaluate the severity of androgenetic alopecia. Diverse classification methods have been developed and modified until now:

In 1950, Beek et al. published a classification system, based on 1,000 Caucasian males. They classified into two categories: frontal and fronto-vertex hair loss.

In the following year, the first systematic classification of androgenetic alopecia was established by Hamilton. In 1975, Norwood refined Hamilton's classification as Norwood–Hamilton classification by emphasizing "frontotemporal" or "vertex only" subcategories of hair loss into seven types with a type A and vertex variant, respectively, and reported the incidence of

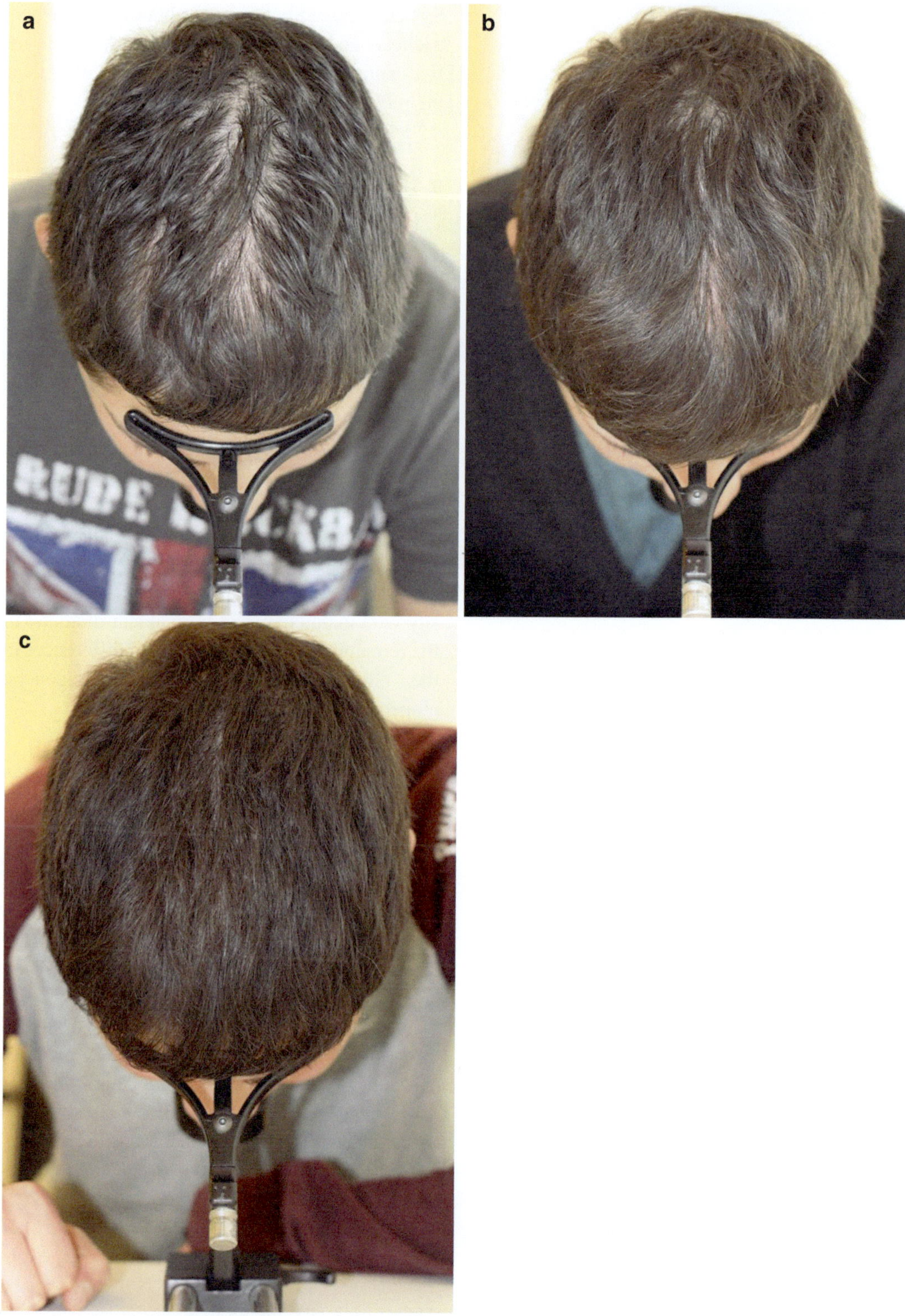

Fig. 3.3 Successful treatment of premature alopecia: (**a–c**) with 2 % topical minoxidil solution twice daily in a 15-year-old boy (**a**) before, (**b**) after 3 months, and (**c**) after 6 months treatment

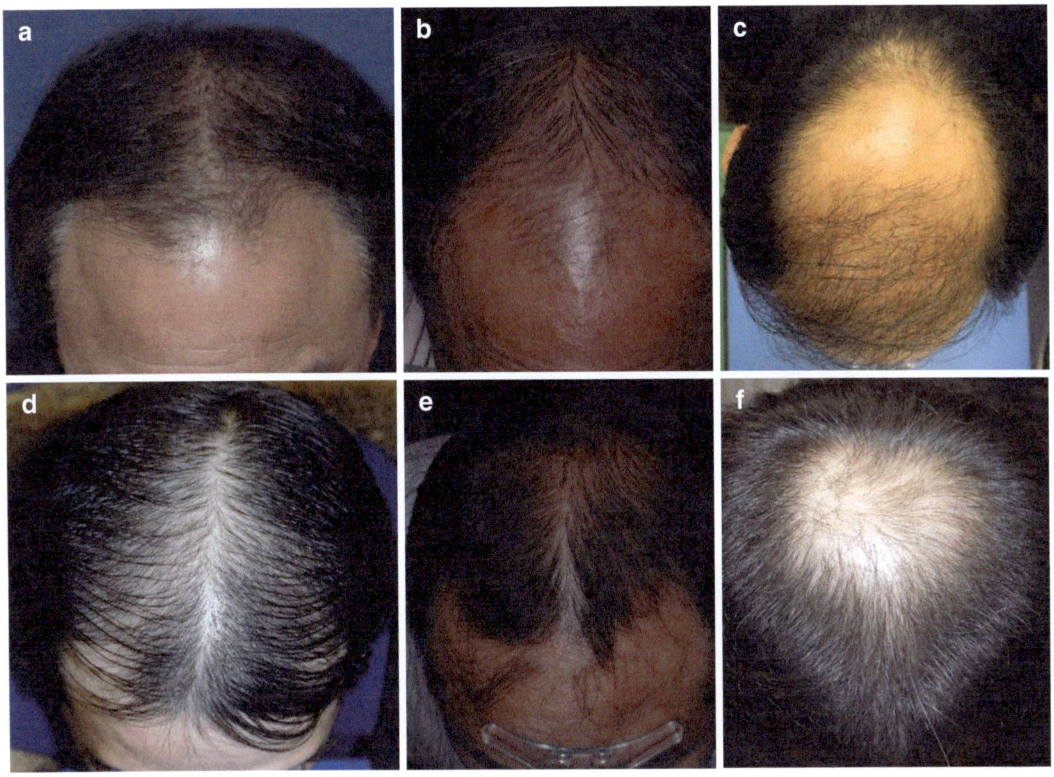

Fig. 3.4 (**a–f**) Clinical presentations of androgenetic alopecia in (Korean) men

androgenetic alopecia at various ages in 1,000 adult Caucasian male subjects.

The Norwood–Hamilton classification has been the most widely used classification system for androgenetic alopecia in men and has been largely used to assess clinically the severity of androgenetic alopecia, especially in clinical research. However, Guarrera et al. challenged the reliability of Norwood–Hamilton classification, even in the hands of experts. They suggested that for obtaining better reliability, the number of groups should be reduced, also it is too detailed, and less stepwise in its explanation, making it hard to memorize for general usage. Ultimately, it proved to be unsatisfactorily reproducible. In addition, Norwood–Hamilton classification does not list some unusual clinical presentations, such as female pattern hair loss in men. Atypical patterns cannot be classified so would have to be designated as an atypical type. Finally, Sehgal et al. found that the range of presentations has relatively stable components for types I, II, III, and VII, while types IV, V, and VI show considerable overlap.

In 1977, Ludwig suggested quite a different presentation of hair loss in women from that described by Hamilton. He emphasized preservation of the frontal hairline despite progressive hair loss over the vertex. There are three types (I, II, III) of hair loss in this classification that represent progressive stages of androgenetic alopecia in females. Birch et al. analyzed the relationship between clinical diagnosis using Ludwig's classification and objective hair measurements and found that mean hair densities were lower in patients classified to have hair loss versus controls. However, women with male pattern hair loss cannot be classified using the Ludwig classification system.

Currently, the most widely accepted standards are the Norwood–Hamilton classification for men and the Ludwig classification for women, with male patients with female pattern hair loss being classified according to the Ludwig classification.

In 2007, Lee et al. newly designed and proposed the basic and specific (BASP) classification system (Fig. 3.5) which provides an improved alternative to the Norwood–Hamilton classification. It is based on observed patterns of hair loss. There are four basic types (L, M, C, and U) and two specific types (F and V).

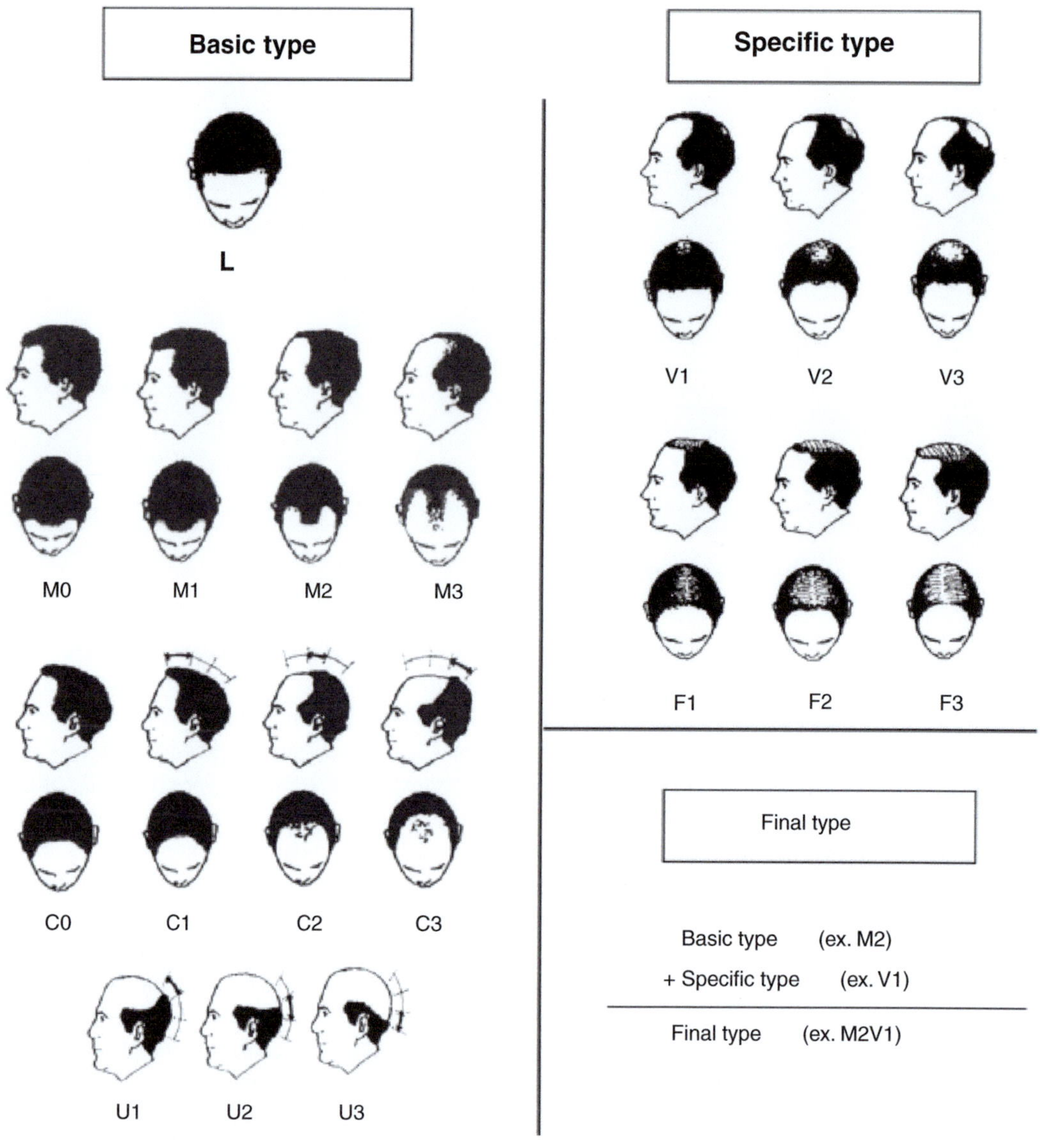

Fig. 3.5 Basic and specific (BASP) classification for pattern hair loss (From: Lee WS, Ro BI, Hong SP et al (2007) A new classification of pattern hair loss that is universal for men and women: basic and specific (BASP) classification. J Am Acad Dermatol 57(1):37–46)

Basic type

The shape of the anterior hairline is divided into four basic types: L, M, C, and U

Type L. No recession is observed along the anterior border in the frontotemporal region. It resembles a linear line and usually means that no hair loss has occurred

Type M. Recession in the frontotemporal hairline is more prominent than the mid-anterior hairline. This type tends to be symmetrical. The hairline resembles the letter M. Type M is further divided into four subtypes depending on the severity of baldness.

Type M0. The original hairline is preserved and represents type M. No hair loss has occurred on clinical history. The subject cannot perceive any changes in the anterior hairline.

Type M1. Frontotemporal recession extends posteriorly but not beyond the anterior third of a virtual line connecting the original hairline and the top of the vertex

Type M2. Frontotemporal recession extends further posteriorly but not beyond the middle third of a virtual line connecting the original hairline and the top of the vertex

Type M3. Frontotemporal recession extends beyond the middle third section into the posterior third of the area of a virtual line connecting the original hairline and the top of the vertex

Type C. Recession in the mid-anterior hairline is more prominent than the frontotemporal hairline. The entire anterior hairline regresses posteriorly in the shape of half circle, resembling the letter C. Type C is further divided into four subtypes depending on the severity of baldness

Type C0. The original anterior hairline is preserved and represents type C. No hair loss has occurred on clinical history

Type C1. The mid-anterior hairline recedes so that it lies within the anterior third of the virtual line connecting the original hairline and the top of the vertex

Type C2. The mid-anterior hairline recedes further so that it lies within the middle third of the virtual line connecting the original hairline and the top of the vertex

Type C3. The mid-anterior hairline recedes further into the posterior third of the virtual line connecting the original hairline and the top of the vertex

Type U. The anterior hairline recedes posteriorly beyond the vertex forming a horseshoe shape, resembling the letter U. Type U is the most severe pattern of androgenetic alopecia. Type U is further divided into three subtypes depending on the severity of baldness. There is no zero grade (UO).

Type U1. The entire anterior border of the hairline lies within the superior third of the virtual line connecting the vertex and the posterior occipital protuberance.

Type U2. The entire anterior border of the hairline lies within the middle third of the virtual line connecting the vertex and the posterior occipital protuberance.

Type U3. The entire anterior border of the hairline lies within the inferior third of the virtual line connecting the vertex and the posterior occipital protuberance.

Specific type

The basic types cannot represent the thinning of hair on the scalp, so additional types representing the degree of thinning need to be introduced. In contrast to the basic types, the specific types may be selectively included when necessary. According to patterns observed at specific areas, there are two specific types: F and V. Each specific type is also subdivided into three subtypes, according to severity. When all the characteristics of both types F and V are observed, both specific types should be selected

Type F. This type only represents a general decrease in the density of hair over the entire top of the scalp, regardless of the anterior hairline. It is usually more marked over the frontal area of the scalp, as observed in females. This type is similar to

Ludwig's classification method but only with regard to thinning hair and is unrelated to the shape of the entire hairline

Type F1. Thinning of the hair on the crown is perceptible (mild change)

Type F2. Thinning of the hair on the crown is pronounced (moderate change)

Type F3. The hair on the crown is very sparse or absent (severe change)

Type V. The hair around the vertex is notably sparser. Hair loss is seen more distinctly in the vertex than in the frontal area. When frontoparietal and vertex regions of alopecia have become confluent, type F2, 3 should not be confused with type V. In this case, the differential point is whether the definite hair loss is primarily on the vertex or not

Type V1. Thinning of the hair around the vertex area is perceptible (mild change)

Type V2. Thinning of the hair around the vertex area is pronounced (moderate change)

Type V3. The hair around the vertex area is very sparse or absent (severe change)

The basic (BA) types represent the shape of the anterior hairline, and the specific (SP) types represent the density of hair on specific areas, which are frontal and vertex.

The final type is decided by the combination of the BA and SP types. One of the basic types must be selected, and the specific type may be selected if it exists. Each of the various types is subdivided into three or four grades (subtypes) according to its severity.

Similarly, Olsen et al. proposed the regional scalp hair density method using the area of the scalp assigned a letter (T, F, M, and V) and the density of hair in that region of the scalp, whereas BASP classification system focuses on the shape of the anterior hairline and scores the density scale of 0–3 which is a simpler method than Olsen's. It also integrated the "specific type V" from modifying Hamilton's, Norwood's, and Koo et al.'s suggested classifications and "specific type F" from Ludwig's proposal.

Albeit comparison of the BASP classification showed that accuracy rate of the BASP method was lower than that obtained by Hamilton, the study about the easy-to-use aspects of this classification revealed that accordance rates accounted for 77.1 % in spite of a study period of only 15 min. This result showed that the BASP classification is easy to learn and practice. Khumalo et al. demonstrated that BASP classification has greater intra-class coefficiency than Norwood–Hamilton classification in both the nurses/secretaries and dermatology residents/consultants. Hong et al. also showed that the BASP classification not only distinguishes all kinds of hair loss patterns, but also has better reproducibility and repeatability than the Norwood–Hamilton classification.

The new BASP classification for pattern hair loss may prove particularly useful in communicating the amount and distribution of hair loss. It can estimate both the further extent of hair loss and the response to therapy. Since the Norwood–Hamilton classification is too detailed and is less stepwise in its description, making it difficult to memorize for common use, BASP classification seems more practical. The Norwood–Hamilton classification also does not list some peculiar types of baldness, such as female pattern hair loss. Additionally, women with male pattern hair loss cannot be classified using Ludwig classification. Clinicians must use distinct methodologies for each gender in order to correctly classify the pattern. The BASP classification not only classifies all kinds of hair loss patterns regardless of sex or race but also has better reproducibility and repeatability than previously used methods. Also, it is easy to memorize, owing to its stepwise and systematical characteristics, with less difficulties in applying the system clinically, and improvement of existing limitations of other classifications.

Finally, the BASP classification was used to analyze familial factors affecting androgenetic alopecia morphology. Parental influences on anterior hairline shape in men were predominantly from the paternal side, whereas these effects were less notable in women.

3.1.8 Comorbidities of Male Androgenetic Alopecia

Recent studies on the relationship between androgenetic alopecia and various systemic diseases have exposed a number of significant findings. As early as 1972, Cotton et al. studied the relationship of androgenetic alopecia with cardiovascular disease and suggested that androgenetic alopecia may be a marker for risk. From that time on, there have been a considerable number of publications stating that the risk of cardiovascular disease, type 2 diabetes mellitus, and metabolic syndrome is increased in males with early-onset androgenetic alopecia. The research results are based predominantly on white males, but do not exclude Asians.

There are many studies on the relationship between androgenetic alopecia and the risk of coronary heart disease, including nonfatal myocardial infarction, angina pectoris, and coronary revascularization.

> The studies indicate that androgenetic alopecia may be a marker for risk of coronary heart disease, with increased risk associated especially with early hair loss (before the 30s). These risks may vary also depending on the type of hair loss (vertex alopecia).

It was stated that vertex pattern baldness appears to be a marker for increased risk of coronary heart disease events, especially among men with hypertension or high cholesterol levels. Lesko et al. reported that men with severe vertex baldness had a three-fold higher risk of myocardial infarction when compared with those without hair loss.

The underlying pathomechanisms for these findings remain for now unknown. Arias-Santiago et al. reported that early-onset (<35 years old) androgenetic alopecia is associated with a higher risk of atherosclerosis, higher blood levels of aldosterone, ESR, CRP, and fibrinogen as compared to controls. Dogramaci et al. reported that the intima–media thickness and CRP are increased in patients with androgenetic alopecia. Recently, there have also been some studies on the association of diabetes mellitus with androgenetic alopecia. The rate of insulin resistance and glucose intolerance was found to be higher in patients with androgenetic alopecia versus controls. Arias-Santiago et al. evaluated the association between early-onset androgenetic alopecia, hyperglycemia, diabetes, and low levels of sex hormone-binding globulin (SHBG). They indicated that low levels of SHBG could be a marker of insulin resistance and hyperglycemia in patients with androgenetic alopecia. Acibucu et al. examined the frequency of insulin resistance, hyperinsulinemia, and metabolic syndrome in individuals with early androgenetic alopecia. According to their study, the prevalence of insulin resistance and metabolic syndrome was significantly higher in the androgenetic alopecia group than in the control group, especially with early-onset androgenetic alopecia. There exists also a series of reports that obesity, dyslipidemia, and hyperlipidemia are increased in patients with androgenetic alopecia. In addition, Su et al. stated that patients with moderate or severe androgenetic alopecia may be at higher risk for metabolic syndrome. Dyslipidemia and systemic inflammatory responses can induce metabolic disease, and in turn, these diseases can induce atherosclerosis to increase the risk of cardiovascular and cerebrovascular diseases. Ultimately, the higher risk of metabolic disease in patients with androgenetic alopecia can be interpreted as increased risk of cardiovascular and cerebrovascular disease.

> Determination of metabolic syndrome and ultrasound study of the carotid arteries may be useful screening methods to detect risk of developing cardiovascular and cerebrovascular disease in patients with early-onset androgenetic alopecia and signal for a potential opportunity for early preventive treatment.

Anterolateral leg alopecia or *peroneal alopecia* (this term is used because the alopecia tends to be distributed along the peroneal nerve, though this association is not substantiated by any clinicopathologic correlation) is a common form of patterned alopecia of the legs in men and once believed to be related to androgenetic alopecia.

> Though anterolateral leg alopecia is frequent with an estimated prevalence of 35 % among males, and preferably occurs in middle-aged and elderly men, Hamilton showed no statistically significant association between male pattern baldness and alopecia of the lower extremities.

The condition is so common that some believe it represents a variant of normal distribution of body hair, the same way others consider male pattern baldness to be a physiological and age-related phenomenon.

Anterolateral leg alopecia presents bilaterally in a symmetrical fashion with sharply demarcated, circumscribed, smooth patches of alopecia confined to the anterior and lateral aspects of the leg (Fig. 3.6). Occasionally, a few hairs may be found to grow within the patches, though broken hairs are not common. Sometimes, alopecia may occur similarly on the thighs.

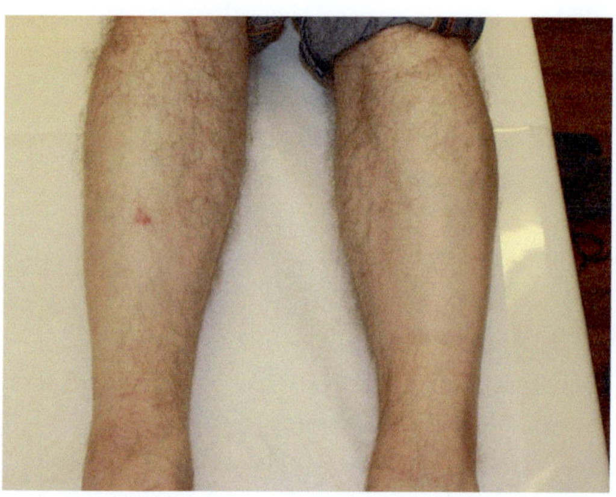

Fig. 3.6 Anterolateral leg alopecia

The etiology of the condition has remained an object of discussion. In the 1920s, Kidd interpreted anterolateral leg alopecia as resulting from "use inheritance" (patients with this condition wore tight-fitting ancestral generation footgear); others have theorized that the habit of leg crossing contributes to the condition, and yet others have pointed to friction and trouser rubbing. In the same line of an exogenous traumatic origin of anterolateral leg alopecia is the more recent report of Adams, who attributed a young male patient's case to friction occurring during recreational water-slide activity and called the condition "water-slide alopecia." Opponents of the proposed connections with trauma and friction have argued that friction alopecia tends to produce truncated hairs and follicular hyperkeratosis. The histopathologic features of anterolateral leg alopecia have scarcely been studied, with only Gupta and Shaw reporting in 2002 their findings in two biopsy specimens that lacked hair follicles but were otherwise unremarkable.

With respect to disease associations, Tommasi suggested in 1940 a possible relation between this pattern of alopecia and an endogenous "neuroarthritic diathesis" with hyperuricemia, but evidence of such a connection is failing; Popkin suggested acute ischemia as a contributing factor in hair loss involving the lower extremities, but Kligman remarked that, aside from the loss of fine hairs on the dorsum of the toes late in severe atherosclerosis obliterans, growth of leg hair is not affected by any kind of atherosclerotic disease.

In summary, various hypotheses and disease associations have been proposed to explain anterolateral leg alopecia, but not have been substantiated so far.

Most men admit to not having noticed the onset of loss of leg hair or never paid serious attention to it. A treatment is not available. Usually, patient education and reassurance are satisfactory.

The most important differential diagnoses are alopecia areata and disseminated lichen planopilaris, which tend to involve other areas and have characteristic clinical and histopathologic findings. With regard to the formerly alleged

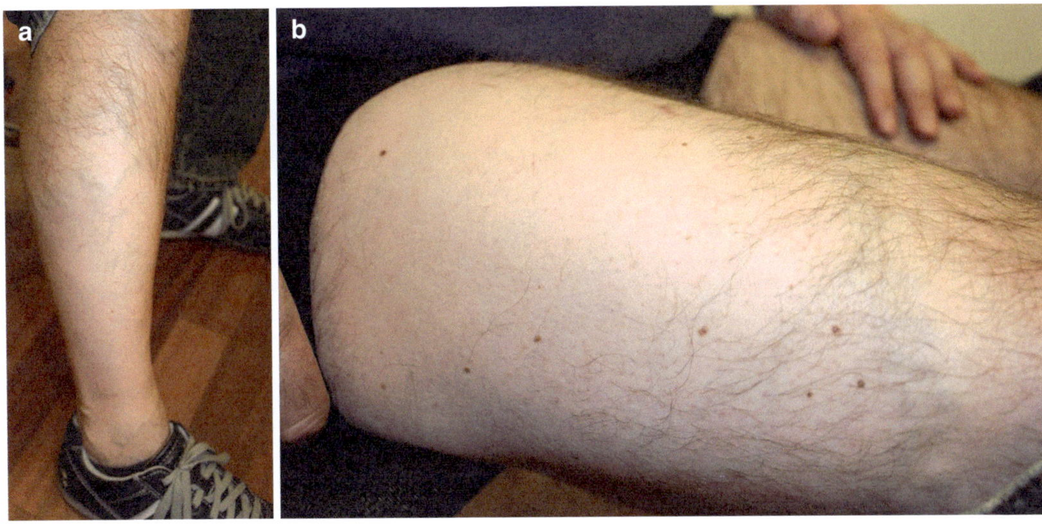

Fig. 3.7 (**a**) Anterolateral leg-like alopecia in male patient with frontal fibrosing alopecia; (**b**) the patient also had loss of hair on the lateral aspects of his thighs

association of anterolateral leg alopecia with male pattern hair loss, it is noteworthy that a similar anterolateral leg-like alopecia (with the characteristics of lichen planopilaris) may be seen in patients with frontal fibrosing alopecia (Fig. 3.7).

3.1.9 Evidence-Based Pharmacologic Treatments

Hair loss in patients with androgenetic alopecia is generally reduced after at least a 6-month period of pharmacologic treatment, and there is a need for continuous treatment for sustained beneficial effect.

> Patients should constantly and continuously take medication to maintain hair density and must understand the limitations of pharmacologic interventions. The main purpose is to prevent further progression of hair loss, although in some patients regrowth of hair can be achieved. Usually, hair density does not completely return to the level before hair loss began.

Currently, topical minoxidil solution and oral finasteride are the only FDA-approved pharmacologic agents for treatment of androgenetic alopecia.

Topical minoxidil is a pyrimidine derivative and the first FDA-approved hair growth-promoting agent for treatment of male androgenetic alopecia. The 2 % topical solution was approved in 1988, followed by approval of 5 % solution in 1997 and 5 % foam in 2006.

> The major action of topical minoxidil on the hair cycle is promotion of initiation of anagen phase followed by shortening of telogen phase and prolongation of anagen by delaying onset of catagen phase.

The mechanism of action of topical minoxidil on hair growth is still unclear, and many hypotheses have been established. Minoxidil is a potassium channel opener and vasodilatator and has been reported to stimulate the production of vascular endothelial growth factor (VEGF) in cultured dermal papilla cells. There is evidence that this effect is mediated by adenosine and sulfonylurea receptors, which are well-known target receptors for adenosine triphosphate-sensitive potassium channel openers. Minoxidil is transformed into minoxidil sulfate by the enzyme sulfotransferase. Minoxidil sulfate is the active metabolite and present in the outer root sheath of anagen hair. Minoxidil acts on adenosine receptor and sulfonylurea receptor and followed by stimulation of adenosine signaling pathway and overexpression of VEGF. Lachgar et al. showed that minoxidil upregulates the expression of VEGF in dermal papilla cells resulting in increase of perifollicular blood supply and hair growth. Wester et al. found that skin blood flow is increased at 10–15 min after applying minoxidil. In addition, hair growth promoters including cytoprotective prostaglandin synthase-1 and hepatocyte growth factor (HGF) m-RNA are increased.

An interesting analogy exists to hypertrichotic osteochondrodysplasia or Cantu syndrome, a genetic disorder characterized by thick scalp hair extending onto the forehead and a general increase in body hair. It is caused by a mutation in the ABCC9 gene on chromosome 12p12 that codes for sulfonylurea receptor 2, involved in ATP-sensitive potassium channels.

> Ultimately, the understanding of the genetic basis of hypertrichosis and the molecules involved may open the venue for the development of targeted treatments for too little hair.

Clinical trials with topical 2, 3, or 5 % minoxidil solution have all shown remarkably rapid increase in hair growth, measured by hair counts or hair weight. The increase is evident within 6–8 weeks of treatment and has generally peaked by 12–16 weeks. Olsen et al. found that twice a day topical minoxidil application was more effective in promoting hair growth than once daily application. Choi et al. showed that hair density and thickness increased in male androgenetic alopecia patients aged 18–54 years old after 1 ml of 3 % minoxidil solution twice a day. They suggested that topical minoxidil must be applied twice a day with recommended dose to gain maximum clinical effect.

> The clinical response to topical minoxidil solution should be evaluated at 6 months after treatment. If it shows favorable effect, treatment needs to be continued.

Olsen et al. also found that effectiveness of topical minoxidil continued after 5 years of application.

> Therefore, 5 % topical minoxidil solution 1 ml twice daily may be recommended to improve or to prevent progression of androgenetic alopecia in male patients.

In an analysis of clinical trial data in 636 males, a therapeutic benefit of topical minoxidil solution was compared to age, duration of balding, diameter of balding vertex area, age, and duration of hair loss: age was found to be the denominator for predicting treatment success. The younger subjects experienced better efficacy than the older subjects although clear treatment effects were noted also in the older age group.

> There was an inverse relationship between effect of topical minoxidil solution and duration of balding. Males with duration of balding <5 years showed a significantly better effect than those with duration of balding >21 years. The diameter of vertex balding showed an inverse relationship with efficacy of minoxidil. Men with <5-cm diameter vertex balding area showed a better effect of treatment than subjects with diameters >15 cm. Finally, duration of hair loss less than 1 year compared to more than 10 years at onset of treatment resulted in a significantly more effective treatment with respect to stabilization of alopecia and new hair growth.

Finasteride is a synthetic azasteroid and type 2 5α-reductase inhibitor. Type 2 isoenzyme activity is predominantly found in the prostate, genitourinary tract, and human hair follicles. Finasteride prevents conversion of testosterone to DHT which results in decreased DHT levels in the scalp. In several studies, 1 mg oral finasteride daily has been shown to be effective in prevention and treatment of hair loss in men: Whiting et al. found that finasteride prevented miniaturization of hair follicles and promoted growth of terminal hair. Drake et al. found that oral administration of 1 mg finasteride decreased scalp DHT levels by 64 % and serum DHT by 68 %. The studies conducted by Kaufman et al. revealed that finasteride decreased serum and scalp DHT and was effective in men with vertex alopecia. Leyden et al. found that 1 mg oral finasteride daily also decreased hair loss and improved hair growth in men with hair loss in the anterior and mid area of the scalp. The finasteride dose ranging studies showed that total hair count was increased with finasteride 0.2, 1, and 5 mg but not with 0.01 mg. Another clinical study found that finasteride 1 and 0.2 mg improved global assessment score by 58 and 54 %, respectively. Van Neste et al. demonstrated that finasteride promoted the conversion of telogen follicle into anagen phase and increased overall anagen hairs.

One milligram oral finasteride decreases serum and scalp DHT and has been shown to be effective in men with androgenetic alopecia in vertex and anterior/mid scalp areas. Finasteride promotes the conversion of telogen follicles into anagen and increases overall anagen hairs.

Clinical studies revealed that both hair weight and hair count increased after administration of oral finasteride, but hair weight increased to a greater extent than hair count. It helps to explain that factors other than the numbers of hairs, such as increased growth rate and thickness of hairs, contribute to the therapeutic effects of oral finasteride in male androgenetic alopecia.

In 2002, the Finasteride Male Pattern Hair Loss Study Group conducted a clinical study over a 5-year period on male androgenetic alopecia in patients aged 18–41 years with 1 mg oral finasteride daily. The hair counts increased in 48 % of patients at 1 year and in 66 % at 2 years. After 5 years of treatment, hair count remained similar to the 1 year level, but patients showed significant improvement in their gross hair appearance using global photography.

It was suggested that maximal number of hairs is obtained by the end of 1-year oral finasteride treatment, and further improvement results from increase in hair length, diameter, and pigmentation.

Kaufman et al. showed that finasteride 1 mg/day over 5 years resulted in marked and sustained reduction of further development of male androgenetic alopecia.

Therefore, 1 mg oral finasteride daily may be recommended to improve or to prevent progression of androgenetic alopecia in male patients.

Dutasteride is a type 1 and 2 5α-reductase inhibitor. Dutasteride is approved by FDA only for treatment of benign prostate hyperplasia and not licensed for treatment of androgenetic alopecia. Its pharmacologic action is similar to finasteride but is more effective in decreasing scalp DHT. Dutasteride reduces serum and scalp DHT level to a greater degree than finasteride. Olsen et al. showed that mean changes in hair counts increased by 11.3 % with dutasteride 2.5 mg and 8.4 % with finasteride 5 mg. In this study, total hair count increased by 8.7 % with 0.1 mg and 10.2 % with 0.5 mg dutasteride. They determined that dutasteride 2.5 mg daily is the most effective dosage for treatment of androgenetic alopecia.

Dutasteride 2.5 mg is five times higher than the dosage for benign prostate hyperplasia which is 0.5 mg. They also found that mean hair counts in the 0.1 and 0.5 mg dutasteride groups were similar to the finasteride 5 mg group. The study conducted by Stough et al. showed that total hair count increased by 6.8/cm^2 at 6 months and 10.5/cm^2 at 12 months after oral administration of dutasteride 0.5 mg. Eun et al. reported that the mean changes of hair counts from baseline to 6 months after treatment start with dutasteride 0.5 mg were 12.21/cm^2 in the dutasteride group and 4.67/cm^2 in the placebo group. In this study, mean changes of hair counts after 3 months of treatment were not significantly different between the two groups.

The use of oral dutasteride for treatment of male androgenetic alopecia is off-label and occurs at the discretion of the prescribing physician.

Olsen et al. compared the prevalence of sexual adverse effects between oral dutasteride and oral finasteride and found no significant differences in total adverse events, serious adverse events, or withdrawals due to adverse events among any of the dutasteride and finasteride groups. In this study, there was no increase of impotence, and decreased libido was noted in a small number of subjects in the 2.5 mg dutasteride group. These events are dose related but commonly disappeared after cessation of dutasteride.

In an attempt to circumvent potential problems related to systemic 5α-reductase inhibition, topical finasteride has been considered for treatment of male androgenetic alopecia. In an original study, Mazzarella et al. used 0.005 % finasteride solution in 52 patients. The clinical outcome, in terms of hair regrowth and balding area reduction, seemed to be encouraging. Hajheydari showed that the therapeutic effects of both 1 % finasteride gel and oral finasteride were relatively similar to each other, while Tanglertsampan did not find any statistically significant difference in hair counts in male patients with androgenetic alopecia treated either with 3 % minoxidil solution or combined 3 % minoxidil/0.1 % finasteride solution. Currently, liposomal systems and finasteride-loaded liquid crystalline nanoparticles are being studied for development of effective topical finasteride applications.

An important issue will be the comparison of finasteride blood levels after topical application as compared to the standard oral therapy.

Finally, there is a considerable interest in the alternative of botanically derived inhibitors of 5α-reductase, such as saw palmetto (*Serenoa repens*), especially in complementary medicine. Widely advertised on the web and sold by direct marketing, it is frequently used as self-medication. Rossi et al. recently performed an open-label study to determine the effectiveness of *Serenoa repens* in treating male androgenetic alopecia compared to oral finasteride. One hundred male patients with clinically diagnosed mild to moderate androgenetic alopecia were enrolled. One group received 320 mg *Serenoa repens* daily, while the other received 1 mg oral finasteride daily for a total study duration of 24 months (2 years). In order to assess the efficacy of the treatments, a score index based on the comparison of the global photos taken at the beginning and at the end of the treatment was used. The investigators found that *Serenoa repens* could lead to an improvement of androgenetic alopecia, while finasteride was more effective for more than half of patients. Moreover, finasteride acts in both the frontal and the vertex area, while *Serenoa repens* prevalently in the vertex.

The role of androgens in the pathogenesis of androgenetic alopecia has led to the consideration also of hormonal agents for its treatment. They are classified into two groups: antiandrogens and estrogenic (or antiestrogenic) drugs, although efficacy studies with these drugs are very limited. Antiandrogens act on androgen receptors and block its effect. There are several drugs for androgen receptor antagonism, including cyproterone acetate (CPA), spironolactone, and flutamide, that are exclusively considered for treatment of female androgenetic alopecia, since they are contraindicated in men due to their feminizing action.

Again, in an attempt to circumvent problems related to systemic hormonal treatments, topical treatment with *17α- and 17β-estradiol* has been studied.

17α-estradiol (alfatradiol) represents a stereoisomer of 17β-estradiol (estradiol) with 100-fold lower estrogenic and two-fold higher 5α-reductase inhibitory action and therefore was also considered for treatment of male androgenetic alopecia, while 17β-estradiol (estradiol) is contraindicated because of its potential in inducing gynecomastia.

In a study involving 103 women with androgenetic alopecia, Blume-Peytavi et al. compared topical alfatradiol with topical minoxidil and found that alfatradiol did not result in an increase in hair density or thickness, in contrast to minoxidil. No data are available for men.

Fluridil is a topical antiandrogen that suppresses the human androgen receptor. While highly hydrophobic and hydrolytically degradable, it is non-resorbable and was therefore considered for treatment of male androgenetic alopecia. To evaluate the safety and efficacy of topical fluridil in male androgenetic alopecia, Sovak et al. evaluated 2 % fluridil versus placebo in 43 men with androgenetic alopecia Norwood grades II–Va, in a double-blind study after 3 months by phototrichograms, hematology, and blood chemistry including analysis for fluridil and at 9 months by phototrichograms. They found that with fluridil anagen rates increased after 3 months from 76 to 85 % and at 9 months to 87 %, while with placebo the average anagen percentage did not change. Sexual functions, libido, hematology, and blood chemistry values remained normal. No fluridil or its decomposition product, BP-34, was detectable in the serum at 0, 3, or 90 days.

Based on preclinical studies in mice in which topical fulvestrant (ICI182,780, an estrogen receptor antagonist used for treatment of breast cancer) caused telogen hair follicles to enter anagen, thereby causing hair growth, a topical formulation of *fulvestrant* was developed for the potential treatment of androgenetic alopecia. A study on the efficacy of fulvestrant by Gassmueller et al. came to the conclusion that topical antiestrogen treatment with fulvestrant is ineffective in treatment of androgenetic alopecia.

3.1.10 Autologous Hair Transplantation

Autologous hair transplantation remains the only treatment option for advanced patterned baldness. With the advent of total micrografting and a sharp decline in scalp reduction procedures, hair restoration surgery has become more satisfying than in the recent past. Modern techniques use the visual qualities of hair and varying design patterns to create the optical illusion of more hair than is actually present. The main advances in hair restoration surgery have been the use of one to four hair grafts, which allows a natural, undetectable hairline and the transplantation of large numbers of these small grafts during a single session.

Careful patient selection and newer techniques are geared toward naturalness and undetectability for the lifetime of the patient.

In the majority of patients, hair transplantation is performed under local anesthesia. Lidocaine is the most commonly used anesthetic. The key to success is superficial infiltration of the dermis, which allows both better pain control and hemostasis for the patient. The patient is placed in either a prone position or a seated position for donor site removal. The amount of hair in the donor area is the only limiting factor in hair transplant surgery. Therefore, efficiency in harvesting follicular groupings is critical. There are two types of methods for harvesting donor hair: strip harvesting and follicular unit extraction.

Strip harvesting has been the standard method for ages. On the posterior scalp, a donor ellipse contains hundreds to thousands of follicular groupings that can be utilized for hair transplantation. Once the donor ellipse is removed, the wound is closed with either staples or sutures. The size of the donor ellipse depends on the amount of grafts that are needed for the particular patient. As with any cutaneous excision, strip harvesting will create a scar on the scalp.

Follicular unit extraction (FUE) utilizes the steel punch technique that was used to extract donor hairs. Recently, 0.75- to 1.25-mm steel punches are used to harvest individual follicular units. These punches are so small that they usually do not leave visible scars. More recently, robotic follicular unit extraction has been introduced into the field. The robot is able to skillfully remove large numbers of follicular units with minimal transection. This technology is a major advance in the harvesting of individual follicular units while minimizing visible scars.

After either method of harvesting, the follicular units obtained must be trimmed under microscopic visualization using a razor blade. Under microscopic visualization, follicles are dissected out in order to produce intact follicular units.

Various techniques are utilized to create and prepare recipient sites for subsequent transplantation of follicular units. Although various types of graft implanter may be conveniently used for the insertion of the grafts, creating slits has been widely used for ages. In creating slits over the recipient area, important considerations include slit size, depth of incision and angle, and direction. Blades may be cut to match the size of the follicular units to be inserted. Hypodermic needles may be used to make incisions for subsequent graft placement. For the frontal hairline, to frame the face well and to create a natural-looking hairline, the slits are made in an irregular pattern to try to mimic the natural hairline, which is mostly very irregular and slightly asymmetric. Twenty five to forty follicular unit grafts per square centimeter are the transplanted densities made by most hair restoration surgeons. This density goal shows a cosmetically acceptable outcome over the recipient area with most patients being satisfied by the results.

Jeweler forceps or similar non-toothed forceps are generally used to gently place the grafts into recipient sites. Transplanted hair follicle viability is maximized by minimizing mechanical trauma to the follicle. This is accomplished by handling the subcutaneous tissue along the base of the graft rather than the graft itself.

> Hair transplantation surgery can be performed in any person with androgenetic alopecia with a good donor area, good general health status, and reasonable expectations.

Caution should be exercised in very young patients whose early alopecia is still evolving, patients with Norwood grade VI or VII with poor density, patients with unrealistic expectations, and patients with significant systemic health problems. Unrealistic expectations or body dysmorphic disorder represents contraindications for hair transplantation surgery.

3.1.11 Miscellaneous Treatments

Since there exists only a very limited number of treatments that have been approved for male androgenetic alopecia, there have been a number of ongoing trials for identifying alternative treatments for androgenetic alopecia:

- Tretinoin in combination with topical minoxidil
- Ketoconazole shampoo

- Prostaglandin analogues (topical bimatoprost and latanoprost)
- Topical melatonin
- Low-level laser therapy (LLLT)
- Mesotherapy
- Platelet-rich plasma (PRP)
- Hair follicle neogenesis and reprogramming

Tretinoin is a synthetic derivative of vitamin A that is commonly used as a topical treatment for acne, sun damage, and wrinkles.

While tretinoin does not significantly induce hair growth, it is used in androgenetic alopecia treatment due to its ability to enhance the effects of topical minoxidil.

Theoretically, tretinoin prevents keratinization of the stratum corneum, allowing better absorption of minoxidil. The therapeutic trial of combining tretinoin with minoxidil showed that when minoxidil was applied along with tretinoin cream, minoxidil absorption was increased nearly threefold, whereas there was only a 1.3-fold increase in the vehicle control cream. Nevertheless, there was no significant change in the stratum corneum thickness as revealed by skin biopsy. Besides skin thickness, however, the transepidermal water loss was increased, supporting a hypothesis that tretinoin increases absorption of minoxidil by increasing stratum corneum permeability. As standard minoxidil therapy is recommended to be applied twice a day, some patients complain of difficulty of using the drug regularly in the morning and at night. A randomized, double-blind, comparative clinical trial was performed in 31 male patients to compare the efficacy of 5 % minoxidil twice daily with combined 5 % minoxidil and 0.01 % tretinoin once daily. In this study, there was no statistical difference in increase of macrophotographic variables of total hair count and non-vellus hair count of both treatment groups. The adverse effects were also similar in both groups.

Therefore, combined topical 5 % minoxidil and 0.01 % tretinoin once daily therapy shares same efficacy and safety with traditional 5 % topical minoxidil twice daily therapy for androgenetic alopecia.

The basis for using *ketoconazole shampoo* in androgenetic alopecia treatment is aimed at the proposed hypothesis of a microbial-driven inflammatory reaction of hair follicles that potentially contribute to hair loss and at a proposed local antiandrogenic action of ketoconazole. Comparable hair growth was observed in an open-label study using 2 % topical minoxidil with 2 % ketoconazole shampoo in treatment of androgenetic alopecia.

Bimatoprost is a prostaglandin analogue (PGF2α) that is currently prescribed to reduce elevated intraocular pressure in glaucoma patients. The observation of eyelash growth in ocular patients using topical bimatoprost has led to the drug's application for cosmetic hair growth. Topical bimatoprost solution has been approved by the FDA in 2008 as eyelash growth enhancer.

Latanoprost is yet another prostaglandin analogue used for treatment of glaucoma. Although higher incidence of eyelash growth has been reported for bimatoprost, latanoprost also possesses ability to lengthen eyelashes. A single center, double-blind, randomized pilot study has been performed for 24 weeks with topical latanoprost 0.1 % in 16 men with mild androgenetic alopecia (Hamilton II–III) by Blume-Peytavi et al. At 24 weeks, there was an increased hair density on the latanoprost-treated site compared to placebo. The number of vellus and terminal hair was increased starting at 8 weeks.

The preliminary study proved a basis for conducting further studies on the positive effects of prostaglandin analogues for treatment of alopecia.

Melatonin possesses abilities of a potent antioxidant and growth modulator. Since androgenetic alopecia is probably not only due to androgen-dependent changes of hair follicles, but also involves follicular microinflammation, fibrosis, and environmental factors with formation of free radicals, melatonin's effect rose to surface as an intriguing treatment modality for androgenetic alopecia. Melatonin is a neurohormone released by the pineal gland that regulates seasonal biorhythms, daily sleep cycles, and the aging process. Along with circadian rhythm function, however, melatonin has a powerful capability to capture free radicals, enabling it to keep the functional integrity of nonneoplastic cells with its antioxidant properties.

Fischer et al. reviewed various studies with topical application of 0.0033 % melatonin for treatment of male and female androgenetic alopecia, including pharmacodynamics and safety studies. The various studies with different designs mostly showed positive effect in early stages of androgenetic alopecia. While the exact mechanism of melatonin for stimulating human hair growth remains elusive, there might be possible effects through MT1 membrane receptor in the dermal papilla, its interaction with androgens and estrogens, or anti-oxidative effects. Since tolerability of topical application of melatonin is good, melatonin may be a possible candidate in early stages of androgenetic alopecia.

> In contrast to topical minoxidil and oral finasteride in the management of male androgenetic alopecia, topical melatonin would seem to represent the first topical "antiaging" product for treatment of aging hair.

Low-level laser therapy (LLLT), also known as red light therapy, cold laser, and photobiomodulation, has been applied in various clinical fields to reduce neurogenic pain and inflammation and to enhance wound healing. The hypothesized mode of action of LLLT is increase in adenosine triphosphate (ATP) production mediated by cytochrome c oxidase. Increased ATP production could change cell metabolism and ultimately increase procollagen synthesis in fibroblasts. The ability of lasers to also induce hair growth was incidentally noted as early as 1967 when Mester et al. used LLLT to treat cancer in mice with shaved backs. Since then, hypertrichosis has been recognized to be a possible side effect of laser treatment. First described in 2002 with IPL therapy, this phenomenon has now been widely acknowledged to occur with an incidence rate ranging from 0.6 to 10 % with low fluences and all laser types. It is thought to be the result of suboptimal fluences that are too low to induce thermolysis, but high enough to stimulate follicular growth. Eventually, LLLT has been developed for treatment of androgenetic alopecia. However, conflicting data on the efficacy of LLLT in hair regrowth have so far been reported.

The HairMax LaserComb® (Lexington International, LLC) is a handheld class 3R low-level laser therapy device that contains a single laser module that emulates (depending on the model) 7–12 beams at a wavelength of 655 nm. The device uses a technique of parting the user's hair by combs that are attached to the device. This improves delivery of distributed laser light to the scalp. The combs are designed so that each of the teeth on the combs aligns with a laser beam. By aligning the teeth with the laser beams, the hair can be parted and the laser energy delivered to the scalp of the user without obstruction by the individual hairs on the scalp. The device received 510(k) clearance from the FDA for the treatment of male androgenetic alopecia.

> This clearance means that the HairMax LaserComb® is considered a moderate-risk medical device by the FDA and is thereby primarily screened for safety.

The HairMax LaserComb® has been tested in a company-sponsored study of 110 male patients with the claim of significant increase in mean terminal hair density when compared to a sham device. Avram and Rogers conducted the first independent blinded study of LLLT on hair growth. A total of seven patients were exposed to treatment for 3–6 months. Videomicroscopic images were taken at baseline, 3, and 6 months and analyzed for changes in vellus hair counts, terminal hair counts, and hair shaft diameter. Both videomicroscopic and global images underwent blinded review for evidence of improvement. The results indicated that on average patients had a decrease in the number of vellus hairs, an increase in the number of terminal hairs, and an increase in hair shaft diameter. However, paired i-testing indicated that none of these was statistically significant. Also, blinded evaluation of global images did not support a recognizable improvement.

Nevertheless, a consensus written by hair loss experts states that based on anecdotal experience, LLLT, particularly 650–900 nm wavelengths at 5 mW, may be an effective treatment option for patients who do not respond to or are not tolerant to topical minoxidil or oral finasteride.

This technology appears to work better for some people than for others. Predictive factors who will most benefit from LLLT are yet to be determined.

Mesotherapy has received much publicity in the media and the Internet, also for treatment of androgenetic alopecia. However, the subject has remained controversial in view of the lack of documented evidence. Moreover, multifocal scalp abscess with subcutaneous fat necrosis and cicatricial alopecia have been reported as complications of scalp mesotherapy.

Platelet rich plasma (PRP) is blood plasma that has been enriched with platelets. As a concentrated source of autologous platelets, PRP contains and releases through degranulation several growth factors and cytokines. These include PDGF, TGFβ, FGF, IGF-1 and 2, VEGF, EGF, IL-8, and KGF. The use and clinical validation of PRP is still in the early stages. Results of basic science and preclinical trials have yet to be confirmed in large-scale controlled clinical trials.

Ultimately, forward-looking developments on the field of hair follicle neogenesis and reprogramming can be followed on the respective commercial websites: www.histogen.com, www.aderanresearch.com, www.replicel.com, and www.follicabio.com.

Among the variety of therapeutic choices given for male androgenetic alopecia, there is no single treatment of choice for such a complex trait. From our experience, it seems best to use combination treatment modalities.

Khandpur et al. enrolled 100 male patients with androgenetic alopecia Hamilton grades II through IV in an open, randomized, parallel-group study, designed to evaluate and compare the efficacy of 1 mg oral finasteride, topical 2 % minoxidil solution, and topical 2 % ketoconazole shampoo alone and in combination. Patients were randomized into four groups: group I (30 patients) was administered oral finasteride alone, group II (36 patients) was given a combination of oral finasteride and topical minoxidil, group III (24 patients) applied topical minoxidil alone, and group IV (10 patients) was administered oral finasteride with ketoconazole shampoo. Treatment efficacy was assessed on the basis of patient and physician assessment scores and global photographic review during the study period of 1 year. At the end of 1 year, hair growth was observed in all the groups with best results recorded with a combination of finasteride and minoxidil (group II) followed by groups IV (oral finasteride and ketoconazole shampoo), I (oral finasteride alone), and III (topical minoxidil along). Subjects receiving finasteride alone or in combination with minoxidil or ketoconazole showed statistically significant improvement over minoxidil-only recipients.

It is important to manage male androgenetic alopecia strategically with the variety of current therapeutic options.

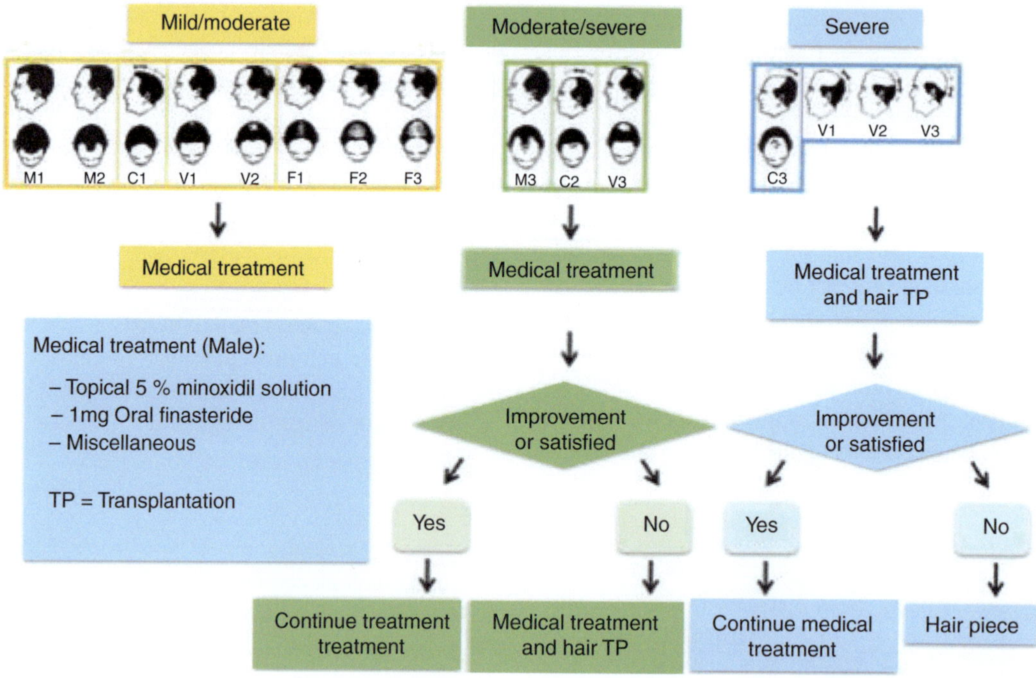

Fig. 3.8 Algorithmic guideline for the management of androgenetic alopecia (AGA). Mild/moderate AGA = BASP type M1-2, C1, F1-3 or V1-2; moderate/severe AGA = BASP type M3, C2-3, U1-3 or V3; severe AGA = BASP type C3 or U1-3 (From: Lee WS, Lee HJ, Choi GS et al (2013) Guidelines for management of androgenetic alopecia based on BASP classification-the Asian consensus committee guideline. J Eur Acad Dermatol Venereol 27:1026–1034)

There have been many treatment guidelines for androgenetic alopecia which are based on Norwood–Hamilton classification for male patients and Ludwig classification for female patients. A new algorithmic treatment guideline for androgenetic alopecia is proposed that is based on the BASP classification system (see Sect. 3.1.7). The main advantage of this guideline is that it is universally applicable regardless of race or sex (Fig. 3.8). Clinicians can utilize this guideline consistently in their practice to monitor treatment response with the goal of securing successful outcomes.

3.2 Effect of Cigarette Smoking and UV Radiation

As the rest of the skin, the scalp and hair are exposed to noxious environmental factors. While cigarette smoking and UV radiation are well appreciated as major factors contributing to extrinsic aging of the skin, their effect on the condition of hair and the natural course of androgenetic alopecia have only later attracted the attention of the medical community.

3.2.1 Effect of Cigarette Smoking on Hair Growth

Besides being the single most preventable cause of significant cardiovascular and pulmonary morbidity and an important cause of death in the general population, tobacco smoking has been associated with various adverse effects on the skin. Premature skin aging has attracted the attention of the medical community only since the 1960s, although a relation between smoking and skin complexion was first suggested as early as 1856. The facial features, designated "smoker's face," were originally defined by Model as one or more of the following: (a) wrinkles typically radiating at right angles from the upper and lower lips or corners of the eyes ("crow's feet"), deep lines on the cheeks, or numerous shallow lines on the cheeks and lower jaw; (b) a gauntness of facial features with prominence of the underlying bony contours, in some cases associated with a leathery, worn, or rugged appearance; (c) an atrophic, slightly pigmented gray appearance of the skin; and (d) a plethoric, slightly orange, purple, and red complexion different from the purply blue color of cyanosis or the bloated appearance associated with alcoholism. In a survey of 116 patients attending a general medical outpatient clinic (for other than dermatologic conditions), Model found that "smoker's face" was present in 46 % of current smokers, whereas 8 % of past smokers and no nonsmokers had "smoker's face." Others have also addressed the topic of smoking as a risk factor for facial wrinkling and come to similar conclusions.

The mechanisms by which smoking causes wrinkling are believed to be multifactorial and related to the effects of cigarette smoke on the microvasculature, cutaneous collagen, and elastic tissue, to pro-oxidant effects of smoking, and to increased hydroxylation of estradiol, as well as inhibition of the enzyme aromatase, which converts androgens to estrogens, creating a relative hypoestrogenic state. Cigarette smoke has been shown to increase plasma neutrophil elastase activity, which may also contribute to abnormal skin elastin, and matrix metalloproteinase (MMP)-1 (collagenase) expression was shown to be increased in the skin of smokers, which may contribute to degradation of collagen. Expression of both MMP-1 and MMP-3 have been shown to be induced in cultured human fibroblasts in a dose-related manner by cigarette smoke extracts, while the expression of tissue inhibitors of metalloproteinases (TIMPPs) was not influenced. The histological features associated with smoking have not been studied as extensively, but have demonstrated increased elastosis.

Given the public's overwhelming quest for a young and pleasing appearance, the consensus is that education about the link between cigarette smoking and skin aging could motivate young people not to smoke or to quit smoking.

> Alike the skin, the hair is subject to intrinsic or physiological aging and extrinsic or accelerated aging due to external factors. Intrinsic factors are related to individual genetic and epigenetic mechanisms with interindividual variations.

Prototypes of intrinsic aging are familial premature graying and androgenetic alopecia; extrinsic factors include exposure to tobacco smoke.

In 1996, Mosley and Gibbs reported in patients visiting a general surgical outpatient clinic in the UK for the first time a significant relationship between smoking and premature gray hair in both men and women and between smoking and baldness in men. Since the number of alopecia in women was very small, no corresponding calculation could be carried out for hair loss in women.

Subsequently, the observation of strikingly dissimilar androgenetic alopecia in a 52-year-old monozygotic male twin pair led to further speculations on the possibility of an association between smoking and hair loss, since studies on the degree of alopecia among monozygotic twins aged over 50 have shown that intrapair differences are negligible in 92 %, slight in 8 %, and striking in none. A salient feature differing the twin brothers in their personal histories was that the balding brother admitted to long-standing, heavy cigarette smoking, while the other was a nonsmoker. A succeeding study failed to confirm this association.

Eventually, a population-based cross-sectional survey among Asian men 40 years or older showed statistically significant positive associations between moderate or severe androgenetic alopecia and smoking status, current cigarette smoking of 20 cigarettes or more per day, and smoking intensity. The odds ratio of early-onset history for androgenetic alopecia grades increased in a dose-response pattern. Risk for moderate or severe androgenetic increased for family history of first-degree and second-degree relatives, as well as for paternal relatives. A reservation to be made is the role of negative psychological effects of androgenetic alopecia on self-esteem and peculiarities of psychological adjustment. Although the study data were collected with respect to age at onset of androgenetic alopecia and age at start of smoking, there is no information on the temporal relationship of these, with respect to the question whether smoking contributes to the development of androgenetic alopecia, or alternatively represents a form of behavioral coping to the impairment in physical appearance resulting from alopecia.

The mechanisms by which smoking accelerates hair loss have not been examined, but it is likely that they are similar to the effects on the skin.

The cutaneous microvasculature is constricted by acute and long-term smoking. Evidence of the consequence of impaired circulation and wound healing is a higher complication rate of hair restoration surgery in smokers versus nonsmokers. Besides inducing local ischemia, the decreased capillary blood flow in the dermal papilla of the hair follicles may focally shunt more toxic substances. Cigarette smoke contains over 4,800 chemicals, many of which are known to be toxic to cells and 69 are known to cause cancer. Both nicotine and cotinine are detected in hair samples of smokers. Apart from cancer, smoking is also a major risk factor in chronic obstructive pulmonary disease, heart disease and cerebrovascular insult, and other disorders such as slowed healing of wounds, impotence, infertility, and peptic ulcer disease.

Smoke genotoxicants metabolized in hair follicle cells may cause DNA damage through the production of DNA adducts, and smoking-associated mitochondrial DNA mutations have been shown in human hair follicles, though the relevance of these for hair follicle pathology is as yet unknown.

Since substantial extracellular matrix remodeling is involved in the hair follicle growth cycle, especially during catagen-associated hair follicle regression, it is conceivable that cigarette smoke-induced imbalance in the intra- and perifollicular protease/antiprotease systems controlling tissue remodeling may also affect the hair follicle growth cycle.

Finally, smoking-induced oxidative stress and a disequilibrium of antioxidant systems may lead to the release of pro-inflammatory cytokines from follicular keratinocytes, which by themselves have been shown to inhibit the growth of isolated hair follicles in culture. Moreover, adjacent fibroblasts are fully equipped to respond to such a pro-inflammatory signal. On the occasion that the causal agent persists, sustained microinflammation of the hair follicle is the result, together with connective tissue remodelling, where again collagenases play an active role and are believed to contribute to perifollicular fibrosis.

The fact that cigarette smoke-associated hair loss is of the androgenetic type indicates that genetic factors contribute. On the other hand, recent studies on the evolution of androgenetic hair loss have focused on oxidative stress.

Naito et al. analyzed the effect of the lipid peroxides on hair follicles and observed that the topical application of linolein hydroperoxides, one of the lipid peroxides, leads to the early onset of the catagen phase in murine hair cycles. Furthermore, they found that lipid peroxides induced apoptosis of hair follicle cells. They also induced apoptosis in human epidermal keratinocytes by upregulating apoptosis-related genes. These results indicate that lipid peroxides, which can cause free radicals, induce the apoptosis of hair follicle cells, and this is followed by early onset of the catagen phase.

Ultimately, Bahta et al. cultured dermal hair papilla cells (DPC) from balding and non-balding scalp and demonstrated that balding DPCs grow slower in vitro than non-balding DPCs. Loss of proliferative capacity of balding DPCs was associated with changes in cell morphology, expression of senescence-associated beta-galactosidase, decreased expression of proliferating cell nuclear antigen and Bmi-1, upregulation of p16(INK4a)/pRb and nuclear expression of markers of oxidative stress and DNA damage including heat shock protein-27, super oxide dismutase catalase, ataxia-telangiectasia-mutated kinase (ATM), and ATM- and Rad3-related protein.

The finding of premature senescence of balding DPC in vitro in association with expression of markers of oxidative stress and DNA damage suggests that balding DPCs are particularly sensitive to environmental stress.

The appearance of hair plays an important role in people's overall physical appearance and self-perception. The well-recognized psychological effects of androgenetic alopecia on affected men and our society's veneration of youth and its attributes, seem to offer a good opportunity for prevention or cessation of smoking.

Increasing public awareness of the association between smoking and hair loss would seem more effective than the link between smoking and facial wrinkles, since the latter can be effectively counteracted by current cosmetic dermatologic procedures, while treatment options for androgenetic alopecia are limited.

3.2.2 Effect of UV Radiation on Hair Growth and Scalp Condition

While the consequences of sustained ultraviolet radiation (UVR) on unprotected skin are well appreciated, mainly photocarcinogenesis and solar elastosis, the effects of UVR on the evolution of androgenetic alopecia have largely been ignored. However some clinical and morphologic observations, as well as theoretical considerations, suggest that UVR has some negative effect.

The number of recognized photosensitive dermatoses that localize to the scalp is essentially limited to light-exacerbated endogenous eczema, dermatomyositis, and cutaneous lupus erythematosus.

Patients with atopic and seborrheic dermatitis occasionally report nonspecific exacerbation of their condition following sun exposure, also on the scalp, where at times it may be difficult to differentiate from exacerbation of itch through heat-induced sweating. A high prevalence of seborrheic dermatitis has been described on the scalp in sun-exposed mountain guides in Austria, Switzerland, and Germany.

While lupus erythematous represents a well-known photosensitive disorder with frequent scalp lesions, localization of dermatomyositis to the scalp is often overlooked or misdiagnosed. Moreover, similar to those with lupus erythematosus, dermatomyositis patients demonstrate a significantly reduced minimal erythema doses (MED) to UV irradiation compared with healthy controls. The inflammation of the scalp may lead to hair loss.

Camacho et al. reported a peculiar type of telogen effluvium following sunburn of the scalp after 3–4 months with hairstyles that left areas of scalp uncovered during prolonged sun exposure. The clinical features were increased frontovertical hair shedding along with a trichogram that disclosed an increase of telogen hairs and dystrophic hairs. In women the hairs on the frontal region appeared unruly, and the frontovertical alopecia showed loss of the frontal hair implantation line. The pathomechanism of this type of telogen effluvium is not clear. It has been proposed that the columns of the cells in the hair shaft act as an efficient fiber-optic type system, transmitting UV light downward into the hair follicle. Morphologically, the keratinocytes within the hair shaft are arranged in compressed linear columns that resemble the coaxial bundles of commercial fiber-optic strands. Thus hair follicular melanocytes located in the region of the hair matrix may function as UV biosensors and respond to photic inputs. Depending on the quantity of UVR exposure, it is conceivable that also photodamage may occur at this site, resulting in telogen effluvium.

Histopathologically, elastosis is regularly found in scalp biopsies, especially in alopecic conditions, but so far has largely been ignored. Up to date, no controlled study has been performed on the degree of scalp elastosis in relation to the pace of development, duration, or grade of androgenetic alopecia, though it would seem to be a good marker for exposure to UVR penetrating the skin. Interestingly, UVB irradiation has been found to stimulate the synthesis of elastic fibers by modified epithelial cells surrounding the hair follicle and sebaceous glands in mice.

> Since all of these disorders of the scalp share the common feature that they are induced or exacerbated by exposure to sunlight, it has been proposed that androgenetic alopecia in particular may be a photoaggravated dermatosis that demands adequate photoprotection.

As a consequence of increased leisure time with a growing popularity of outdoor activities and holidays in the sun, awareness of sun protection has become important. Topically applied chemicals that act as sun protectors are widely utilized and offer the most convenient means of protecting the glabrous skin against acute (sunburn) and chronic pathologic effects of UVR. Out of cosmetic reasons their use on the hair-bearing scalp is problematic, unless complete baldness is present. Although hats provide the best protection of the scalp from UVR, not all patients find it convenient or acceptable for this purpose.

While protection of the hair against photodamage has been extensively studied, there are no data on photoprotection of the hair-bearing scalp: It has been found that hair dyes may protect hair against photodamage; experimental work indicates that cinnamidopropyltrimonium chloride, a quaternized UV absorber, delivered from a shampoo system, is suitable for photoprotection of hair, while simultaneously providing an additional conditional benefit on hair; and solid lipid nanoparticles have been developed as novel carriers of UV blockers for the use on skin and hair, while offering photoprotection on their own by reflecting and scattering UV radiation.

Finally, systemic photoprotection has been the focus of more recent investigation, in as much as this would overcome some of the problems associated with the topical use of sunscreens: Preclinical studies illustrate photoprotective properties of supplemented antioxidants, particularly beta-carotene (provitamin A), α-tocopherol (vitamin E), and L-ascorbate (vitamin C). However, clinical evidence that these prevent, retard, or slow down solar skin damage is still impending. The same applies to topical melatonin, which has been found to suppress UV-induced erythema and UV-induced reactive oxygen species in a dose-dependent manner. Nevertheless, these results suggest the probable utility of combining these compounds with known sunscreens to maximize photoprotection.

3.2.3 Diffuse Red Scalp Disease

Red scalp was first been described by Thestrup-Pedersen and Hjorth in 1987 and subsequently commented on by Moschella in 1992, who stated on the difficult problem of *diffuse red scalp disease which can also be itchy and burning. …. It is non responsive to any therapy including potent topical steroids or anti-seborrhoeic therapy.* Patients frequently report aggravation in the sun or report repeated episodes of sunburn of the scalp.

Grimalt et al. presented their findings in 18 patients with "red scalp syndrome" at the 2000 Annual Meeting of the European Hair Research Society: The majority were middle-aged females consulting for hair loss. By definition no specific dermatologic disease was found. The scalp redness was associated with androgenetic alopecia in 13 out of 18 patients, and 3 of 10 biopsies performed were compatible with a cicatricial alopecia (not otherwise specified). Some patients reported associated discomfort of the scalp. The most prevalent speculations with respect to the pathogenesis of scalp discomfort in the absence of a specific dermatologic disease are perifollicular inflammation and increased expression of the neuropeptide substance P in the vicinity of affected hair follicles.

In our published series of 403 patients complaining of hair loss examined for trichodynia, the dermatoscopic finding of scalp telangiectasia was found to strongly correlate with presence of trichodynia.

An interesting analogy exists to rosacea, where patients with the telangiectatic variant of rosacea reported stinging sensation to the topical application of 5 % lactic acid on the cheeks more frequently than patients with the papulopustular type of rosacea or normal controls.

On the one hand, these findings suggest a connection between sensory or subjective irritation and cutaneous vascular reactivity. On the other hand, dilated and tortuous vessels are typically found in photodamaged skin.

Oberholzer et al. recently described patients with red scalp disease with clinical and histopathologic findings consistent with rosacea and response to oral tetracycline therapy (Fig. 3.9a–f). On the basis of the observation of clinical and histopathologic features of rosacea, and response to oral tetracycline therapy, patients complaining of red scalp accompanied with scalp discomfort were suggested to suffer of a rosacea-like dermatosis of the scalp.

Careful examination of the affected scalp, including dermoscopy, invariably reveals erythema, telangiectasia, follicular papules, and pustules.

Histology demonstrates ectatic venules and a usually sparse perivascular infiltrate, in the case of papules a more pleomorphic perifollicular infiltration with granuloma formation, including neutrophils. Intrafollicular collections of neutrophils are found when pustules are observed.

Rosacea is a chronic inflammatory disorder usually affecting the central parts of the face with flushing, persistent erythema, and telangiectasia, in combination with episodes of swelling, papules, and pustules. It typically presents either as erythematotelangiectatic rosacea or as the papulopustular type. Eye involvement (ocular rosacea) is common; other extrafacial locations may be involved more frequently then appreciated because of failure to search; in particular, rosacea affecting the upper forehead and bald scalp has previously been reported.

Demodex infestation of the scalp (Fig. 3.10a–c) has previously been put forward as a possible etiologic factor in scalp rosacea. However, demodex mites are common commensals of the pilosebaceous unit. In humans, *Demodex folliculorum* and *D. brevis* have been identified and implied to play a role in pustular folliculitis of the face, papulopustular scalp eruptions, perioral dermatitis, and blepharitis. In general, the clinical presentations of demodicidosis have been classified into three main groups: "pityriasis folliculorum," "rosacea-like demodicidosis," and "granulomatous rosacea-like demodicidosis gravis." Methods used for diagnostic purposes include cyanoacrylic adhesives, comedone extractor, cellophane tape preparations, skin scraping, punch biopsy, and standardized surface skin biopsy.

However, there is no consensus to what degree demodex mites are causative of skin pathology and how they might contribute to disease in humans.

3.2.4 Erosive Pustular Dermatosis of the Scalp

Erosive pustular dermatosis of the scalp is observed as a distinct disorder peculiar to the balding scalp. Erosive pustular dermatosis of the scalp was first described by Burton and subsequently delineated by Pye, Peachey, and Burton as a distinctive clinical entity producing chronic extensive pustulation confined to the scalp of elderly individuals and leading to erosion and scarring alopecia (Fig. 3.11).

A high incidence of antecedent local trauma strongly suggests that scalp injury may be important in initiating erosive pustular dermatosis of the scalp in a susceptible elderly person with atrophic skin changes of the scalp, particularly due to prolonged exposure of long-standing androgenetic alopecia to UVR.

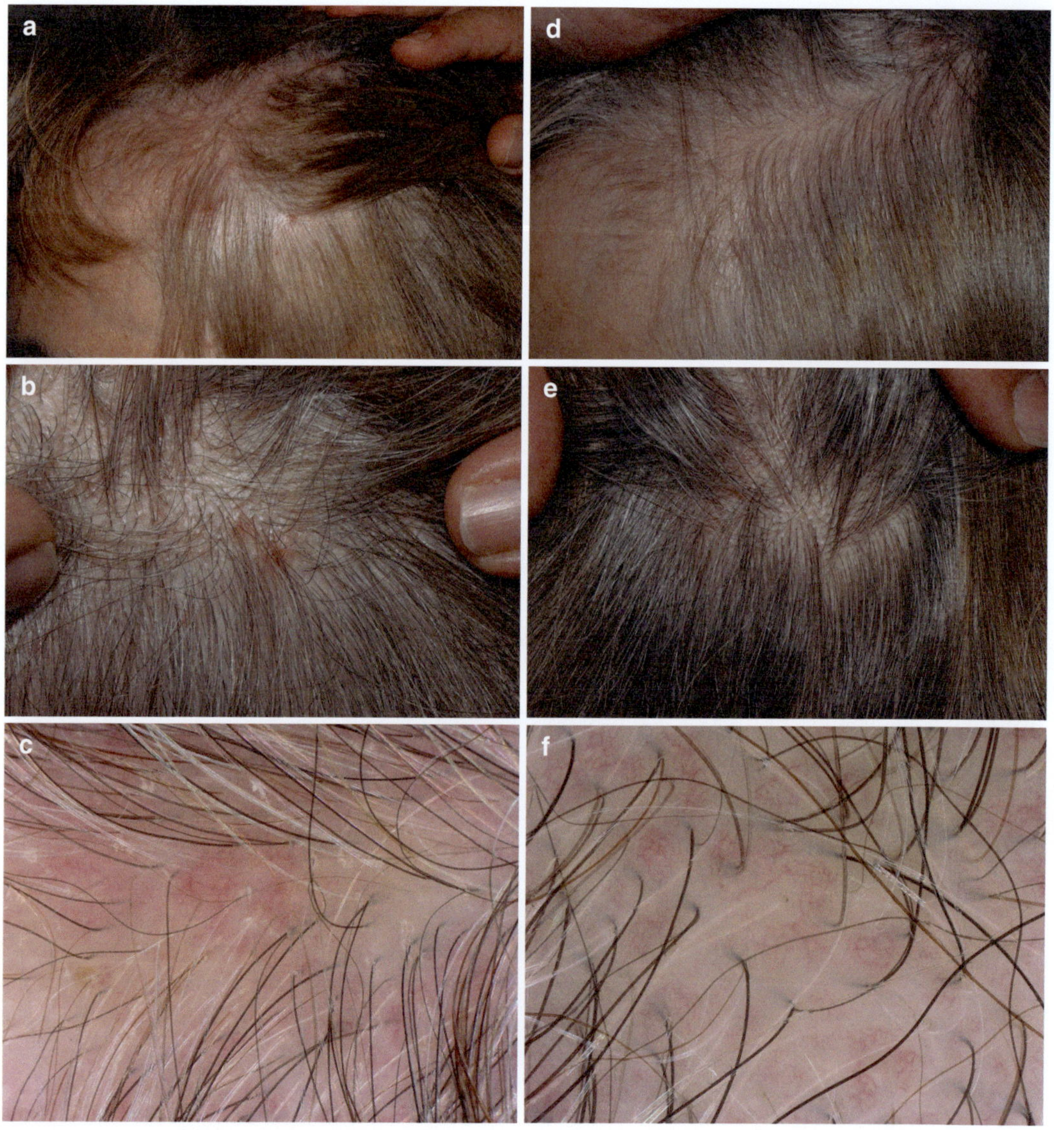

Fig. 3.9 (**a–f**) Red scalp or rosacea-like dermatosis of scalp. Clinical and dermoscopic findings (**a–c**) before and (**d–f**) following successful therapy with oral tetracycline

No recognized cause of pustulation is present, and the histology is nonspecific. Response to antibiotics is poor, but the condition is suppressed by potent topical steroids, suggesting an inflammatory rather than an infective etiology. The condition has been observed following contusion, laceration, blistering sunburn, shingles, synthetic fiber implantation, craniotomy, and skin grafting of the scalp, as well as following treatment of solar keratoses with 5 % topical fluorouracil cream, cryotherapy and topical tretinoin, and soft x-ray therapy.

> Therefore, one must think of the possibility of erosive pustular dermatosis of the scalp in cases of delayed wound healing following treatment of actinic keratoses on the scalp.

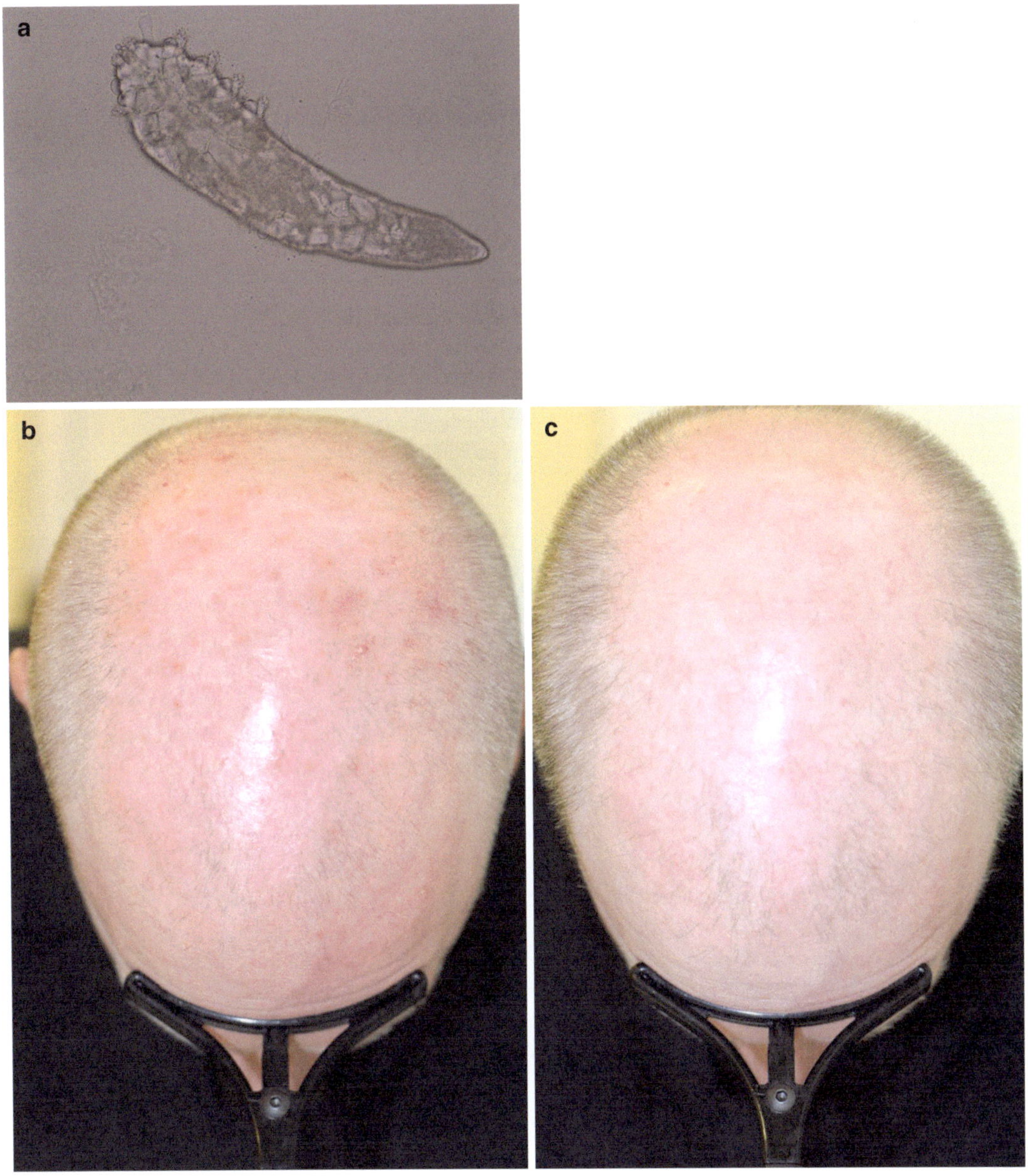

Fig. 3.10 (**a–c**) Rosacea-like demodicidosis of the scalp (**a**) light microscopy of *demodex* extracted from an inflammatory follicular lesion (**b**) before and (**c**) after 30 days treatment with oral metronidazole 250 mg bid and 5 % topical permethrin cream

Response to therapy has been variable, with best responses reported to potent topical steroids and more recently to topical 0.1 % tacrolimus. Anecdotal reports describe partial response to nimesulide, a phenoxymethane sulfonanilide that inhibits the respiratory burst of human granulocytes. Long-term follow-up is advised, since neoplastic change has been reported.

3.2.5 Actinic Field Cancerization of the Bald Scalp

Terrestrial solar UVR ranges from approximately 290–400 nm. UVB (290–315 nm) reaches the upper dermis only, while UVA (315–400 nm) penetration into the dermis increases with wavelength. The two most important chronic effects of

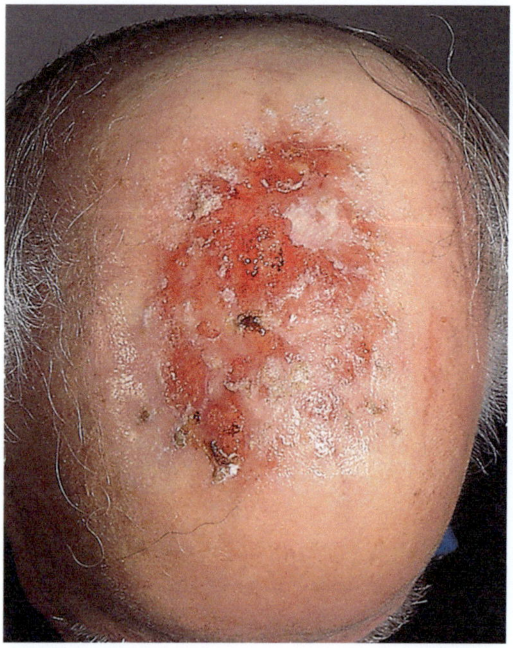

Fig. 3.11 Erosive pustular dermatosis of the scalp

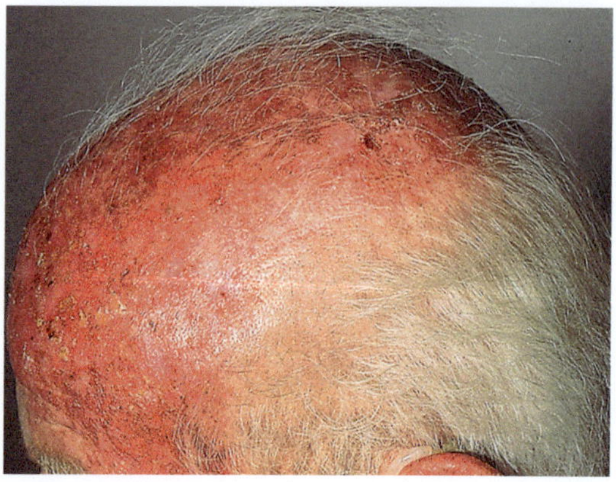

Fig. 3.12 Actinic keratoses of the scalp (actinic field cancerization)

UVR on the skin and bald scalp are photocarcinogenesis and solar elastosis. The mechanisms by which UVR plays a role in the development of skin cancer are varied and represent a multistep process involving alterations in DNA structure, resulting from purine photoproducts, cytosine photohydrates, single-strand breaks, and sister chromatid exchange, as well as from reactive oxygen species that are generated during exposure of cells to UVR. Theoretically, any alteration capable of causing a mutation in specific target genes could contribute to carcinogenesis, since there is a close correlation between mutation and transformation by UVR. Recent progress has been made in identifying specific genes that control cellular growth that may be involved in photocarcinogenesis. Also, UVR induces deviations of tumor immunosurveillance mechanisms that eventually aid the survival and progressive growth of UVR-induced malignancies. Finally, it has been found that telomerase activity plays a crucial role in the immortalization of human cells: Telomerase activity is found in plucked hair follicles, which is associated with the presence of stem cells in the follicle, and is found in a high percentage of skin tumors. Evidence of UVR-associated activation of telomerase in human skin further suggests that telomerase activation is involved in skin photocarcinogenesis.

Actinic keratoses of the scalp are often multiple, and although usually asymptomatic, the patient may note mild local tenderness. At times multiple, confluent lesions of the centroparietal scalp with androgenetic alopecia may be misinterpreted as refractory seborrheic eczema of the scalp.

Actinic keratosis is the most common epidermal precancerous lesion resulting from chronic UVR exposure, usually on sun-exposed body regions of middle-aged or older people, including the balding scalp or bald scalp area. It presents as a skin-colored to reddish, ill-defined macule with a dry adherent scale (Fig. 3.12).

Topical therapies include 5-fluorouracil cream (5, 1, 0.5 %), imiquimod cream (5 and 3.75 %), diclofenac sodium gel 3 % with 2.5 % hyaluronic gel, ingenol mebutate gel (0.05 and 0.015 %), and cryotherapy. Aminolevulinic acid photodynamic therapy is a procedural field therapy.

A deeper understanding of the pathophysiology underlying the development of actinic keratosis to squamous cell carcinoma of the scalp, combined with an increasing global prevalence of actinic keratoses, underscores the importance of combining local treatments that remove individual lesions with topical or procedural field therapies that treat the entire actinically damaged field.

Sunlight damage of the hair causes discoloration and irregular surface, resulting in reduced tensile strength and vulnerability toward additional environmental damage. Therefore, hair fibers should be protected from the sunlight.

3.2.6 Hair Photoaging

Among environmental factors contributing to hair damage, photoaging due to sunlight is especially unavoidable. In addition to sunlight, water, dust, friction, hair combing, and cosmetic hair treatments (dyeing or permanent waving) can cause hair damage. These external factors are collectively termed "hair weathering." Among these factors, sunlight and particularly ultraviolet (UV) rays play a significant role in photoaging. Hair photoaging is the natural process of various reactions which result in chemical and physical changes in the hair fiber.

As the outer layer of the hair fiber gets higher intensities of light, cuticle cells are damaged to greater degree than cortical cells by sunlight.

Photodamaged hair shaft results in dryness, increased breakage, split ends, coarse feel, lack of manageability, and lack of luster. It becomes paler in color and weakens in strength and shine with the respective alterations in cosmetic properties.

Chemical reactions occur in hair protein, lipids, and pigments. Lipid oxidation, disulfide bond cleavage, tryptophan degradation, and cysteic acid formation make the hair fiber increase in porosity and surface roughness and weaken the mechanical strength. These chemical reactions mainly depend on melanins and chromophores in hair. Detailed examination of the structure of damaged hair reveals irregular cuticle layer, especially toward the hair end, as well as increased oxidation of hair.

Once the hair is exposed to sunlight, the light penetrates through several layers of the hair. Intact hair cuticles are composed of 6–10 layers, each 0.3–0.5 μm thick, with combined thickness of nearly 5 μm. UVB can penetrate approximately 5 μm of thickness, mainly affecting the cuticle layer; UVA and visible light (VIS), which have longer wavelengths, completely penetrate the entire cuticle and influence the cortex as well. According to Jeon et al., UVB results in greater destruction of cuticle compared to UVA, while the destruction of intercellular lipid layer is not different between UVA and UVB. UV light is the main cause of hair damage, but VIS also results in hair damage. The ratio of UV, VIS, and infrared (IR) in sunlight is approximately 6, 52, and 42 %, respectively, with VIS being the main component. Sunlight mainly destroys protein, melanin, and lipid components of hair; according to Hoting et al., UV light dissolves protein, melanin, and lipid, while VIS reacts with melanin and lipid. In other words, protein is mainly destroyed by UV, and melanin is destroyed by both VIS and UV. Whether VIS or UV causes greater damage is under great debate.

Long-term ultraviolet exposure causes physical and chemical changes to greater extent than short-term exposure.

These changes usually occur from the periphery with higher levels of damage with progression to deeper portions of fiber with lower levels of damages. Longer exposure of these photodamaged hairs to oxidizing solution (aqueous alkaline solution or peroxide solution) results in dissolution or removal of cuticle scale and melanin.

The main protein component of human hair is keratin. The cortex, which is mainly involved in mechanical property of the hair, takes up to 65–95 % of total hair mass. The cuticle layer surrounding the cortex protects the hair from environmental and chemical damage. The cuticle layer is more vulnerable to UV damage due to its external location compared to the cortex. Among the various proteins that constitute keratin, tryptophan, cysteine, tyrosine, and histidine are particularly more sensitive.

Cysteine shows the most conspicuous alteration since it better absorbs 254- to 350-nm wavelength that matches with UV range. Cysteine is mainly damaged through break down of C–S fission. As concentration of cysteine is the highest in hair cuticle, the photodegradation especially occurs in the cuticular region.

Oxidative reactions caused by singlet oxygen occur more frequently in photodamaged hair. It results in increased cuticle fragility, fiber porosity, and surface roughness of the hair, as well as decreased mechanical strength, leading to further vulnerability of the hair to additional mechanical or chemical treatment. Robbins and Bahl et al. have reported that the oxygen radicals created by UV light breaks down the disulfide bonds of structural units, forming carbonyl groups and new intra- and intermolecular cross-links that reduce structural integrity. The amino acid components show individual variability. Cysteine is more frequently found in male than in females and in dark hair compared to light hair. Tryptophan is also found in greater quantity in black hair than in light hair and in old age, suggesting that the amount of tryptophan increases with age. Interestingly, photodegradation of tryptophan results in elevated photosensitivity of other amino acids. Carbonyl group is better formed in dry hair than in wet hair and is more vulnerable to oxidative damage. On the other hand, application of mineral oil reduces the destruction of amino acids.

Ubiquitin is a stable protein existing in normal hair. However, once exposed to UV light, it becomes a heat-labile and soluble protein, making it a useful indicator of hair damage. In addition, S100A3 is a protein belonging to calcium-binding S100 family that is present in the inner endocuticle of hair fiber. It is connected to hair keratin through disulfide bridge, maintaining the structural integrity of the hair. Hair washing, rinsing, UVB irradiation, and other damages to the hair release S100A3 from the hair fiber, weakening the hair structure.

Recently Marsh et al. investigated the role of low levels of redox metals such as copper in accelerating damage to hair on exposure to UV irradiation. The methods used were proteomics to measure the protein damage via protein loss after different periods of exposure and mass spectroscopy methods to identify marker peptides that are specifically created by this type of damage. They identified for the first time in hair the role of exogenous copper in increasing UV damage both in terms of total protein degradation and increased formation of the marker peptide.

This work provides evidence for the role of copper in water for UV-induced damage to hair and strategies to reduce copper levels in hair using a chelant such as *N,N′*-ethylenediamine disuccinic acid (EDDS).

There are two types of melanin: pheomelanin and eumelanin. The former is mainly degraded by VIS, while the latter is degraded by all components of sunlight, particularly by UVA and VIS. Images by transmission electron microscopy showed that melanin pigments are released from their envelope and some disappear. This phenomenon results in the loss of hair color in photodamaged hair. Melanin is degraded once it absorbs light. During the degradation, melanin absorbs and filters light, protecting proteins from further degradation. Since melanin is present only in the cortex, this protection occurs only in the cortex and frequently occurs with low wavelength UV light.

The cuticle layer does not contain melanin and therefore is not protected; meanwhile, the cortex is protected from UV by melanin, resulting in less degradation of amino acids.

Eumelanin is less prone to degradation by sunlight compared to pheomelanin, therefore offering better protection. Black hair is composed of 99 % eumelanin and 1 % pheomelanin: brown and blond hair consists of 95 and 5 % eumelanin, respectively. In other words, dark hair has higher ratio of eumelanin.

The destruction of melanin leads to photoyellowing or photobleaching.

According to Hoting et al., photobleaching more frequently occurs in light brown hair compared to black hair: the former also shows elevated degradation of cysteine, proline, and valine.

The intercellular layer of hair cuticle is composed of cell membrane cortex (CMC), which is a laminar structure containing protein and lipid layer. Lipid consists in 0.7–1.3 % of total hair. Two types of hair lipid exist: surface lipid (external lipid) and integral lipid (internal lipid, IL). IL is located between the keratinized cells in inner root sheath and Henle layer.

The hair cuticles are composed of thin integral lipid layer which is covalently attached to proteins. Unlike the keratin layer of the epidermis or sebaceous gland of the hair, the major component of this lipid layer is fatty acid, with 18-methyl eicosanoic acid composing 40 % of all fatty acid. Also unlike the lipids of the keratin layer of the epidermis, it is a branched form of fatty acid. IL can be analyzed by three compartments: hair shaft, inner root sheath, and whole hair follicle. Lee et al. showed that IL is composed of fatty acid, phytosphingosine, ceramide, cholesterol, and cholesterol sulfate in decreasing order in whole hair follicle. They also found that composition of hair lipid in IRS and hair shaft

Table 3.2 Chemical composition of integral hair lipid

	Hair shaft (%)	Inner root sheath (%)	Whole hair follicle (%)
Fatty acid	29.60	49.90	49.10
Phytosphingosine	37.20	23.30	26.30
Ceramide	26.90	23.20	20.20
Cholesterol	5.10	2.50	3.70
Cholesterol sulfate	1.10	0.20	0.30
Cholesterol oleate	0.20	0.80	0.30

Lee WS, Oh TH, Chun SH et al (2005) Integral lipid in human hair follicle. J Investig Dermatol Symp Proc 10:234–237

was varied from that of whole hair follicle (Table 3.2). IL is essential in providing hydrophobicity and stiffness of the hair that protects the hair.

Visible range of light destroys integral hair lipid to a greater extent than UVB and UVA light. Also, integral hair lipid is known to be degraded in greater quantity in blond hair compared to black hair.

Weakening of the CMC occurs in multiple steps when exposed to light. UV light destroys approximately 25 % of cholesterol in blond hair, compared to 60 % degraded by VIS and global radiation. In black hair, light exposure does not significantly alter lipid composition: only about 24 % is degraded. The reason for this phenomenon is attributed to melanin, particularly eumelanin, found in greater quantity in black hair, which protects IL from photodegradation.

3.3 Telogen Effluvium

Diffuse shedding of hair has originally been called "defluvium capillorum." In 1932, Sabouraud restricted the term to sudden diffuse loss of hair following shortly after a severe emotional shock, while others applied it to all forms of alopecia. In 1961, Kligman revealed the pathodynamics of one common pattern of response of hair follicles to a variety of insults and named it telogen effluvium.

> Whatever the cause, the follicle tends to behave in a similar way. To grasp the meaning of this generalization requires understanding of the hair cycle and its derangements.

3.3.1 Pathologic Dynamics of Hair Loss

In general, disease states that cause hair loss are categorized according to whether the hair loss is diffuse or localized and to whether the follicle remains intact or is destroyed and replaced by a scar.

> Except for the scarring alopecias, hair loss represents a disorder of hair follicle cycling.

As originally proposed by Mildred Trotter, the hair follicle is subject to constant turnover in the course of perpetual cycles through phases of proliferation in anagen, involution in catagen, and resting in telogen, with regeneration in the successive hair cycle (Fig. 3.13).

It is a major characteristic of *anagen* (duration: 2–6 years) that not only the hair shaft is growing but that most epithelial hair follicle compartments undergo proliferation, with the hair matrix keratinocytes showing the highest proliferative activity.

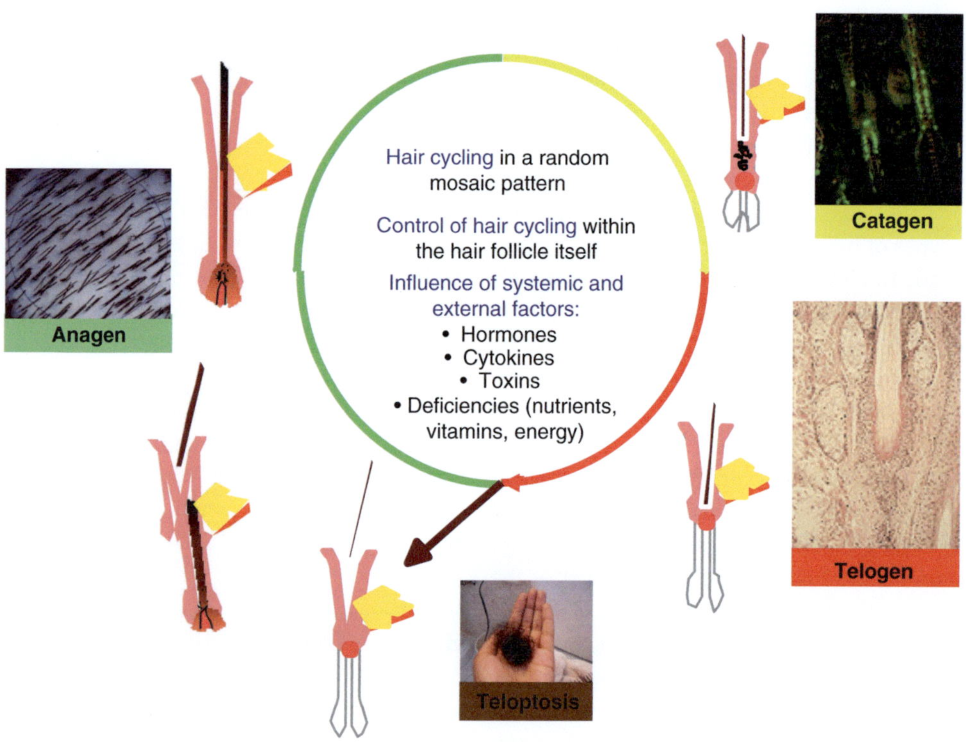

Fig. 3.13 Hair cycle

During *catagen* (duration: 2 weeks), hair follicles enter a process of involution that is characterized by a burst of programmed cell death (apoptosis) in the majority of follicular keratinocytes. The resulting shortening of the regressing epithelial strand is associated with an upward movement of the follicle.

In *telogen* (duration: 3 months), the hair shaft matures into a club hair, which is held tightly in the bulbous base of the follicular epithelium, before it is eventually shed. It was unresolved, whether shedding of the telogen hair (*teloptosis*) is an active, regulated process or represents a passive event that occurs at the onset of subsequent anagen, as the new hair grows in.

Cyclic hair growth activity occurs in a random mosaic pattern with each follicle possessing its own individual control mechanism over the evolution and triggering of the successive phases, though systemic factors as well as external factors linked to the environment, have influence, such as:

- Hormones
- Cytokines and growth factors
- Toxins
- Deficiencies of nutrients, vitamins, and energy (calories)

Finally, there are considerable variations in length of these phases depending on the body site location, with the duration of anagen determining the type of hair produced, particularly its length. On the scalp, hairs remain in anagen for a 2- to 6-year period of time, whereas that of telogen is approximately 100 days, resulting in a ratio of anagen to telogen hairs of 9:1. On average, the amount of new scalp hair formation matches the amount that is shed, thereby maintaining a consistent covering. With a range of 75,000–150,000 hairs on the head, the reported average daily telogen hair shedding varies from 35 to 180 hairs.

In general, the anagen phase is shorter in men than in women.

Since the original description of the hair growth cycle, additional phenomena relevant to hair growth and shedding have been recognized:

In 1996, Guarrera et al. observed that anagen hairs may fail to replace telogen hairs in androgenetic alopecia. By using the phototrichogram, a novel phenomenon was discovered: emptiness of the hair follicle following teloptosis. Rebora chose to call this phenomenon *kenogen*, deriving from the Greek word for "empty." During kenogen, the hair follicle rests physiologically, but duration and frequency were shown to be greater in androgenetic alopecia, possibly accounting for baldness. In addition to the classical cycle, the hair follicle may follow an alternative route during which the telogen phase, not accompanied by a coincident new early anagen, ends with teloptosis leaving the follicle empty.

In 2002, Stenn et al. recognized the shedding phase of the hair growth cycle, then renamed *exogen*, to be a uniquely controlled final step in the hair cycle involving a specific proteolytic step.

Finally, in 2013, Bernard et al. from L'Oréal Research and Innovation laboratories identified hypoxia markers in the human hair follicle stem cells and proposed hypoxia signaling mediated by the hypoxia-inducible transcription factor HIF1 to be important for reentry of the follicle into a new hair cycle in the course of a novel neomorphogenic hair cycle phase, named *neogen*. Ultimately, it was further hypothesized that molecules that mimic hypoxic signaling may figure as a new approach to sustain hair growth and cycling.

Many factors can lead to pathologically increased hair loss. The pathologic dynamics of hair loss can be related to disorders of hair cycling.

Telogen effluvium is by far the most common cause of hair loss and results from increased shedding of hairs from the telogen phase of the hair cycle.

An increase in the percentage of follicles in telogen >20 % leads to increased shedding of normal club hairs. This can either be due to synchronization phenomena of hair cycling or to shortening of the anagen phase, resulting in a higher percentage of hairs in telogen.

On the basis of changes in different phases of the follicular cycle, Headington proposed classification of telogen effluvium into five functional types depending on changes in different phases of the hair cycle (Table 3.3).

In Kligman's original description, telogen effluvium is an acute and diffuse hair loss brought about by a variety of triggers. Clinical experience, however, proves that chronic telogen effluvium also exists. It is defined as diffuse telogen hair loss that persists longer than 6 months.

Table 3.3 Functional types of telogen effluvium

In *immediate anagen release*, follicles that would normally complete a longer cycle by remaining in anagen prematurely enter telogen. It is a very common form of telogen effluvium, typically occurring after periods of physiological stress including episodes of high fever. In fever, the pyrogens, basically circulating cytokines, drive the hair follicle keratinocytes into apoptosis initiating catagen with following telogen. Because the shedding is dependent on transition from anagen through catagen and telogen with subsequent release of telogen hairs, hair loss occurs 3–4 months after the inciting event.
In *delayed anagen release*, hair follicles remain in prolonged anagen rather than cycling into telogen. When finally released from anagen, the clinical sign of increased shedding of telogen hair will be found. This type of telogen effluvium underlies postpartum hair loss.
In *immediate telogen release*, hair follicles normally programmed for release of the club hair after an interval of usually 100 days after the end of anagen are prematurely stimulated to cycle into anagen. There is premature teloptosis. This type of telogen effluvium underlies the shedding of hair upon initiation of therapy with topical minoxidil (shedding phase).
In *delayed telogen release*, hair follicles remain in prolonged telogen rather than being shed and recycling into anagen. When finally teloptosis sets in, again the clinical sign of increased shedding of club hairs is observed. This process underlies moulting in mammals and probably also seasonal shedding of hairs in humans or mild telogen effluvia following travel from low-daylight to high-daylight conditions.
Finally, a *short anagen phase* (without synchronization) results in a slight but persistent telogen effluvium in association with decreased hair length: this may occur in hereditary hypotrichosis, ectodermal dysplasia (trichodental syndrome), and as an isolated disorder in otherwise healthy children, as originally described by Barraud-Klenovsek and Trüeb. Far more frequent is acquired progressive shortening of anagen due to androgenetic alopecia.

Headington JT (1993) Telogen effluvium. New concepts and review. Arch Dermatol 129:356–363

3.3.2 Seasonal Hair Shedding

In 2009, Kunz et al. published a study of 823 otherwise healthy women with telogen effluvium observed over a period of 6 years and demonstrated the existence of overall annual periodicity in the growth and shedding of hair, manifested by a maximal proportion of telogen hairs in July. A second peak seemed to exist, although less pronounced, in April (Fig. 3.14a). The telogen rate was lowest toward the beginning of February. These results confirmed the findings of authors who had formerly demonstrated seasonal changes in human hair growth: Orentreich originally reported three women in New York who experienced maximum hair loss in November. Studying a group of 14 men during 18 months, Randall and Ebling showed that the proportion of telogen hair and of hair shedding were maximal in September. Finally, Courtois et al. observed ten men, with or without alopecia, for a period of between 8 and 14 years and also demonstrated a maximal proportion of telogen hairs at the end of summer. Some subjects also exhibited a periodicity approximately corresponding to two annual peaks.

In 2012, a 39-year-old long-haired male presented at the Center for Dermatology and Hair

Diseases Professor Trüeb with early androgenetic alopecia. He had counted his hairs shed in the course of hair washing every 3 days from the years 1996–2011 and plotted their mean value against the month of the year (Fig. 3.14b). There was a striking congruence with the graphic formerly demonstrated for women by Kunz et al., which proves that men are subject to the same seasonal changes of hair growth and shedding as women. The difference is that the hair shedding is less noticeable in men, who commonly wear their hair shorter. Moreover, men usually have a lesser sensitivity than women for the condition of their hair. Nevertheless, this fluctuation may also reflect in subsequent clinical images taken of patients (Fig. 3.14c, d).

The cyclical activities of the hair follicle are the mechanism by which mammals change their coat of hair to meet the exigencies of growth, seasonal changes in the ambient environment, and, perhaps, normal wear and tear. It seems likely that environmental factors, such as the photoperiod, mediate through the optic pathway and the neuroendocrine system coat phenotype and function to match environmental changes. The fact that human hair follicles, just as those of other mammals, undergo cyclical activity and are influenced by hormones implies that human hair is not unaffected by these phenomena.

> From an evolutionary point of view, the maintenance of the low winter level of hair shedding and the postponement of hair fall until the end of summer might, perhaps, be postulated as having a selective advantage with respect to isolation of the head against the cold in winter and protection of the scalp against the midday sun in summer, respectively.

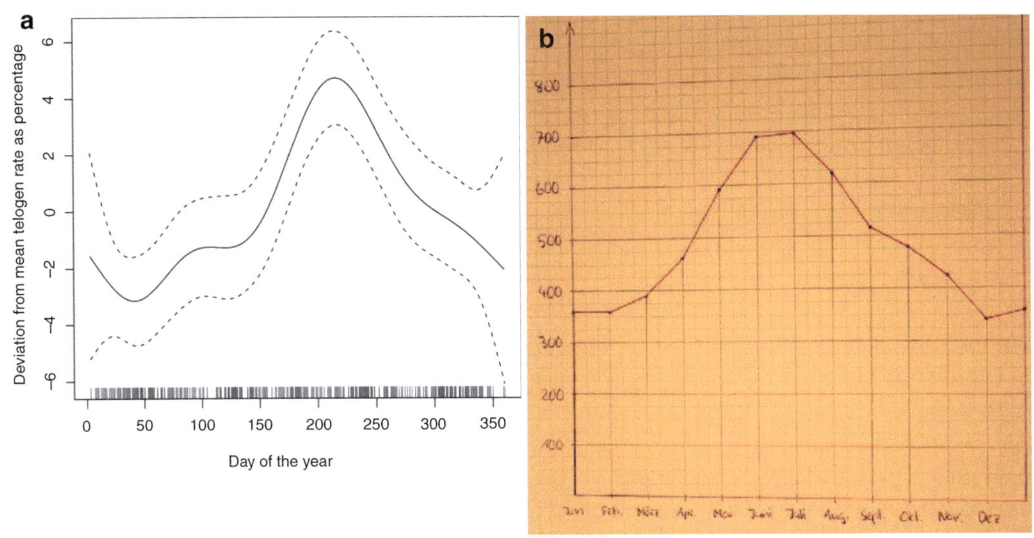

Fig. 3.14 (**a**–**d**) Seasonality of hair growth and shedding: (**a**) fluctuations in frontal telogen rates ($n = 823$) in relation to the day of the year in women complaining of hair loss (From: Kunz M, Seifert B, Trüeb RM (2009) Seasonality of hair shedding in healthy women complaining of hair loss. Dermatology 219:105–110), and (**b**) fluctuations of shed hair in a 39-year-old healthy male, counted between 1996 and 2011. The mean counted values were plotted in relation to the month of the year, (**c**) subsequent images taken in February 2013 and (**d**) August 2013 in a 40-year-old male. Note: larger hair part width in late summer

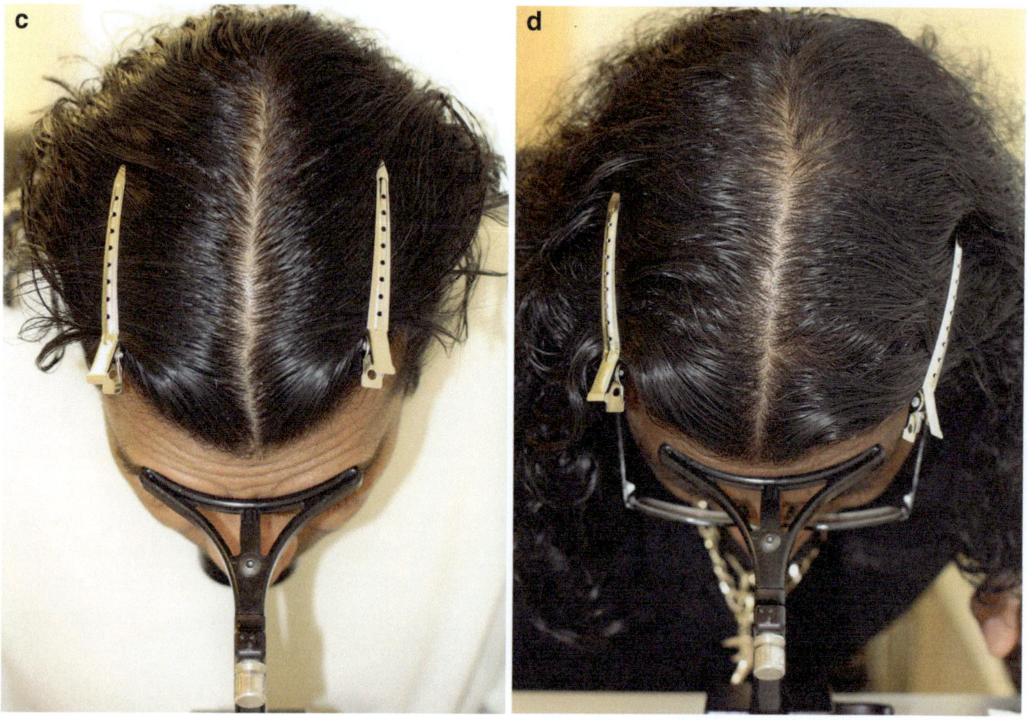

Fig. 3.14 (continued)

The existence of seasonal fluctuations in hair growth and shedding may complicate the assessment of pharmacologic effects when treating hair loss:

Awareness of these fluctuations is prerequisite to providing the correct cause and prognosis to the patient, ensuring patient compliance with therapy.

Ultimately, seasonal fluctuations of hair growth and shedding may have potentially serious implications for investigations with new hair growth-promoting agents: Depending on the stage of periodicity in growth and shedding of hair for a particular subject, the heterogenicity of included subjects may be enough to distort the clinical efficacy results and the perceived benefit of an investigational agent. In the active stage of seasonal telogen effluvium, the involved hair follicles would probably fail to respond to the therapeutic agent, which may cause a false-negative result. In the recovery stage, the increased amounts of spontaneously regrowing hair might be interpreted falsely as a positive result.

3.3.3 General Medical Problems Affecting the Condition of Hair

Most patients with general medical problems affecting the condition of hair seen in clinical practice present with diffuse telogen effluvium.

> Acute telogen effluvium presents as a diffuse, non-patterned hair loss from the scalp that occurs around 3 months after a triggering event and is usually self-limiting within 6 months by definition. Therefore, a careful patient history with respect to the chronology of events usually reveals the diagnosis and the cause.

A host of different triggers has been implicated and identifies the clinical species of the genus, e.g., postfebrile, posttraumatic, postinterventional, and psychogenic effluvium. Severe febrile illness, accidental trauma or surgical operations with a large hemorrhage, a crash diet, and severe emotional distress are among the most common causes. Most are self-limiting and will undergo normal reversal.

Chronic telogen effluvium is a diffuse shedding of telogen hairs that persists >6 months secondary to a variety of systemic disorders:

> Iron deficiency, thyroid disease, systemic lupus erythematosus, syphilis, HIV infection, and drugs are frequent culprits in diffuse telogen effluvium and therefore must be systematically investigated.

In comparison, other dietary deficiencies, metabolic diseases, connective tissue disorders, and malignant or chronic infectious diseases are infrequent causes of hair loss in office-based clinical practice.

Thyroid hormones have influence on the growth and differentiation of many tissues and total energy expenditure of the organism and on the turnover of many substrates, vitamins, and other hormones. Thyroid activity affects oxygen consumption, protein synthesis, and mitosis and is therefore essential for the formation and growth of hair. Expression of the thyroid hormone receptor beta1 was demonstrated in the human hair follicle, and it was shown that triiodo-l-thyronine significantly enhances human hair survival in vitro. The impact of thyroid hormone activity on the hair is most notable during deficient or excess states. Schell et al. demonstrated for the first time by means of DNA flow cytometry the influence of thyroid hormones on in vivo cell cycle kinetics of human scalp hair bulbs.

> Clinically, the effect of thyroid disorders on hair is nonspecific; nevertheless, the associated symptoms and signs of thyroid hormone deficiency or excess may provide an important clue to the diagnosis in instances of unsuspected thyroid disease.

Hypothyroidism results from a deficiency of thyroid hormones. It is caused most commonly by chronic autoimmune thyroiditis (Hashimoto's disease) or by iatrogenic thyroid ablation (I131 therapy or surgical thyroidectomy). Iodine deficiency is rare in developed countries, but is common in some regions of the world. Hypothyroidism is about ten times less frequent in men than in women and is therefore less thought of in men complaining of hair loss. Early hypothyroidism is often asymptomatic and can have very mild symptoms (Table 3.4). Dull, coarse, brittle hair or diffuse alopecia may be present with particular thinning of the lateral eyebrows. The hair growth rate is slowed, with an increase in the proportion in telogen. The alopecia is of very gradual onset. Long-standing hypothyroidism may be associated, in the genetically predisposed, with androgenetic alopecia. The mechanism is presumed to be due to an increase in plasma free androgens. Such symptoms may easily be overlooked or ascribed merely to aging.

Hyperthyroidism is due to excessive quantities of circulating thyroid hormones. Graves' disease is by far the most common cause with an estimated prevalence of 5.9 % in a population of patients 60 years and older. Again, it is a disease of autoimmune origin affecting women much more frequently than men. The most common symptoms of hyperthyroidism are systemic rather than cutaneous and due to a hypermetabolic state known as thyrotoxicosis. Hyperthyroidism usually begins slowly. At first, the symptoms may be mistaken for simple nervousness due to stress. If one has been trying to lose weight by dieting, one may be pleased with weight loss success until the hyperthyroidism, which has quickened the weight loss, causes other problems. Diffuse hair loss is present in 20–40 % and axillary hair loss in 60 %. The hair itself is fine, soft, straight, and allegedly unable to retain a permanent wave.

> In hyperthyroidism, the severity of alopecia does not correlate with the severity of thyrotoxicosis; moreover, hair loss may alternatively be related to the treatment of hyperthyroidism with thyreostatics.

Table 3.4 List of clinical symptoms of hypothyroidism

Early
Cold intolerance, increased sensitivity to cold
Constipation
Weight gain and water retention
Bradycardia (low heart rate – fewer than sixty beats per minute)
Fatigue
Decreased sweating
Muscle cramps and joint pain
Dry, itchy skin
Thin, brittle fingernails
Depression
Poor muscle tone (muscle hypotonia)
Late
Goiter
Slow speech and a hoarse, breaking voice – deepening of the voice can also be noticed
Dry puffy skin, especially on the face
Thinning of the outer third of the eyebrows (sign of Hertoghe)
Low basal body temperature
Uncommon
Impaired memory
Impaired cognitive function (brain fog) and inattentiveness
A slow heart rate with ECG changes including low-voltage signals. Diminished cardiac output and decreased contractility
Sluggish reflexes
Hair loss
Difficulty swallowing
Shortness of breath with a shallow and slow respiratory pattern
Increased need for sleep
Irritability and mood instability
Yellowing of the skin (carotoderma)
Acute psychosis (myxedema madness) (a rare presentation of hypothyroidism)
Decreased sense of taste and smell (anosmia)
Puffy face, hands, and feet (late, less common symptoms)
Deafness
Enlarged tongue

Lupus erythematosus is a systemic autoimmune disorder associated with polyclonal B-cell activation, resulting in diverse patterns of autoantibody production and a heterogeneous clinical expression constituting a spectrum extending from cutaneous disease (cutaneous lupus erythematosus) to a life-threatening systemic disease process (systemic lupus erythematosus). The clinical characteristics of cutaneous lupus erythematosus are well defined in terms of morphology, and for the classification of systemic lupus erythematosus, clinical and laboratory criteria are available. The American College of Rheumatology (ACR) established eleven criteria as a classificatory instrument to operationalize the definition of systemic lupus erythematosus in clinical trials (Table 3.5). For the purpose of identifying patients for clinical studies, a person has systemic lupus erythematosus if any 4 out of 11 symptoms are present simultaneously or serially on two separate occasions.

The many different types of skin lesions encountered in patients with lupus erythematosus have been classified into those that are histologically specific for lupus erythematosus and those that are not; this also applies to the involvement of the scalp and hair. The typical skin lesion of lupus erythematosus-specific disease on the scalp is discoid lupus erythematosus. Scalp involvement occurs in 60 % of discoid lupus erythematosus patients and is the only area involved in approximately 10 %. Patients with systemic disease may also have discoid lesions, including the scalp, though less frequently. Nevertheless, because of the high specificity of the discoid lesion, it has been included in the criteria for the classification of systemic lupus erythematosus.

Of patients presenting with discoid lesions of lupus erythematosus, 5–10 % develop clear-cut evidence of systemic disease, with the extent and distribution of the discoid lesions determining the risk: patients with lesions both above and below the neck (generalized discoid lupus erythematosus) have a higher rate of immunological abnormalities and risk for progression to systemic disease compared to patients with discoid lesions restricted to the head and neck area (localized discoid lupus erythematosus).

Patients with only discoid lesions of lupus erythematosus of the scalp very uncommonly progress to systemic disease.

Table 3.5 Systemic lupus erythematosus ACR criteria

Criteria	Sensitivity (%)	Specificity (%)
1. *Malar rash* (rash on cheeks)	57	96
2. *Discoid rash* (red, scaly patches on skin that cause scarring)	18	99
3. *Serositis*: pleurisy or pericarditis (pleural is more sensitive; cardiac is more specific)	56	86
4. *Oral ulcers* (includes oral or nasopharyngeal ulcers)	27	96
5. *Arthritis*: nonerosive arthritis of two or more peripheral joints, with tenderness, swelling, or effusion	86	37
6. *Photosensitivity* (exposure to ultraviolet light causes rash or other symptoms of disease flare-ups)	43	96
7. *Hematologic disorder*: hemolytic anemia (low red blood cell count) or leukopenia (white blood cell count <4,000/μl), lymphopenia (<1,500/μl), or thrombocytopenia (<100,000/μl) in the absence of offending drug	59	89
8. *Renal disorder*: more than 0.5 g per day protein in urine or cellular casts seen in urine under a microscope	51	94
9. *Antinuclear antibody test positive*	99	49
10. *Immunological disorder*: positive anti-Smith, anti-ds DNA, antiphospholipid antibody, and/or false positive serological test for syphilis. Presence of anti-ss DNA in 70 % of cases (hypocomplementemia is also seen, due to consumption of C3 and C4 by immune complex-induced inflammation or to congenitally complement deficiency, which may predispose to systemic lupus erythematosus)	85	93
11. *Neurologic disorder*: seizures or psychosis	20	98

In addition to the focal and scarring form of alopecia associated with the discoid lupus erythematosus lesion, systemic lupus erythematosus patients may experience a diffuse, non-scarring, and transient hair loss associated with exacerbations of their lupus disease process. This diffuse hair loss seen in systemic disease is usually the result of a telogen effluvium. The telogen effluvium is in all probability the result of both severe catabolic effects and elevated levels of circulating pro-inflammatory cytokines of the lupus disease flare on hair growth cycling.

3.3.4 Drug-Induced Hair Loss

Adverse drug reactions on the hair are common. Drugs are capable of producing a wide spectrum of hair loss, ranging from barely detectable shedding to frank and irreversible baldness. Other side effects observed are the stimulation of hair growth with hypertrichosis or induction or worsening of hirsutism, as well as changes in hair structure or color.

Drug-induced hair loss is usually a diffuse non-scarring alopecia which is reversible upon withdrawal of the drug. Only a few drugs, mainly antimitotic agents, regularly cause hair loss, whereas many drugs may be the cause of isolated cases of alopecia. There is a long list of drugs that on occasion has been cited as causing hair loss (Table 3.6), and diagnosis of drug-induced alopecia remains a challenge. The only way to confirm it is to see if an improvement occurs after cessation of the suspected drug. This side effect must be recognized because it may be a source of poor compliance in some patients.

In general, the incidence of drug-related adverse events increases with age, due to a higher susceptibility to drug-related side effects, a higher frequency of medications, co-medications, and comorbidities in older patients.

Table 3.6 Drugs responsible for telogen effluvium (selection)

Telogen effluvium with known or assumed mechanism	
Interference with keratinization process in the hair follicle: retinoids	
Vitamin A (>50,000 I.E. daily)	
Acitretin	
Isotretinoin	
Interference with blood flow in follicular papilla: anticoagulants	
Heparin	
Warfarin	
Interference with cholesterol synthesis: lipid-lowering agents	
Fibrates (Clofibrate, Bezafibrate, Fenofibrate)	
Lovastatin	
Complexation of zinc (thiol moiety): ACE inhibitors	
Captopril	
Enalapril	
Interference with thyroid metabolism: thyreostatics and others	
Propylthiouracil	
Levothyroxine	
Amiodarone (antiarrhythmic)	
Lithium (antipsychotic)	
Androgen effect: androgens, anabolics	
Mesterolone	
Testosterone	
Danazol	
Cytokine effect: interferons	
Alpha interferon	
Gamma interferon	
Telogen effluvium with unknown mechanism (in order of indications)	
Blood pressure-lowering agents (beta-blocking agents)	
Acebutolol	Nadolol
Atenolol	Pindolol
Labetalol	Propanolol
Metoprolol	
Topical beta-blocking agents for therapy of glaucoma	
Betaxolol	Timolol
Levobunolol	
Analgesics/nonsteroidal anti-inflammatory agents	
Acetaminophen	Piroxicam
Ibuprofen	Indomethacin
Ketoprofen	Penicillamine
Naproxen	Gold and gold compounds
Psychotropic agents/antidepressives	
Amitriptyline	Haloperidol
Desipramine	Imipramine
Doxepin	Nortriptyline
Fluoxetine	Trimipramine
Antiepileptics	
Carbamazepine	Paramethadione
Clonazepam	Phenytoin
Ethotoin	Trimethadione
Mephenytoin	Valproic acid
Antibiotics/tuberculostatics	
Thiamphenicol	Isoniazid
Gentamicin	Ethambutol
Nitrofurantoin	
Varia	
Chloroquine, hydroxychloroquine (antimalarials)	
Albendazole, mebendazole (anthelmintic agents)	
Cimetidine, famotidine, ranitidine (antacids)	
Allopurinol (uricostatic agent)	
Sulfasalazine (antiphlogistic/sulfonamide)	
Bromocriptine (prolactin inhibitor/antiparkinson agent)	
Levodopa (antiparkinson agent)	
Halothane (inhalation anesthetic)	

3.3.5 Antitumor Necrosis Alpha Therapy-Induced Alopecia

Tumor necrosis factor (TNF) alpha inhibitors (infliximab, etanercept, adalimumab) are increasingly being used for the treatment of a variety of autoimmune diseases, such as rheumatoid arthritis, ankylosing spondylitis, Crohn's disease, and plaque psoriasis. During these treatments adverse effects involving the hair and scalp have been reported.

The most consistent among the anti-TNF alpha therapy-induced adverse effects affecting the condition of the scalp has been a psoriasis-like dermatitis with diffuse alopecia and the potential of irreversible, scarring hair loss. Joyaux et al. have pointed out that psoriasis occurring during anti-TNF alpha therapy is de novo psoriasis and not an aggravation of a preexisting psoriasis. To this day, several hypotheses have been proposed to explain the underlying immunological mechanisms. It appears to be a class effect.

In contrast, the reported associations with alopecia areata may be fortuitous, since alopecia areata represents a common condition. Not until the incidence of alopecia areata in patients treated with anti-TNF alpha agents has been shown to be higher than in the general population can alopecia areata be definitely regarded as a potential side effect. On the other hand, the observation of alopecia areata during anti-TNF alpha therapy proves the inefficacy of anti-TNF alpha therapy for alopecia areata. Finally, Doyle et al. have demonstrated that anti-TNF alpha therapy-related alopecia may closely mimic alopecia areata, but is histologically distinguished by epidermal psoriasiform changes.

3.4 Hair Aging

Hair length, color, and cosmetic properties play an important role in people's physical appearance and self-perception. Civilized mankind's ancient preoccupation with hair is heightened as today's increasing life expectancy fuels the desire to preserve youthfulness. This attention reflects a hair care market that is a multibillion dollar enterprise. The development of safe and effective means for the treatment of age-related hair changes indicates strategies for maintenance of healthy and beautiful hair in the young as well as the old.

The study of hair aging focuses on two main streams of interest: On one hand, the *aesthetic* problem of aging hair and its management, in other words everything that happens outside the skin; on the other hand, the *biological problem* of aging hair, in terms of microscopic, biochemical (hormonal, enzymatic), and molecular changes, in other words the "secret life" of the hair follicle in the depth of the skin.

> Aging of hair affects hair color, hair production, and structural properties of the hair fiber with its consequence for manageability and overall appearance of hair.

Most literature on age-related hair changes focuses on alopecia, but it is equally important that the hair fibers that emerge from the scalp exhibit significant age-related changes that have an equal impact on the overall cosmetic properties of the hair. It is these changes that are ultimately experienced by subjects that have retained their hair as they age.

> Age-related deterioration of cosmetic properties of the hair is related to changes in hair pigmentation (graying), diameter, curvature, structural properties (stretching, bending, torsional rigidity), lipid composition, and the interdependence of these changes.

Depending on the individual's original hair color, quantity, quality, and hair care habits, there is a great variability in the age of onset of the first signs of hair aging. Hair graying is closely related to chronologic age, and the age of its onset is largely controlled by genetics. The perception of graying is dependent on the original hair color, with the perception of "any gray" occurring earlier in dark hair and later in light hair. Vice versa, the perception of "completely gray" is perceived to occur earlier in light hair and later in dark hair. Diameter changes with age are likely to impart the largest impact on overall perception of hair aging. In Japanese men, Otsuko and Nemoto found scalp hair fiber diameter to increase to a maximum in the late teenage years and then to decrease relatively rapidly with increasing age. Trotter and Dawson found similar effects in a study on 82 male French Canadians. Courtois et al. studied 10 French male subjects aged 25–49 over a period of 14 years and demonstrated that the diameter of hair shafts decreased with increasing age beginning at age 25. In contrast, female hair diameter does not have a linear relationship with age, but rather displays a curve increasing to a maximum near the age of 40 and decreasing thereafter.

> Age has a larger effect on hair fiber diameter in men than in women.

Changes in hair fiber diameter with age also affect structural properties of hairs increasing combing forces and therefore breakage. The same applies to age-related increase of hair fiber curvature. Increase of hair fiber curvature also results in loss of hair luster and frizziness, whereby frizziness has been explained as a lack of synchronization in the curvature of neighboring hair fibers in an assembly of hair. Finally, hair lipid levels and hair lipid composition change with age: the two major sources for hair lipids are the hair matrix cells (cholesterol, cholesterol sulfate, ceramides, covalent fatty acids, 18-methyl eicosanoic acid) and the hair follicle-associated sebaceous glands (squalene, wax esters, triglycerides, total fatty acids). The amount of sebum produced varies with the size of sebaceous glands, being low before puberty, rapidly increasing at puberty, and remaining at a high level until 45–50 where it declines. The decline is greater in females than in males. Age-related lipid changes affect hair greasiness, shine, softness, and smoothness.

> Finally, basic scientists interested in the biology of hair growth and pigmentation have exposed the hair follicle as a highly accessible and unique model that offers important opportunities also to the gerontologist for the study of aging.

Its complex multicell-type interaction system involving epithelium, mesenchyme, neuroectoderm, and its unique cyclical activity of growth, regression, rest, and regrowth provides the investigator with a range of stem, differentiating, mitotic and postmitotic terminally differentiated cells, including cells with variable susceptibility to apoptosis, for study. A number of intrinsic and extrinsic modulating factors for hair growth and pigmentation have been identified and are being further tested in vitro.

Aging is a complex process involving various genetic, hormonal, and environmental mechanisms. Much like the skin, the hair is subject to intrinsic or chronologic aging and extrinsic aging due to environmental factors. Both occur in conjunction with the other and are superimposed on each other. Intrinsic factors are related to individual genetic and epigenetic mechanisms with interindividual variation. Examples are familial premature graying and androgenetic alopecia. Extrinsic factors include ultraviolet radiation (UVR), smoking, and nutrition. Extrinsic aging of the hair fiber has also been designated as hair weathering and is related to physical and chemical stressors, as well as photoaging.

Experimental evidence supports the hypothesis that oxidative stress plays a major role in the aging process. As early as 1956, Harman et al. first proposed the "free radical theory of aging." Today it is one of the most widely accepted theories used to explain mechanisms underlying the aging process. Free radicals are highly reactive molecules with unpaired electrons that can directly damage various cellular structural membranes, lipids, proteins, and DNA. The damaging effects of these reactive oxygen species are induced internally during normal metabolism and externally through exposure to various oxidative stresses from the environment. The body possesses endogenous defense mechanisms, such as anti-oxidative enzymes (superoxide dismutase, catalase, glutathione peroxidase) and nonenzymatic anti-oxidative molecules (vitamin E, vitamin C, glutathione, ubiquinone), protecting it from free radicals by reducing and neutralizing them. With age, the production of free radicals increases, while the endogenous defense mechanisms decrease. This imbalance leads to the progressive damage of cellular structures, presumably resulting in the aging phenotype.

3.4.1 Rare Premature Aging Syndromes

From a clinician's perspective, age-dependent progressive hair loss occurs in the following fundamentally different settings: as a symptom of one of the rare premature aging syndromes (progerias), as a consequence of androgenetic alopecia, or with onset of senescence.

> Scientists are particularly interested in the premature aging syndromes because these might reveal clues about the normal process of aging.

Hutchinson–Gilford progeria and *Werner's syndrome* (Fig. 3.15) are repeatedly given as examples of premature aging and as evidence for the genetic basis of aging. However, the analogy of these syndromes with physiological aging has been challenged. These pathologic conditions should rather be viewed as deviations from normal development. Since the mesenchymal tissue is severely affected in both diseases, and the inductive phenomena necessary for the differentiation and development of the different organs take place through the interaction of connective tissue with other tissues, it is conceivable that defects in the connective tissue lead to a variety of deviations in the whole organism. Symptoms of accelerated aging of the hair include premature loss and graying of hair.

Nevertheless, these rare syndromes and others with premature hair loss, such as myotonic dystrophy Curschmann–Steinert and the Laron syndrome, give insights into the roles of telomeres, mitochondrial function, human growth hormone (hGH), and insulin-like growth factor 1 (IGF-1) for the growth and aging of hair.

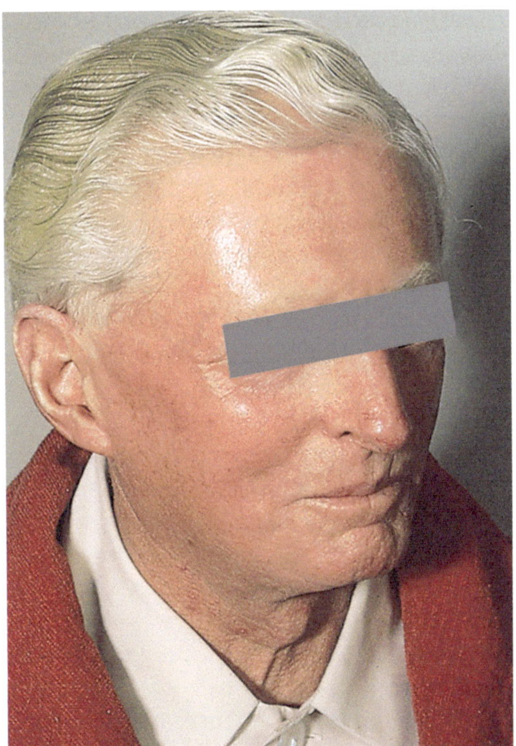

Fig. 3.15 Werner's syndrome: typical facies (prematurely aged face with a beaked nose) and canities (*gray hair*)

3.4.2 Graying

Hair graying (canities) is a natural age-associated feature. The hair graying trait correlates closely with chronologic aging and occurs to varying degrees in all individuals.

> The normal incidence of hair graying is 34 ± 9.6 years in Caucasians and 43.9 ± 10.3 years in Africans, and, by 50 years of age, 50 % of people have 50 % gray hair.

This graying incidence appears irrespective of sex and hair color. In men graying usually begins at the temples and in the sideburns. Women will usually start around the perimeter of the hairline. Gradually, the gray works its way back through the top, sides, and back of the hair.

Although graying is understood as a loss of pigment in the shaft, its cellular and molecular origins are incompletely understood. Theories for the gradual loss of pigmentation include exhaustion of enzymes involved in melanogenesis, impaired DNA repair, loss of telomerase, antioxidant mechanisms, and antiapoptotic signals.

The color of hair mainly relies on the presence or absence of melanin pigment. Skin and hair melanins are formed in cytoplasmic organelles called melanosomes, produced by the melanocytes, and are the product of a complex biochemical pathway (melanogenesis) with tyrosinase being the rate-limiting enzyme. So far, the process of hair graying has been attributed to the loss of the pigment-forming melanocytes from the aging hair follicle. The net effect of this reduction is that fewer melanosomes are incorporated into cortical keratinocytes of the hair shaft. In addition, there appears also to be a defect of melanosome transfer, as keratinocytes may not contain melanin despite their proximity to melanocytes with remaining melanosomes. This defect is further corroborated by the observation of melanin debris in and sometimes around the graying hair bulb. This anomaly is due to either defective melanosomal transfer to the cortical keratinocytes or melanin incontinence due to melanocyte degeneration. Eventually, no melanogenic melanocytes remain in the hair bulb. This decrease of melanin synthesis is associated with a decrease in tyrosinase activity. Ultrastructural studies have shown that remaining melanocytes not only contain fewer melanosomes, but the residual melanosomes may be packaged within autophagolysosomes. This removal of melanosomes into autophagolysosomes suggests that they are defective, possibly with reactive melanin metabolites. This interpretation is supported by the observation that melanocytes in graying hair bulbs are frequently highly vacuolated, a common cellular response to increased oxidative stress.

By analogy with the free radical theory of aging, a "free radical theory of graying" has been proposed.

The extraordinary melanogenic activity of pigmented bulbar melanocytes, continuing for up to 10 years in some hair follicles, is likely to generate large amounts of reactive oxygen species via the hydroxylation of tyrosine and the oxidation of DOPA to melanin. If not adequately removed by an efficient antioxidant system, an accumulation of these reactive oxidative species will generate significant oxidative stress. It is possible that the antioxidant system becomes impaired with age leading to damage to the melanocyte itself from its own melanogenesis-related oxidative stress. Since mutations occur at a higher rate in tissue exposed to high levels of oxidative stress, and these accumulate with age, the induction of replicative senescence with apoptosis is likely to be an important protective mechanism against cell transformation.

Wood et al. have recently demonstrated for the first time that human white scalp hair shafts accumulate hydrogen peroxide (H_2O_2) in millimolar concentrations and almost absent catalase and methionine sulfoxide reductase (MSR) protein expression in association with functional loss of methionine sulfoxide repair in the entire gray hair follicle. Accordingly, methionine sulfoxide formation of methionine residues (Met), including Met 374 in the active site of tyrosinase, the key enzyme in melanogenesis, limits enzyme functionality, which eventually leads to loss of hair color. While the entire hair follicle is subject to H_2O_2-mediated stress, it is tempting to assume that, besides tyrosinase and MSR, other proteins and peptides, including antiapoptotic Bcl-2 protein, are targets for oxidation, which in turn could explain melanocyte apoptosis in the gray hair follicle. Moreover, H_2O_2-mediated oxidation has been documented for many other important regulators of pigmentation, including the proopiomelanocortins α-melanocyte-stimulating hormone (MSH) and β-endorphin, the prohormone convertases, and the synthesis and recycling of the ubiquitous cofactor 6-tetrahydrobiopterin.

Although as yet little published data is available on the hair follicle melanocyte stem cell population, it is tempting to speculate that these cells may well also be target to oxidation. Since the discovery of unpigmented melanocyte stem cells located within the hair follicle, the question has arisen whether the process underlying hair graying arises specifically from changes in differentiated, pigmented melanocytes or the unpigmented progenitors which provide them. Utilizing melanocyte-tagged transgenic mice and aging human hair follicles, Nishimura et al. recently demonstrated that hair graying may be caused by defective self-maintenance of melanocyte stem-cells, and not of differentiated melanocytes. This process was dramatically accelerated with Bcl-2 deficiency, which causes selective apoptosis of melanocyte stem cells.

The rate at which an individual turns gray depends on genetics. It is not uncommon to observe kinships with marked early graying throughout.

Hair is said to gray prematurely if it occurs before the age of 20 in Caucasians and before 30 in Africans.

While premature canities more commonly appear without underlying pathology, presumably inherited in an autosomal dominant manner (familial premature graying), it has been linked to a similar cluster of autoimmune disorders observed in association with vitiligo, i.e., pernicious anemia and autoimmune thyroid disease and several rare premature aging syndromes, such as Hutchinson–Gilford and Werner's syndrome. In Curschmann–Steinert's myotonic dystrophy, onset of gray hair may precede myotonia and muscle wasting.

Reports linking cigarette smoking with premature gray hair have drawn on the one hand the attention to the role of oxidative stress on hair growth and pigmentation, on the other to canities as a marker for the general health status.

A possible explanation of the observation may be that smoking-related diseases increase aging in general, including pigmentation. However, more direct effects, e.g., via smoke genotoxin-induced apoptosis, may also be involved. Whether canities, premature or otherwise, is a predictor or risk marker for disease remains controversial, mainly due to poor epidemiologic study design. Moreover, if it exists at all, it is more likely to reflect associated genetic effects rather than direct linkage.

Anecdotal evidence indicates that gray hair becomes coarser and less manageable than pigmented hair.

Gray hair is said to often fail to hold a temporary or permanent set, and to be more resistant to incorporating artificial color, both of which suggest changes to the underlying substructure of the hair fiber. Gray hair has been found to have increased sensitivity to weathering, increased cysteic acid residues and decreased cystine, and increased fiber reactivity to reducing and oxidizing agents. Moreover, gray hair is more sensitive to UVR. Photochemical impairment of the hair includes degradation and loss of hair proteins as well as degradation of hair pigment. UVB radiation is responsible for hair protein loss, and UVA radiation is responsible for hair color changes. Absorption of radiation in photosensitive amino acids of the hair and their photochemical degradation is producing free radicals. They have adverse impact on hair proteins, especially keratin, while melanin can partially immobilize free radicals and block their entrance in keratin matrix.

Given the close interaction of melanin transferring-melanocytes with hair shaft-forming pre-cortical keratinocytes, it is conceivable that other functions of these cell types are affected by this activity. One possibility is that melanin transfer decreases keratinocyte turnover and increases keratinocyte terminal differentiation. Indeed, white beard hair has been shown to grow up to four times the rate of adjacent pigmented hair. In this way, aging hair follicles may reprogram their matrix keratinocytes to increase production of medullary, rather than cortical, keratinocytes. In fact the medulla is often enlarged and collapsed, forming a central cavity in gray and white hairs. An evolutionary basis for this increased medullation in senile white hair may reflect the enhanced insulation provided by these hairs which would confer an important benefit for temperature regulation. In this way, it may compensate for the loss the sunlight-absorbing and thus heat-trapping properties of melanized dark hair.

3.4.3 Senescent Alopecia

Senile involutional or senescent alopecia has been defined as non-androgen-dependent hair thinning found in those over 60 years of age. Much like androgenetic alopecia, it involves a progressive decrease in the number of anagen follicles and hair diameter. It frequently occurs together with androgenetic alopecia, further complicating its delineation from the latter.

In their study on aging and hair cycles over an exceptionally long duration of 8–14 years, Courtois et al. found a reduction in the duration of hair growth and in the diameter of hair shafts and a prolongation of the interval separating the loss of a hair in telogen and the emergence of a replacement hair in anagen (latency phase). These phenomena resemble those observed in the course of androgenetic alopecia, although their development is less marked, suggesting androgenetic alopecia to represent a premature aging phenomenon. This aging process was evidenced by a reduction in the number of hairs per unit area and deterioration in the quality of scalp hair. The reduction in density was manifested to different degrees in different individuals. It amounted to less than 10 % in 10 years in the individuals with the least alopecia and was much more pronounced in the balding subjects. The maximal length of hair diminished as the subjects aged; in parallel the hairs became finer. However, among non-balding subjects, there was a tendency for the proportion of thicker hairs to increase. Finally, aging did not appear to follow a perfectly regular course over time. Periods of stability, or even partial remission, alternated with periods of more marked evolution, reflecting perhaps the influence of individual factors such as the subject's general health, lifestyle, and risk factors for accelerated aging.

Eichmüller et al. proposed that senescent alopecia may result from cumulative physiological degeneration of selected hair follicles. In healthy murine skin they described clusters of perifollicular macrophages as perhaps indicating the existence of a physiological program of immunologically controlled hair follicle degeneration by which malfunctioning follicles are removed by programmed organ deletion. On the other hand, Price et al. did not identify any "dropout" of follicles in senescent alopecia upon staining biopsies for elastin, whereas there was less 5α-reductase enzyme activity in comparison to androgenetic alopecia.

> Recent data comparing androgenetic alopecia and senescent alopecia using microarray analysis have demonstrated significant differences in the gene expression patterns suggesting they represent different entities.

In androgenetic alopecia, genes required for anagen onset (Wnt-beta-catenin, TGF-alpha, TGF-beta, Stat-3, Stat-1), epithelial signal to dermal papilla (PPARd, IGF-1), hair shaft differentiation (Notch, Msx2, KRTs, KAPs), and anagen maintenance (Msx2, Activin, IGF-1) were downregulated, and genes for catagen (BDNF, BMP2, BMP7, VDR, IL-1, ER) and telogen induction and maintenance (VDR, RAR) were upregulated. In senescent alopecia, genes involved in epithelial signal to dermal papilla (FGF5), actin cytoskeleton (DST, ACTN2, TNNI3, PARVB), and mitochondrial function (JAK2, PRKD3, AK2, TRAP1, TRIO, ATP12A, MLL4, STK22B) were downregulated, while oxidative stress and inflammatory response genes were upregulated.

More recently, Nishimura found mouse hair follicles to age through defective renewal of hair follicle stem cells much in the manner as maintenance of melanocyte stem cells becomes incomplete with aging. Aging-related loss of hair follicle stem cell marker expression starts well before hair follicles have shortened. Using genomic instability syndromes and exposure to ionizing radiation as models, Nishimura proposed an accumulation of DNA damage to be involved in the aging process (oral communication, 7th World Congress for Hair Research, 4–6th May 2013, Edinburgh, Scotland).

3.4.4 Age-Related General Medical Problems Affecting the Condition of Hair

The quantity and quality of hair are closely related to the nutritional, general, and mental health state of the individual, while older patients increasingly suffer from a variety of conditions that affect the hair, i.e., nutritional deficiency, endocrine disorders, psychological problems, and drug-related adverse effects. Sometimes symptoms of overt pathologic conditions are misinterpreted as signs of normal aging, ignored and left untreated.

> In taking care of older patients with hair problems, it is important to be suspicious of the possibility of a more general problem underlying the patient's complaint.

3.4.4.1 Nutritional Deficiencies

Vitamin and nutritional deficiencies are common in the elderly population. As many as 50 % have a vitamin and mineral intake less than the recommended dietary allowance, and as many as 30 % of the elderly population have subnormal levels of vitamins and minerals. In general, malnutrition is due to one or more of the following factors: inadequate food intake, food choices that lead to dietary deficiencies, and illness that causes increased nutrient requirements, increased nutrient loss, poor nutrient absorption, or a combination of these factors. Nutritional inadequacy in the elderly can be the result of one or more of the following factors: A physiological decline in food intake is seen in people as they age, regardless of illness, and is often referred to as "anorexia of aging." It probably involves alterations in neurotransmitters and hormones that affect the central feeding drive and the peripheral satiation system. Moreover, sensory decline in both olfaction and taste decreases the enjoyment of food and dietary variety. Socioeconomic status and functional ability have an important influence on nutritional status. When financial concerns are present, meals are skipped, and food that is purchased may not provide a nutritionally adequate diet. Declines in both physical and cognitive functional status affect an individual's ability to shop for food and to prepare meals. Nutritional problems are further compromised by social isolation, which commonly leads to apathy about food and decreased intake. The older person has experienced change and loss through retirement, disability, and death of friends and family, as well as change in financial, social, and physical health status. These changes may lead to depression. Depression is often unrecognized in older persons. Malnutrition may be a presenting symptom of depression in the elderly. Ultimately, underlying pathology and medical treatment can cause anorexia and malnutrition. Problems with dentition and disorders of the gastrointestinal system are related to poor intake and malabsorption of nutrients. Many diseases (i.e., thyroid, cardiovascular, and pulmonary disease) lead to an increased metabolic demand and at the same time decreased appetite and caloric intake. Drugs may affect nutritional status through side effects (i.e., anorexia, nausea, and altered taste perception) and through alteration of nutrient absorption, metabolism, and excretion.

> At present, the only scientifically documented means of slowing aging through dietary changes is by caloric restriction. It must be kept in mind though that an antiaging diet is significantly different than a weight loss diet. The key efforts of an antiaging diet focus more importantly on altering body composition to keep the organism at near-peak performance during the advancing years.

The approach covers a decrease of calorie intake by approximately 30 % daily, addition of high-density nutrients, and improvement of digestion and gastrointestinal function. Moreover, there is evidence that with age, the needs for types and quantities of nutrients may change. Since an important commercial interest lies in the nutritional value of various vitamin and amino acid supplements, finally, another question that arises is whether increasing the content of an already adequate diet with specific amino acids, vitamins, and/or trace elements may further promote hair growth in the elderly.

3.4.4.2 Endocrine Disorders

Antiaging medicine is concerned with discovering and applying therapies to modify, alleviate, or slow the progressive afflictions associated with age. Besides nutrition, vitamins, and supplements, the antiaging marketplaces focus on hormone replacement therapies under the assumption that a decline of hormone production with age is closely related to the aging process. In both sexes, growth hormones, melatonin, dehydroepiandrosterone (DHEA), and its sulfate compound DHEAS reach their maximum levels in the third decade of life and then decline progressively. In addition, a constant decrease in the production of biologically active free testosterone of approximately 1 % per year is observed in men.

> Hormones relevant for the condition of the hair are androgens, estrogens, thyroid and parathyroid hormones, prolactin, corticosteroids, GH/IGF-1, and melatonin.

Deficient androgen activity may result in decrease of sexual desire and arousability, loss of muscle tone, diminished vital energy, and dry skin. With the development of androgen deficiency after puberty, sexual hair remains present but grows slowly, since maintenance of sexual hair is less dependent on androgen than is the development of sexual hair.

Hypoparathyroidism is seen most commonly in the geriatric population following inadvertent removal of the parathyroid glands during thyroid surgery or radical neck dissection for cancer. Patients suffer attacks of hypocalcemia with tetany. Thinning of the hair or complete alopecia may be seen. The nails commonly develop horizontal grooves on the nail (Beau's lines) that appear at the base of the nails approximately 3 weeks following a tetanic attack. Enamel defects of the teeth may be misinterpreted as from poor oral hygiene especially in the elderly. Chronic disease manifestations as visual blurring from cataracts, Parkinson's disease, lethargy, and personality changes may again falsely be attributed to aging by the patient and physician.

Growth hormone deficiency is the medical condition of inadequate production of growth hormone (GH). Deficiency of GH produces significantly different problems at various ages. In newborn infants the primary manifestations may be hypoglycemia or micropenis. In later infancy and childhood, growth failure may be the major effect. Though growth ends with sexual maturity, GH continues to be secreted throughout life. In adults, GH contributes to maintenance of muscle and bone mass and strength as well as quality and productivity in life. GH deficiency in adults is rare; its causes include damage to the pituitary from intracranial disease (e.g., hydrocephalus), intracranial tumors in or near the sella turcica, especially craniopharyngioma, damage to the pituitary from radiation therapy to the head for leukemia or brain tumors, surgery in the area of the pituitary, autoimmune inflammation (hypophysitis), severe head trauma, ischemic or hemorrhagic infarction from low blood pressure (Sheehan syndrome), or hemorrhage pituitary apoplexy. GH secretion declines progressively with aging, and many age-related changes resemble those of the adult GH deficiency syndrome, including decrease in lean body mass, increase in body fat, especially in the visceral/abdominal compartment, adverse changes in lipoproteins, and a reduction in aerobic capacity. GH replacement is effective in reversing many of these changes in adult GH deficiency, and GH is FDA approved for treatment of adults with documented GH deficiency or hypopituitarism. This experience with GH deficiency has led to speculation that replacing GH may also be beneficial in normal aging and to widespread off-label use of GH in this context. However, its safety, efficacy, and role in healthy elderly individuals have remained highly controversial.

Melatonin, the chief secretory product of the pineal gland, is known to modulate hair growth and pigmentation, presumably as a key neuroendocrine regulator that couples coat phenotype and function to photoperiod-dependent environmental and reproductive changes. Important extrapineal melatonin synthesis has recently been demonstrated in human scalp hair follicles in anagen, where melatonin may functionally play a role in hair cycle control, as it downregulates apoptosis. Because of melatonin's additional property as a free radical scavenger and DNA repair inducer, the metabolically and proliferatively highly active anagen hair bulb may also exploit melatonin synthesis in loco as a self-cytoprotective strategy.

3.4.4.3 Drug-Related Problems

In general, the incidence of drug-related adverse events increases with age, due to a higher susceptibility to drug-related side effects, a higher frequency of medications, co-medications, and comorbidities in older patients.

3.4.4.4 Dementia

Dementia (from: "de-" = apart, away + "mens" (genitive: "mentis") = mind) is the progressive decline in cognitive function due to damage or disease in the body beyond what might be expected from normal aging. It represents a nonspecific set of symptoms in which affected areas of cognition may be memory, attention, language, and problem solving. Higher mental functions are affected first in the process; in the later stages of the condition, affected persons may be disoriented in time, in place, and in person.

Some cases of dementia are due to different specific disease processes that may be reversed with treatment. Out of this reason, routine blood tests are recommended to rule out treatable causes. These include vitamin B12, folic acid, thyroid-stimulating hormone (TSH), C-reactive protein (CRP), full blood count, electrolytes, calcium, renal function, liver enzymes, and syphilis serology.

Abnormalities may suggest vitamin deficiency, infection, or other problems that commonly cause confusion or disorientation in the elderly. The problem is complicated by the fact that these cause confusion more often in persons who have early dementia, so that "reversal" of such problems may ultimately only be temporary.

Also mental illnesses, including depression and psychosis, may produce symptoms which must be differentiated from dementia (pseudodementia). Chronic abuse of substances, such as alcohol, can also predispose to cognitive changes suggestive of dementia.

Manifestations of dementia on the scalp is neglect of hair and hair care.

3.4.4.5 Multimorbidity

With technologic advances and improvements in medical care, an increasing number of patients survive medical conditions that used to be fatal. This fact combined with the aging of the population means that a growing proportion of patients have multiple concurrent medical conditions. The term "multimorbidity" means several concurrent medical conditions within one person. According to a survey done in Canada in 1998, 30 % of the population reported suffering from more than one chronic health problem, and the percentage increased with age. In the USA, the prevalence of multimorbidity among those 65 and older has been estimated at 65 %. Numerous pharmacologic treatments, practice guidelines, and educational programs have been developed for managing chronic diseases. With few exceptions, the interventions address isolated chronic diseases and take little account of the multimorbidity experienced by patients.

The increasing number of chronic conditions per patient and the increasing amount of multimorbidity in the elderly population lead to a more complex approach to successful treatment of hair problems in the elderly.

3.4.5 Possibilities and Limitations for Reversal of Age-Related Pigment Loss

Reports of spontaneous repigmentation of white hair are very scant in the medical literature, though this phenomenon may not be as rare as assumed (Fig. 3.16a, b). In fact, it is not too uncommon to see spontaneous repigmentation along the same individual hair shaft in early canities. Moreover, melanocytes taken from gray and white hair follicles can be induced to pigment in vitro.

The most dramatic cases of return of normal hair color from gray are probably examples of pigmented hair regrowth following alopecia areata.

The reported repigmentation of gray hair in association with Addison's disease has also been connected to a mechanism similar to that in alopecia areata or vitiligo, in view of the known association between these diseases. Alternatively, it may be explained through the effect of elevated levels of MSH, which also applies to darkening of skin and hair in Nelson's syndrome and ectopic ACTH syndrome. Since the stimulation of

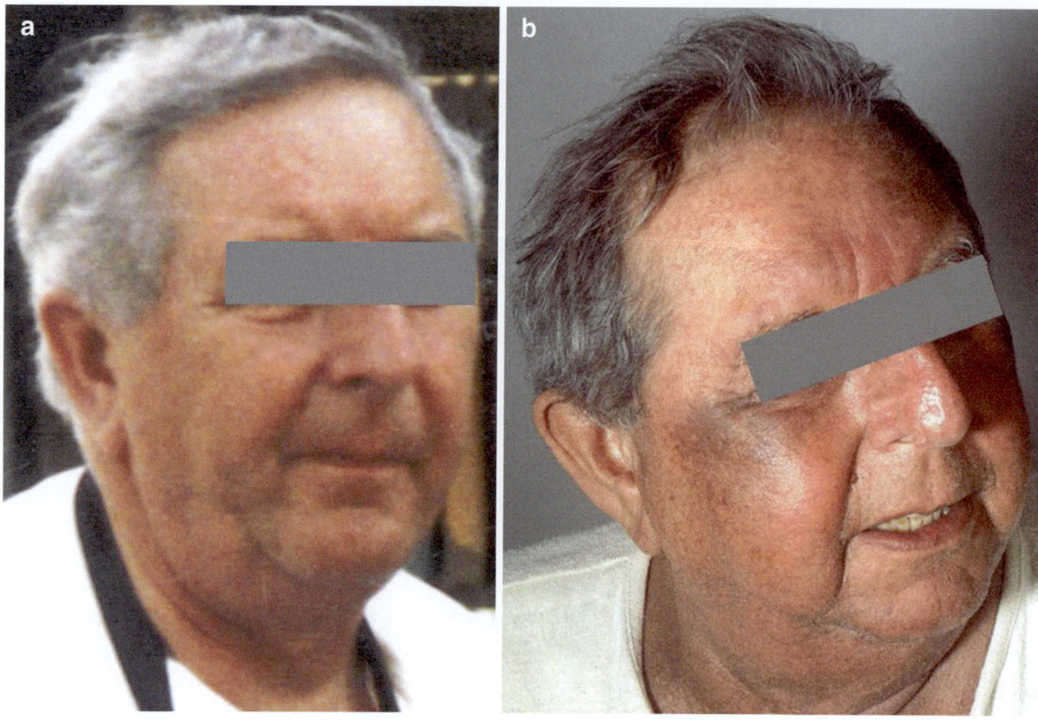

Fig. 3.16 (**a**, **b**) Spontaneous repigmentation of hair

pigment formation may also affect the hair, a conspicuous darkening of the hair should suggest the possibility of these disorders.

Temporary hair darkening has been reported after ingestion of large doses of p-aminobenzoic acid (PABA): Sieve gave 100 mg three times daily to 460 gray-haired individuals and noted a response in 82 %. Darkening was obvious within 2–4 months of starting treatment. The hairs turned gray again 2–4 weeks after stopping therapy. The mechanism of action has remained unclear. A major drawback are gastrointestinal side effects. For this reason, PABA is usually incorporated in smaller doses in commercially available oral dietary supplements for hair growth and color.

> Darkening of hair has been observed in the course of treatment of androgenetic alopecia with the topical hair growth-promoting agent minoxidil. The mode of action is probably prolonged anagen and follicular enlargement, enhancing normal melanogenesis.

In the absence of another way to reliably reverse hair graying, hair colorants have remained the mainstay of recovering lost hair color, reaching back as far as to the ancient Egyptians who colored their hair with henna and indigo and the ancient Romans who used lead combs dipped into vinegar.

Possibilities for prevention or reversal of senile graying of human hair are the subject of current intense research into the underlying biology of hair pigmentation and its derangements, respectively. Since reactive oxygen species have been implicated in hair follicle melanocyte apoptosis and DNA damage, and under in vitro conditions, Met oxidation of tyrosinase could be shown to be prevented by L-methionine; it will be interesting whether L-methionine could be useful for intervention or reversal of the hair graying process.

There is also an increasing interest in the hair follicular route for delivery of active compounds affecting the hair. Research activities also focus on topical liposome targeting for melanins, genes, and proteins selectively to hair follicles for therapeutic and cosmetic modification of hair.

Finally, tissue engineering with cells of hair follicular origin with stem cell properties represents yet another line of research in the quest of new treatments for loss of pigmentation. Advances in the identification and characterization of stem cell populations have led to substantial interest in understanding the precise triggers that would operate to induce activation of quiescent stem cells. Melanocyte stem cells that reside in the bulge region of murine hair follicles are characterized by reduced expression of the microphthalmia-associated transcription factor (Mitf) and its target genes implicated in differentiation. As Mitf is implicated in control of proliferation, Saha et al. explored the possibility that inducing Mitf expression via lipid-mediated activation of the p38 stress-signaling pathway may represent a repigmentation strategy. They isolated from placental extract a C18:0 sphingolipid able to induce Mitf and tyrosinase expression via activation of the p38 stress-signaling pathway. Strikingly, in age-onset gray-haired C57BL/6 J mice that exhibit decaying Mitf expression, topical application of placental sphingolipid led to increased Mitf in follicular melanocytes and fresh dense black hair growth.

3.4.6 Possibilities and Limitations for Reversal of Age-Related Hair Loss

Current available treatment modalities with proven efficacy for treatment of hair loss in men with androgenetic alopecia are topical minoxidil, oral finasteride, and autologous hair transplantation.

It has been known for over 30 years that minoxidil stimulates hair growth, and clinical trials of topical 5 % minoxidil solution in male hair loss have all shown remarkably rapid increase in hair growth, measured by hair counts or hair: The increase is evident within 6–8 weeks of treatment and has generally peaked by 12–16 weeks. However, topical minoxidil has not been studied in the specific perspective of aging and senescent alopecia. In an analysis of clinical trial data in 636 males, a therapeutic benefit of topical minoxidil solution was compared to age, duration of balding, and diameter of the balding vertex area: Age was found to be the denominator for predicting treatment success. The younger subjects experienced better efficacy than the older subjects, although clear treatment effects were noted also in the older age group (Fig. 3.17a–c). Males showed an inverse relationship between effect and duration of balding. Males with duration of balding <5 years showed a significantly better effect of topical minoxidil than those with duration of balding >21 years. The diameter of vertex showed an inverse relationship with efficacy of minoxidil. Men with <5 cm diameter vertex balding area showed a better effect of treatment than subjects with diameters >15 cm. Finally, duration of hair loss less than 1 year compared to more than 10 years at onset of treatment resulted in a significantly more effective treatment with respect to stabilization of alopecia and new hair growth.

One milligram oral finasteride daily has also proven to be effective in aging male, though to a lesser degree and with a higher frequency of sexual adverse effects compared to men between 18 and 40 years. The lesser effect may be attributed to the fact that in senescent alopecia scalp thinning is not DHT dependent.

Finally, in the course of hormonal antiaging protocols containing recombinant human growth hormone (hGH) at the Palm Springs Life Extension Institute, Chein reported improvement of hair thickness and structure in 38 % of patients, in some cases darkening of hair, and in few increased hair growth.

Autologous hair transplantation remains the only treatment option for advanced patterned baldness. With the advent of total micrografting and a sharp decline in scalp reduction procedures, hair restoration surgery has become more satisfying than in the recent past. Modern techniques use the visual qualities of hair and varying design patterns to create the optical illusion of more hair than is actually present. The main advances in hair restoration surgery have been the use of one to four hair grafts, which allows a natural, undetectable hairline, and the transplantation of large numbers of these small grafts during a single session. Careful patient selection and these newer techniques are geared toward naturalness and undetectability for the lifetime of the patient.

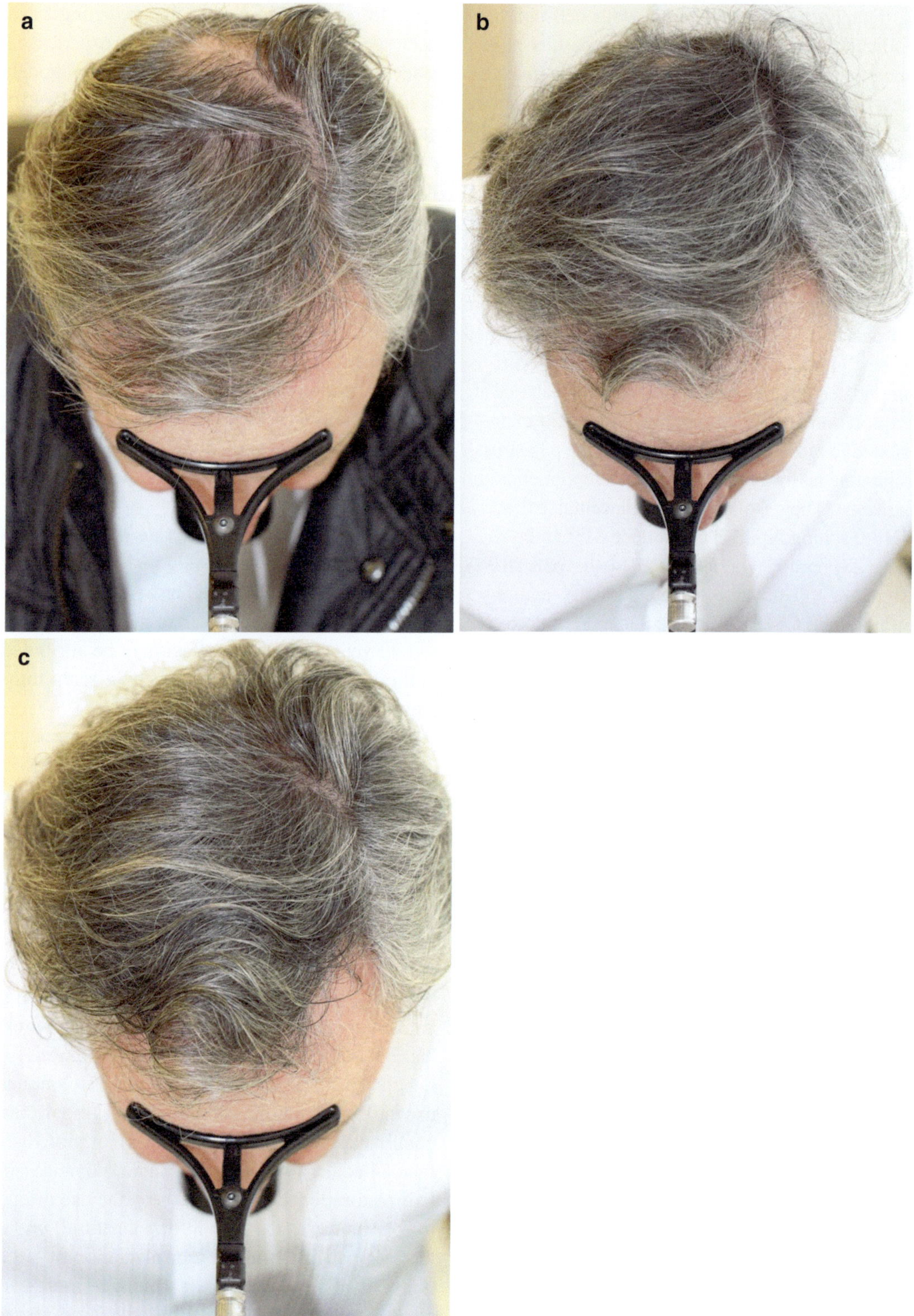

Fig. 3.17 (**a–c**) Successful treatment of pattern hair loss in a 71-year-old male with 5 % topical minoxidil solution twice daily, (**a**) before, (**b**) after 3 months, and (**c**) 6 months treatment

3.4.7 Dorian Gray Syndrome

The recently proposed *Dorian Gray syndrome* denotes a cultural and societal phenomenon characterized by extreme pride in one's own appearance accompanied by difficulties coping with the aging process. Sufferers of Dorian Gray syndrome are by definition users of cosmetic medical procedures and products in an attempt to preserve their youth, including hair growth restorers.

The syndrome was first described on the occasion of a symposium on lifestyle drugs and aesthetic medicine and is named after Oscar Wilde's famous gothic horror novel "The Picture of Dorian Gray," in which the protagonist, a beautiful young aesthete, exclaims in front of his portrait:

> Why should it keep what I must lose? Every moment that passes takes something from me, and gives something to it. Oh, if it were only the other way! If the picture could change, and I could be always what I am now! For that - for that - I would give everything! Yes, there is nothing in the whole world I would not give! I would give my soul for that!

The syndrome probably represents a variant of body dysmorphic disorder. Body dysmorphic disorder represents a condition in which sufferers are intensely preoccupied with an imagined or grossly exaggerated defect in some aspect of their physical appearance. They are more likely to consult physicians for correction of the "defect" than to seek help from mental health professionals. The particularity of the Dorian Gray syndrome is that patients wish to remain forever young and seek lifestyle drugs and surgery to deter the natural aging process (Table 3.7).

An estimated 3 % of the total population in Western society displays features of the syndrome. Disastrous results of excessive plastic surgery and cosmetic dermatologic procedures are found under www.oddee.com/item_96587.aspx. Among the ten worst male celebrity examples are Michael Jackson (1958–2009) and Pete Burns (of "Dead or Alive"). If the defensive "acting out" character of the syndrome is not understood properly and the patient incessantly uses lifestyle products without understanding the underlying psychodynamics, a chronic state of narcissistic emptiness may develop. Depressive episodes and suicidal crisis are often observed if medical and surgical lifestyle treatments as means of defense are not sufficient to preserve the patient's idea of beauty.

Table 3.7 Criteria for the diagnosis of Dorian Gray syndrome

Criteria
Signs of body dysmorphic disorder
Inability to mature and to progress in terms of psychological development
Use of at least two of the following medical/surgical lifestyle treatments (different groups required):
1. Hair growth-promoting agents
2. Weight-reducing agents
3. Agents to treat erectile dysfunction
4. Mood-modifying agents
5. Minimal invasive cosmetic dermatologic procedures
6. Cosmetic surgery

From: Brosig B, Kupfer J, Niemeier V et al (2001) The "Dorian Gray Syndrome": psychodynamic need for hair growth restorers and, other "fountains of youth". Int J Clin Pharmacol Ther 39:279–283

Beauty is an abstract concept and has been an object of interest and discussion both of philosophers since ancient Greece and of evolutionary scientists. The earliest Western theory on beauty can be found in the records of early Greek philosophers from the pre-Socratic period, such as Pythagoras (570–495 BC). The Pythagorean school believed in a strong association between mathematics and beauty; in particular, they noted that objects proportioned according to the *golden ratio* seemed more attractive. Plato (428–348 BC) considered beauty to be the idea (form) above all other ideas. Aristotle (384–322 BC) saw a relationship between the beautiful and virtue, arguing that "virtue aims at the beautiful." The classical Greek noun for beauty was *kállos*, and the Koine Greek word for beautiful was *hōraios*, an adjective etymologically coming from the word *hōra,* meaning "hour." In Koine Greek, beauty was thus associated with "being of one's hour."

Therefore, a ripe fruit (of its time) was considered beautiful, whereas a young being trying to appear older or an older being trying to appear younger would not be considered beautiful.

Contemporary research has attempted to identify the physical features that account for the attractiveness of an individual and has recognized several factors: facial and body symmetry, averageness of appearance (koinophilia), body size ratios, and youthfulness.

Beauty has been understood as an individual's subjective appraisal of attractiveness that is influenced by cultural standards. Sociocultural images of beauty are best reflected in a variety of popular beauty icons. However, despite some unique cultural variabilities in aesthetic judgments, evidence has shown that similar patterns emerge across different cultures. Moreover, a set of convincing studies confirm that our perception of attractiveness predates cultural influences. Studies in infants have suggested that the ability to discriminate attractive from unattractive faces may be innate abilities, or at least one acquired at an earlier age than previously believed. For the International Mate Selection Project, 50 scientists studied 10,047 people in 37 cultures located on 6 continents and 5 islands and found that without exception, physical signs of youth and health were perceived as attractive. In his seminal "The Descent of Man and Selection in Relation to Sex," Charles Darwin (1809–1882) reflected on the physical characteristics that seemed to act as open lures to predators and therefore interfere with survival. For example, how could the brilliant plumage of peacocks have evolved? Darwin's answer was *sexual selection*, that is, that certain characteristic evolved because of reproductive advantage rather than survival advantage. The evolutionary argument hypothesizes that physical signs of youth and health, such as full lips, smooth skin, clear eyes, lustrous hair, good muscle tone, animated facial expression, and high energy level, are at the top of every culture's beauty list, simply because they are the most reliable physical signals for fertility.

Youthfulness in particular marks an extended period of reproductive potential. Looking young may be more important than actually being young, and altering facial features in the direction of youth results in higher ratings of attractiveness.

In the 1990s, *body image* became one of the hottest topics covered by numerous professional textbooks and hundreds of journal articles. In a landmark publication, "Exacting Beauty" Thompson et al. pointed out that at least 14 terms are used with reference to body image and that body image is akin to *self-esteem*. Thompson et al. suggested that body image has come to be accepted as the internal representation of our own outer appearance and plays a significant role in how people feel about both their appearance and themselves. While there is little agreement to the exact definition of body image, there is a consent that body image is a multidimensional construct: *perceptual influences* account for an individual's capacity to determine the physical features of a specific body part; *developmental influences* take the influence of childhood and adolescent experiences, such as appearance-related teasing, into consideration; and *sociocultural influences* relate to the interaction of the mass media and cultural ideas of appearance, which frequently portray unrealistic or exaggerated iconic images of beauty.

Finally, the issue of *body image dissatisfaction* determines behaviors to improve body image, from cosmetic to cosmetic surgical procedures.

Body image dissatisfaction falls into a continuum from a dislike of a specific appearance feature to psychopathologic dissatisfaction.

Sarwer et al. suggested that attitudes toward the body condition have two dimensions: The first consists of *valence*, defined as the degree of importance of body image to one's self-esteem; the second consists of *value*, which is understood as the degree of satisfaction or dissatisfaction with the body image. The theory of body image can be used to understand physical appearance concerns and the relentless pursuit of an improved body image through respective behaviors.

In contrast to the substantial literature on the psychology of physical appearance and attractiveness, relatively little has been published on the impact of androgenetic alopecia. In the earliest study, published in 1971, sketches of balding men were rated as weak, inactive, and least potent and those of bald men as most unkind, bad, ugly, and hard, while men with a full head of hair were seen as most handsome, virile, and active. Because of the limited validity of a study design with sketches of men, Cash subsequently conducted a controlled study on the first impressions brought forth by photographs of 18 men with visible androgenetic alopecia compared with 18 men with a full head of hair, who were matched on age, facial expression, attire, and other physical features. Adults of both sexes judged balding men as older and less physically and socially attractive that their non-balding peers. When the physical attractiveness differences between balding and non-balding men were statistically removed, all other perceived differences disappeared as well.

Further research corroborated that baldness diminishes perceived attractiveness and youthfulness.

Although, androgenetic alopecia may initially influence social perceptions, the more important issue is whether hair loss affects the individual's own psychological well-being and quality of life. Patients' reactions to their hair loss relate more to self-perceptions of their alopecia than to objective clinical ratings. Extreme distress in some patients may involve body dysmorphic disorder, a condition in which sufferers are intensely preoccupied with an imagined or grossly exaggerated defect in some aspect of their physical appearance.

Hair thinning and the fear of baldness are a focal preoccupation in 50 % of body dysmorphic disorder cases, second only to the skin at 65 %.

3.5 Alopecia with Scarring Phenomena

The scarring alopecias represent a diverse group of disorders that cause permanent destruction of the pilosebaceous unit and irreversible hair loss, characterized by visible loss of follicular ostia and destruction of the hair follicle on histopathologic examination. There is substantial evidence that follicular inflammation and fibrosis may also contribute to the pathogenesis of androgenetic alopecia: on histological examination of scalp biopsies, the miniaturization of terminal hairs is frequently associated with perifollicular lymphocytic infiltration and eventually fibrosis. It is therefore conceivable that the role of this microscopic follicular inflammation causing fibrosis below the shortened balding follicle has so far been underestimated, though it seems likely that this would prevent the follicle to reform a terminal hair follicle.

Bernard et al. proposed the term follicular microinflammation, because the process involves a slow, subtle, and indolent course, in contrast to the inflammatory and destructive process in the classical inflammatory scarring alopecias.

3.5.1 Inflammatory Phenomena and Fibrosis in Male Androgenetic Alopecia

The implication of microscopic follicular inflammation in the pathogenesis of androgenetic alopecia has emerged from several independent studies: an early study referred to an inflammatory infiltrate of activated T cells and macrophages in the upper third of the hair follicles, associated with an enlargement of the follicular dermal sheath composed of collagen bundles (perifollicular fibrosis), in regions of actively progressing alopecia. Horizontal section studies of scalp biopsies indicated that the perifollicular fibrosis is generally mild, consisting of loose, concentric layers of collagen that must be distinguished from cicatricial alopecia.

The significance of follicular microinflammation and fibrosis in androgenetic alopecia has remained controversial.

Nevertheless, morphometric studies in male patients with androgenetic alopecia treated with topical minoxidil showed that 55 % of those with microinflammation had regrowth in response to treatment, in comparison to 77 % in those patients without inflammation and fibrosis.

An important question is how the inflammatory reaction pattern is generated around the individual hair follicle. Inflammation is regarded a multistep process which may start from a primary event. The observation of a perifollicular infiltrate in the upper follicle near the infundibulum suggests that the primary causal event for the triggering of inflammation might occur near the infundibulum. On the basis of this localization and the microbial colonization of the follicular infundibulum with *Propionibacterium* spp., *Staphylococcus* spp., *Malassezia* spp., or other members of the transient flora, one could speculate that microbial toxins or antigens could be involved in the generation of the inflammatory response. The production of porphyrins by *Propionibacterium* spp. in the pilosebaceous duct has also been considered to be a possible cofactor of this initial pro-inflammatory stress.

Alternatively, keratinocytes themselves may respond to chemical stress from irritants, pollutants, and UV irradiation, by producing radical oxygen species and nitric oxide and by releasing intracellularly stored IL-1 alpha. This pro-inflammatory cytokine by itself has been shown to inhibit the growth of isolated hair follicles in culture. Moreover, adjacent keratinocytes, which express receptors for IL-1, start to engage the transcription of IL-1 responsive genes: mRNA coding for IL-1 beta, TNF alpha, and IL-1 alpha, and for specific chemokine genes, such as IL-8, and monocyte chemoattractant protein-1 (MCP-1) and MCP-3, themselves mediators for the recruitment of neutrophils and macrophages, have been shown to be upregulated in the epithelial compartment of the human hair follicle. Besides, adjacent fibroblasts are also fully equipped to respond to such a pro-inflammatory signal. The upregulation of adhesion molecules for blood-borne cells in the capillary endothelia, together with the chemokine gradient, drives the transendothelial migration of inflammatory cells, which include neutrophils through the action of IL-8, T cells, and Langerhans cells at least in part through the action of MCP-1. After processing of localized antigen, Langerhans cells, or alternatively keratinocytes, which may also have antigen-presenting capabilities, could then present antigen to newly infiltrating T lymphocytes and induce T-cell proliferation. The antigens are selectively destroyed by infiltrating macrophages or natural killer cells.

On the occasion that the causal agents persist, sustained inflammation is the result, together with connective tissue remodeling, where

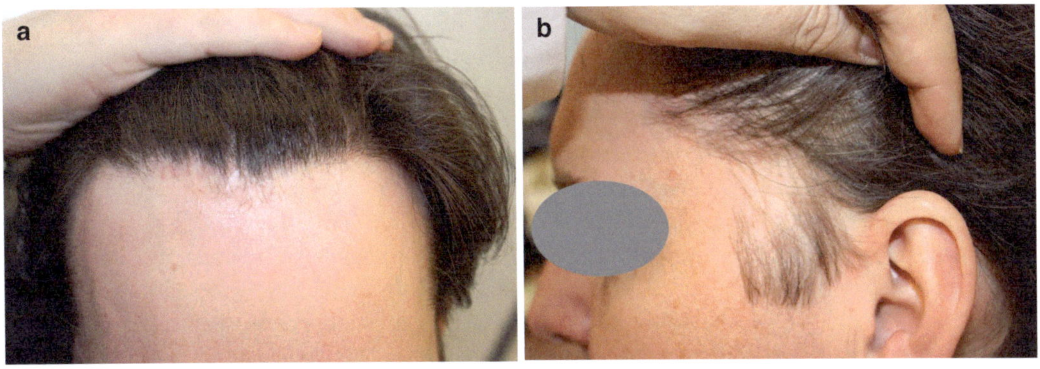

Fig. 3.18 (**a**, **b**) Male frontal fibrosing alopecia, with (**b**) loss of sideburns

collagenases, such as matrix metalloproteinase (also transcriptionally driven by pro-inflammatory cytokines), play an active role. Collagenases are suspected to contribute to the tissue changes in perifollicular fibrosis.

3.5.2 Male Frontal Fibrosing Alopecia

Frontal fibrosing alopecia represents a peculiar condition originally described by Kossard in women in the postmenopause. The condition presents with a symmetric, marginal alopecia along the frontal and frontal–temporal hairline, often with concomitant thinning or complete loss of the eyebrows. Affected women typically present with the complaint of asymptomatic, progressive recession of their frontal hairline. The affected scalp skin is pale and smooth with loss of follicular orifices, often perifollicular erythema, and follicular keratinization is observed, marking the underlying inflammatory process.

Histopathologic examination of affected scalp shows a reduced number of hair follicles, which have been replaced by fibrous tracts, and a perifollicular, lymphocytic, lichenoid infiltrate that is typical of lichen planopilaris.

Since Kossard's original description in 1994, the number of cases of frontal fibrosing alopecia has exploded exponentially worldwide, while its etiology remains obscure. The condition has meanwhile also been described in men (Fig. 3.18a) with the typical presentation of scarring alopecia of the sideburns (Fig. 3.18b). Moreover, it has been recognized to represent a more generalized rather than localized process of inflammatory scarring alopecia, with extension beyond the frontotemporal hairline and loss of peripheral body hair.

3.5.3 Fibrosing Alopecia in a Pattern Distribution (Cicatricial Pattern Hair Loss)

Alopecia in a pattern distribution is a common event associated with androgenetic hair loss and aging. Although it is regarded as a pathologic process by some physicians and many affected patients, by others it is considered a genetically determined physiological event in the lives of most men and women. The same controversy applies to the histological finding of inflammatory cells in the vicinity of the upper hair follicle in androgenetic alopecia inasmuch as it remains uncertain whether this phenomenon is still a physiological event or already reflects a pathologic process. Remarkably, in healthy murine skin clusters of perifollicular macrophages have been described as perhaps indicating the existence of a physiological program of immunologically controlled hair follicle degeneration by which malfunctioning follicles are removed by programmed organ deletion. It has been proposed that forms of clinically perceptible, permanent alopecia might represent pathologic exaggeration of this type of programmed organ deletion, resulting in a lichenoid tissue reaction pattern and true scarring alopecia.

In general, androgenetic alopecia is understood to be a noninflammatory and non-scarring process that eventually leads to permanent hair loss of the affected scalp. In our original description of *fibrosing alopecia in a pattern distribution*, patients displayed progressive scarring alopecia in a pattern distribution (Fig. 3.19a). Close clinical examination reveals obliteration of follicular orifices, perifollicular erythema (Fig. 3.19b), and follicular keratosis limited to the area of androgenetic hair loss (Fig. 3.19c). Histological findings of androgenetic alopecia, i.e., increased numbers of miniaturized hair follicles with underlying fibrous streamers, are evident in the majority of patients and associated with a perifollicular lymphocytic infiltrate. A pattern of follicular interface dermatitis targeting the upper follicle is found in early lesions, whereas perifollicular lamellar fibrosis and the presence of selectively fibrosed follicular tracts characterize late lesions.

The pattern distribution and histological findings share features with Kossard's original description of postmenopausal frontal fibrosing alopecia. Kossard et al. later interpreted this type of alopecia as a frontal variant of lichen planopilaris on the basis of histopathologic and immunohistochemical studies. Considerable overlap exists among frontal fibrosing alopecia, lichen planopilaris, and fibrosing alopecia in a pattern distribution: postmenopausal frontal fibrosing alopecia has been described in association with lichen planus elsewhere, including the oral cavity, and frontal fibrosing alopecia-type changes can also be observed in patients with fibrosing alopecia in a pattern distribution.

> In 2005, Olsen ultimately acknowledged existence of clinically significant inflammatory phenomena and fibrosis in androgenetic alopecia and proposed the term *cicatricial pattern hair loss* for these conditions.

Follicular microinflammation and fibrosis, frontal fibrosing alopecia, and fibrosing alopecia in a pattern distribution seem to represent a continuum from microscopic inflammation and fibrosis to localized resp. more generalized forms of clinically perceptible inflammatory scarring alopecia.

Further studies are required in patients with cicatricial pattern hair loss to elucidate a presumable role of androgenetic factors in addition to that of the lymphohistiocytic infiltrate, perifollicular lamellar fibrosis, and apoptosis-mediated follicular regression. An important question to be addressed is how the lichenoid tissue reaction pattern is generated around the individual androgenetic hair follicle. Follicles with some form of damage or malfunction might express cytokine profiles that attract inflammatory cells to assist in damage repair or in the initiation of apoptosis-mediated organ deletion. Alternatively, an as yet unknown antigenic stimulus from the damaged or malfunctioning hair follicle might initiate a lichenoid tissue reaction in the immunogenetically susceptible individual. The possible role of microbial antigens or superantigens in this context remains to be elucidated.

3.5.4 Inflammatory Scarring Alopecias

> The irreversibility and the possible important cosmetic consequences of scarring alopecia demand special diagnostic attention in order to promptly attain a precise diagnosis and specific treatment.

Loss of follicular orifices in an area of alopecia points to an irreversible loss of hair, either due to permanent damage to essential parts of the hair follicle or destruction of the entire hair follicle. Where there is no obvious physical/chemical injury or acute infectious etiology, clinical differential diagnosis of scarring alopecia is often

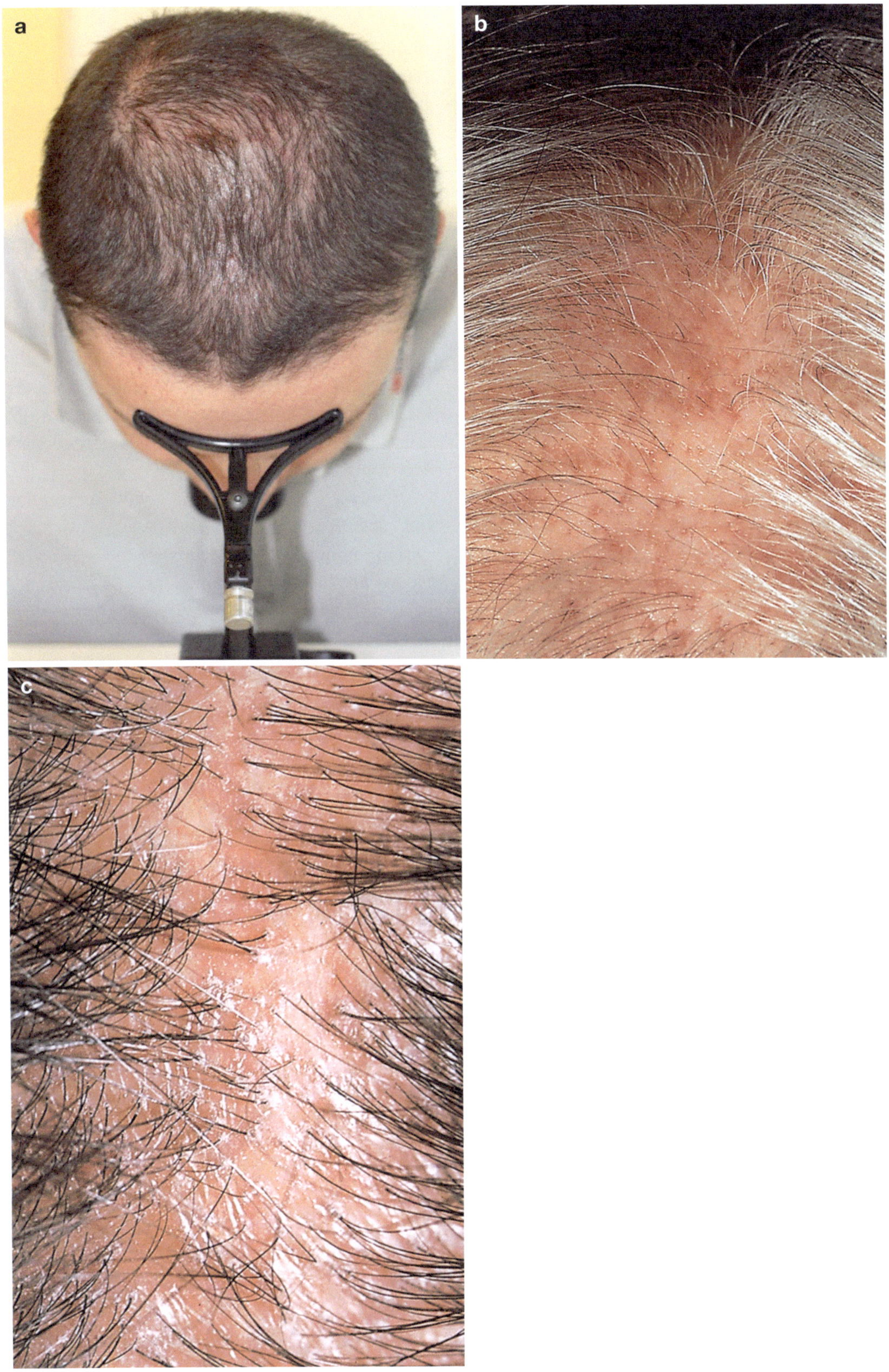

Fig. 3.19 (**a–c**) Fibrosing alopecia in a pattern distribution. (**a**) Patterned scarring alopecia, (**b**) follicular erythema, and (**c**) follicular keratosis

difficult. The clinical inspection is of limited usefulness in establishing a diagnosis. Overlapping features may blur the distinction between different diseases; moreover, these share the common final pathway of replacement of follicle by fibrous tissue. Finally, there is no characteristic biological marker for most entities.

> The scarring alopecias are both a diagnostic and therapeutic challenge to the practitioner. A fortiori, accurate diagnosis based on a careful patient history, clinical examination, microbiological studies, and scalp biopsy is a prerequisite to therapy.

Problems inherent to scalp biopsies are a reluctance of many practitioners in performing them and a lack of familiarity of many pathologists with scalp histopathology. Ultimately, it must be borne in mind that the hair follicle and its derangements are complex and dynamic. A biopsy gives only a momentary snapshot of the underlying pathology.

Scarring alopecias may be due to hereditary or developmental defects. Examples of these rare conditions are aplasia cutis congenita, organoid nevi (Fig. 3.20a), hereditary epidermolysis bullosa, alopecia ichthyotica (Fig. 3.20b), and the follicular keratosis syndromes.

More frequently they are due to acquired, irreparable destruction of critical hair follicle structures (follicular sheath, stem cells, follicular papilla, and their interaction) or of the whole hair follicle. The acquired scarring alopecias are further differentiated into primary and secondary scarring alopecias:

Primary scarring alopecia is due to preferential destruction of the follicle. Well-defined, chronic inflammatory diseases of the scalp amenable to specific therapies are differentiated microscopically from a morphologic point of

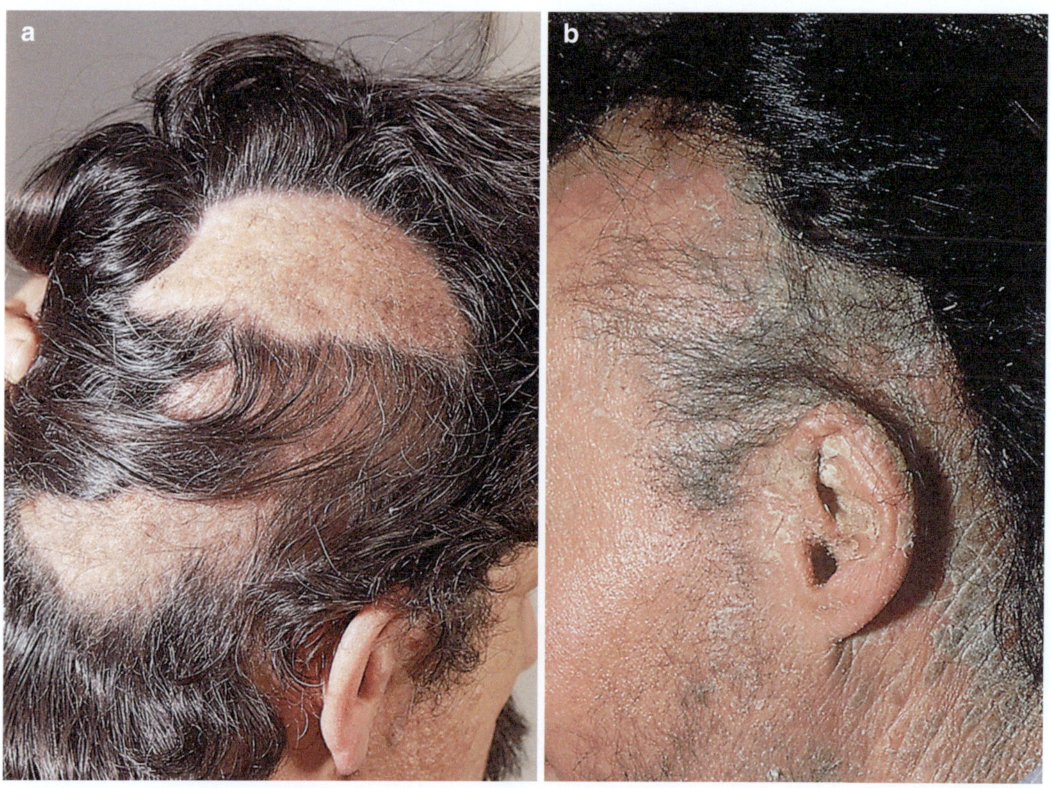

Fig. 3.20 (**a**, **b**) Examples of congenital scarring alopecia: (**a**) organoid nevus and (**b**) alopecia ichthyotica

Table 3.8 Primary cicatricial alopecias: proposed working classification of NAHRS

Lymphocytic group
(Classic) Lichen planopilaris and variants:
Disseminated (Lassueur–Graham Little syndrome)
Patterned:
Frontal fibrosing alopecia (Kossard)
Fibrosing alopecia in a pattern distribution (Zinkernagel and Trüeb)
Chronic cutaneous lupus erythematosus
(Classic) pseudopelade of Brocq
Central centrifugal cicatricial alopecia?
Neutrophilic group
Folliculitis decalvans (Quinquaud) and variants:
Tufted hair folliculitis (Sanderson and Smith)
Cicatrising seborrheic eczema (Laymon)
Dissecting cellulitis of the scalp (perifolliculitis capitis abscedens et suffodiens Hoffmann)
Mixed group
Keratosis follicularis spinulosa decalvans (Siemens)/ folliculitis spinulosa decalvans
Folliculitis (acne) keloidalis (nuchae)/dermatitis papillaris capillitii
Folliculitis (acne) necrotica (varioliformis/miliaris)
Erosive pustular dermatosis (of the scalp)
End-stage nonspecific group
Pseudopeladic state (Degos)

Modified from: Olsen EA, Bergfeld WF, Cotsarelis G et al. (2003) Summary of North American Hair Research Society (NAHRS) – sponsored Workshop on Cicatricial Alopecia. J Am Acad Dermatol 48:103–110

view on the basis of the pattern of inflammation and the type of inflammatory cell that predominates (Table 3.8).

In a study of 136 scalp biopsies obtained for histopathology and direct immunofluorescence studies, Trachsler and Trüeb found lichen planopilaris (28 %), folliculitis decalvans (23 %), chronic cutaneous lupus erythematosus (21 %), and pseudopelade of Brocq (10 %) to be the most prevalent.

Lichen planopilaris is the most common cause of scarring alopecia in the adult. It presents with pruritic central or multifocal alopecic patches with follicular hyperkeratosis and erythema at the hair-bearing margin (Fig. 3.21a). Histopathology reveals a lymphocytic primary scarring alopecia. Non-scalp involvement (mucous membranes, glabrous skin, nails) may be present. The Lassueur–Graham Little syndrome is considered a disseminated variant, Kossard's frontal fibrosing alopecia, and Zinkernagel and Trüeb's fibrosing alopecia in a pattern distribution as patterned variants of lichen planopilaris. With regard to its pathogenesis, lichen planopilaris may be regarded as a T-cell-mediated autoimmune reaction. This autoimmune process triggers apoptosis of the epithelial cells. Several cytokines are involved, including tumor necrosis factor alpha, interferon gamma, interleukin-1 alpha, interleukin 6, and interleukin 8. This autoimmune, T-cell-mediated process is thought to be in response to some antigenic change, but a specific antigen has yet not been identified. Where a causal or triggering agent is identified, this is termed a lichenoid reaction rather than lichen planus. These may include drug reactions, with the most common inducers including gold salts, beta blockers, antimalarials, thiazide diuretics, furosemide, spironolactone, metformin, and penicillamine; hepatitis, specifically hepatitis B and hepatitis C infection; and cutaneous graft-versus-host disease.

Chronic cutaneous or discoid lupus erythematosus presents as symptomatic, erythematous scaly plaques with follicular plugs, telangiectases, atrophy, and depigmentation with time (Fig. 3.21b). In contrast to lichen planopilaris, activity tends to be in the center of alopecic patches. Histopathology again reveals a lymphocytic primary scarring alopecia. Non-scalp involvement may be present, since lupus erythematosus may represent a systemic autoimmune inflammatory disease.

Folliculitis decalvans represents a chronic and recurrent pustulofollicular scalp inflammation resulting in scarring alopecia. It usually presents in the central scalp area with exudative crusted areas and grouped follicular pustules at the hair-bearing margin with centrifugal progression (Fig. 3.21c). Histopathology reveals a neutrophilic primary scarring alopecia. Invariably pathogenic strains of *Staphylococcus aureus* can be detected. Only very rarely there may be an association with immune deficiency. A recent study provided evidence of the presence of bacterial biofilms in the infrainfundibular part of human scalp hair follicles to be pathogenic. A biofilm is any group of microorganisms in which cells stick to each other on a surface. These adherent cells are frequently embedded within a self-produced matrix of extracellular polymeric substance. Biofilms form on living or nonliving surfaces and in the case of folliculitis decalvans on the surfaces of the hair shaft. Bacteria living in a biofilm usually have significantly different properties from free-floating bacteria of the same species, as the dense and protected environment of the film allows them to cooperate and interact in various ways. One benefit of this environment is increased resistance to antibiotics, as the dense extracellular matrix and the outer layer of cells protect the interior of the community. Biofilms have been found to be involved in a wide variety of microbial infections in the body, and more recently it has been noted that bacterial biofilms may impair cutaneous wound healing and reduce topical antibacterial efficiency in healing or treating infected skin wounds.

Pseudopelade as first described by Brocq in 1888 and redefined by Bergner and Braun-Falco presents with asymptomatic, noninflamed, ivory-white or flesh-colored small oval-round, reticulate, or large, irregular patches of the central scalp area (Fig. 3.21d). Non-scalp involvement is absent. It is considered a lymphocytic primary scarring alopecia with selective destruction of hair follicles. It is clinically and histologically indistinguishable from end-stage lichen planopilaris.

Two other conditions of primary scarring alopecias predominantly seen in men are dissecting cellulitis of the scalp and folliculitis (or acne) keloidalis nuchae.

Dissecting cellulitis of the scalp also known as perifolliculitis capitis abscedens et suffodiens, or Hoffmann's disease, is a rare but well-characterized chronic inflammatory disease of the scalp leading to scarring alopecia. Most of those

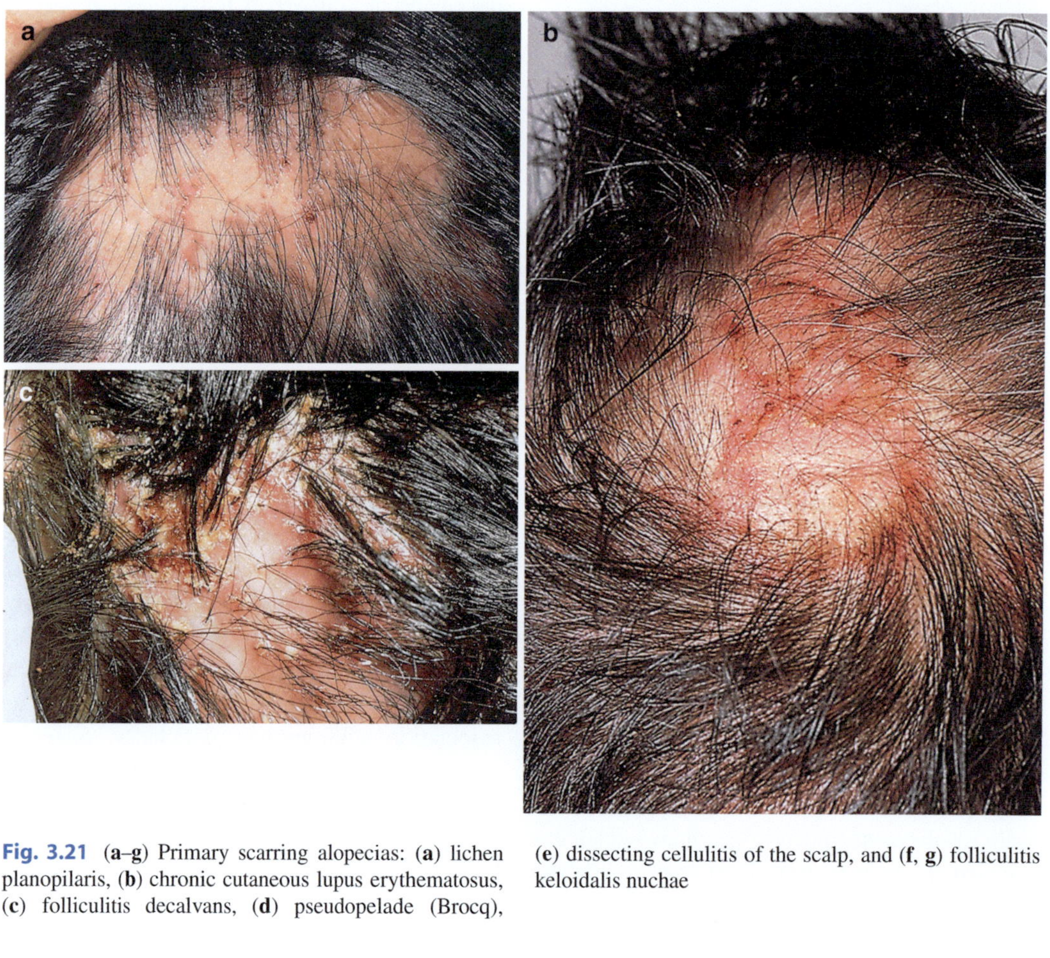

Fig. 3.21 (**a–g**) Primary scarring alopecias: (**a**) lichen planopilaris, (**b**) chronic cutaneous lupus erythematosus, (**c**) folliculitis decalvans, (**d**) pseudopelade (Brocq), (**e**) dissecting cellulitis of the scalp, and (**f, g**) folliculitis keloidalis nuchae

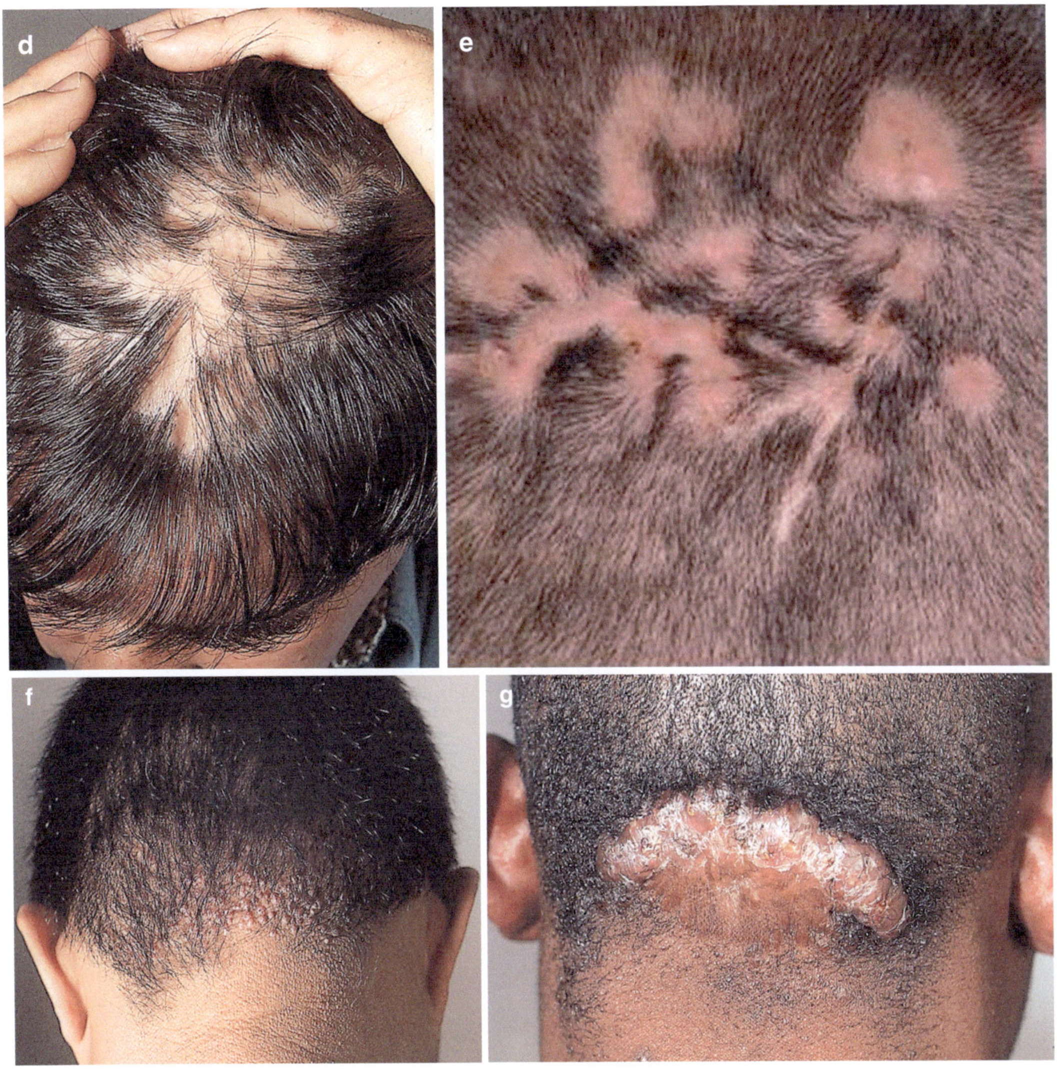

Fig. 3.21 (continued)

affected are young black males; about 10 % of cases involve white males. Association with acne conglobata was described as early as in 1903. Today, the condition is considered to be part of the follicular occlusion triad, along with acne conglobata and hidradenitis suppurativa (acne inversa), although isolated scalp disease occurs. Deep inflammatory nodules develop on the occipital scalp or vertex and can evolve to extensive confluent boggy plaques with sinus tract formation. Hairs overlying the nodules can be easily plucked, and sinus tracts may discharge purulent material. Ultimately, a multifocal scarring alopecia ensues that is potentially disfiguring (Fig. 3.21e). Histopathology reveals a neutrophilic primary scarring alopecia. Pathogenetically, a defect in follicular keratinization is blamed, leading to poral obstruction and accumulation of sebaceous and keratinous material within dilated pilosebaceous units. Subsequently, follicles burst, and an intense neutrophilic inflammatory reaction with abscess and sinus tract formation follows.

Folliculitis keloidalis nuchae represents yet another form of chronic inflammatory folliculitis. Again, the condition tends to occur preferentially in young black men, although white men may also be affected. The disease involves the occipital scalp. Lesions start as firm follicular papules (Fig. 3.21f), a condition that has also been synonymously named *Dermatitis papillaris capillitii*. Especially in black men, these may coalesce into larger, keloid-like plaques (Fig. 3.21g). Histopathology reveals a mixed cellular primary scarring alopecia.

Secondary scarring alopecia results from events outside the follicle, which eventually

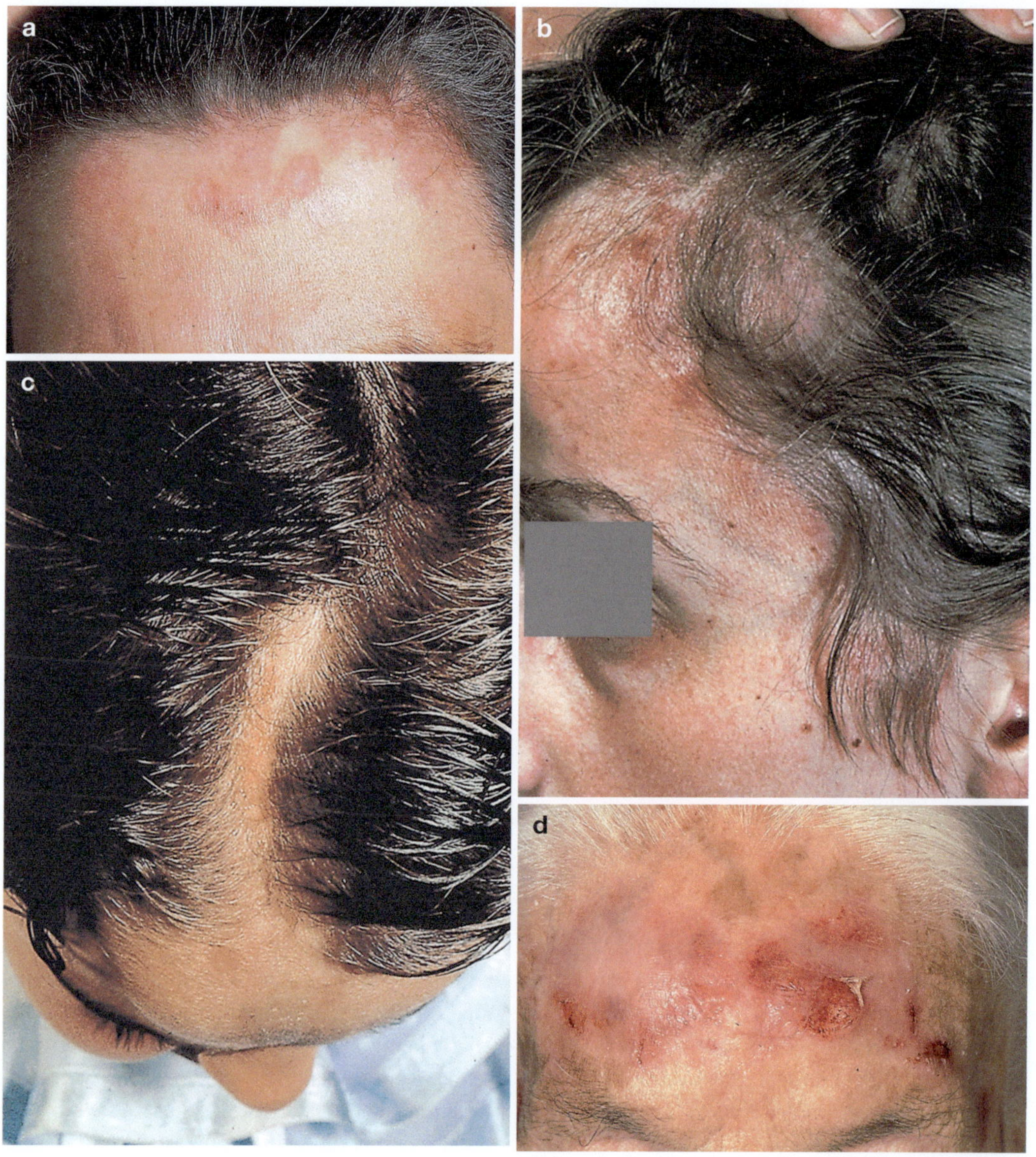

Fig. 3.22 (**a**–**e**) Secondary scarring alopecias: (**a**) sarcoidosis, (**b**) necrobiosis lipoidica (Miescher's granulomatosis disciformis progressiva), (**c**) circumscribed scleroderma (en coup de sabre), (**d**) cicatricial pemphigoid (Brunsting–Perry), and (**e**) necrotizing temporal arteritis (Horton's disease)

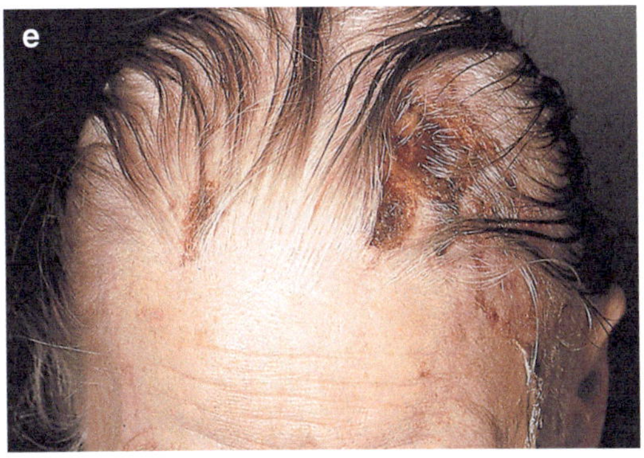

Fig. 3.22 (continued)

impinge upon and eradicate the follicle. These include physical or chemical injury, infectious diseases (fungal, bacterial, viral), granulomatous disease (sarcoidosis, Fig. 3.22a; necrobiosis lipoidica/Miescher's granulomatosis disciformis progressiva, Fig. 3.22b) or neoplastic processes (primary or metastatic solid tumors, malignant lymphoma), and autoimmune diseases, such as circumscribed scleroderma (Fig. 3.22c), cicatricial pemphigoid (Fig. 3.22d), and necrotizing temporal arteritis (Fig. 3.22e).

Finally, *pseudopeladic state of Degos* (1954) represents the nonspecific end stage of a variety of at least 60 types of primary or secondary cicatricial alopecias, whereby *pseudopelade of Brocq* (1905) probably represents the end stage or a variant of lichen planopilaris; *Sperling's central centrifugal scarring alopecia* (2000) with its predilection for African-Americans and close relationship to LoPresti's hot comb alopecia (1968), a USA-specific perspective of Degos' pseudopeladic state due to peculiarities of African-American hair grooming habits and hair anatomy; and *alopecia parvimaculata Dreuw* (1911) possibly the pediatric variant of Degos' pseudopeladic state. The relationship of the different groups of scarring alopecia is graphically summarized in Fig. 3.23.

3.5.5 Treatment

So far, the inflammatory component has not been included in treatment protocols for androgenetic alopecia. Also, no treatment has convincingly been found to significantly alter the course of frontal fibrosing alopecia, in part due to the patients' delay in consulting a physician for the condition, or the doctor's delay in making the diagnosis.

Basically, frontal fibrosing alopecia is very much treated in the same way as lichen planopilaris (see Table 3.9). Regrowth of eyebrow can be induced with intralesional triamcinolone acetonide. In a retrospective review of 19 female patients with frontal fibrosing alopecia seen at Duke University, Olsen et al. found dutasteride to be the most effective in halting disease progression, although no therapy was associated with significant hair regrowth. Autologous hair transplantation may be considered, where permanent loss of hair causes significant cosmetic embarrassment.

The goal of therapy in the scarring alopecias is mostly to halt further progression. Problems related to the treatment of the scarring alopecias include patients' delay, when irreversible scarring has already occurred. Since the causes are mostly unknown, therapy has remained empiric and nonspecific. Published data on recommended therapies have usually low levels of evidence. Recommended treatment regimens for the most prevalent among the inflammatory scarring alopecias are summarized in Table 3.9.

Management of less well-classified entities, such as pseudopelade of Brocq, alopecia parvimaculata of Dreuw, and pseudopeladic state of Degos, is problematic, since the etiologies are varied or not understood, and hair loss is permanent. Where end-stage fibrosis is established, surgical treatment or prosthetic help is taken into consideration.

With the expanding knowledge of the biology of hair growth and immunological phenomena, specifically of the molecular controls of immune-mediated hair follicle degeneration by apoptosis-mediated organ deletion, there is hope for the feasibility of therapeutic interventions that interfere early in the course of the pathogenetic processes ultimately leading to permanent hair loss from follicular inflammation and fibrosis, either due to androgenetic alopecia, cicatricial patterned hair loss, or the inflammatory scarring alopecias.

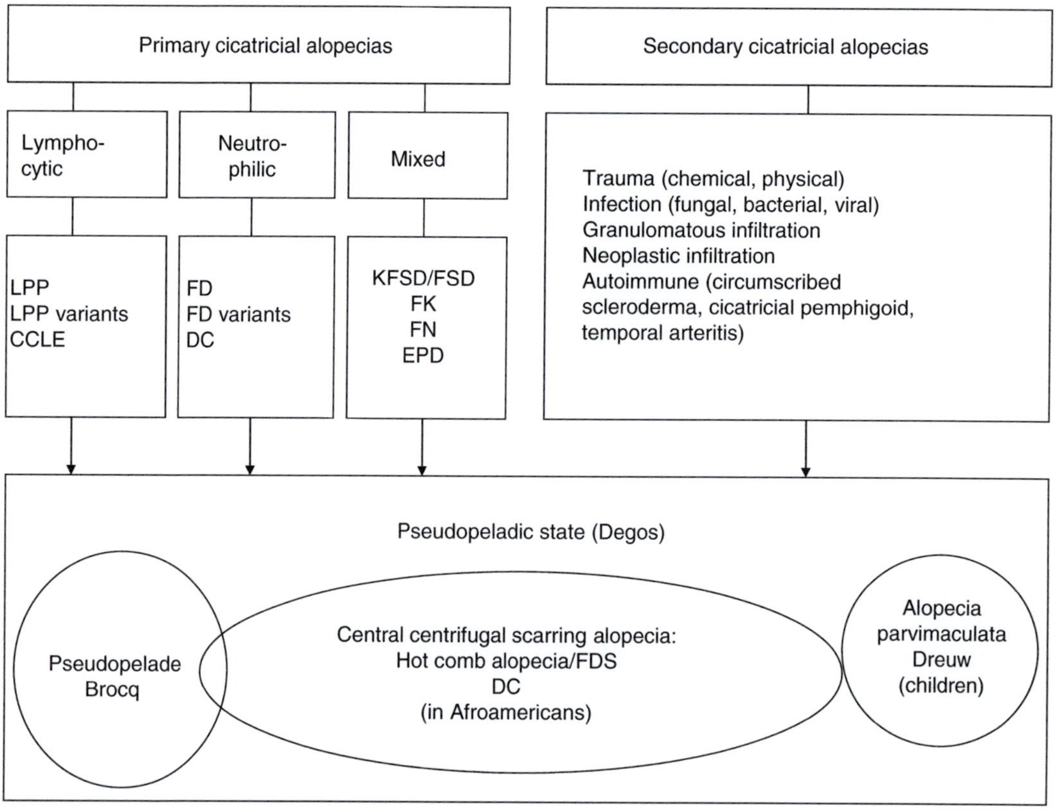

Fig. 3.23 Overview of scarring alopecias. *Abbreviations*: *LPP* lichen planopilaris, *CCLE* chronic cutaneous lupus erythematosus, *FD* folliculitis decalvans, *DC* dissecting cellulitis, *KFSD* keratosis follicularis spinulosa decalvans, *FSD* folliculitis spinulosa decalvans, *FK* folliculitis keloidalis, *FN* folliculitis necrotica, *EPD* erosive pustular dermatosis

Table 3.9 Inflammatory scarring alopecias. Recommended treatment regimens

Lichen planopilaris
Topical clobetasol propionate first month twice daily, 3 months daily, thereafter every second day, in combination with
Oral doxycycline 100–200 mg daily for 3–6 months
If unsuccessful, may be combined with oral hydroxychloroquine 200 mg daily
If unsuccessful, oral pioglitazone 15 mg daily
If unsuccessful, oral cyclosporine A 3–5 mg/kg body weight daily for 4 months, may be combined with
Surgical reduction of patches of scarring alopecia (during immunosuppression with oral cyclosporine A)
or
Trial with low-dose excimer 308-nm laser
Frontal fibrosing alopecia
Same may be tried as in lichen planopilaris
As an alternative to topical corticosteroids, topical calcineurin inhibitors (pimecrolimus, tacrolimus) may be tried at the frontotemporal hairline or in the eyebrow area
Intralesional triamcinolone acetonide 10 mg/ml is effective for (early) treatment of eyebrows
Autologous hair transplantation surgery may be effective both at the frontotemporal hairline and for the eyebrows (Fig. 3.24a, b)

Table 3.9 (continued)

Chronic cutaneous lupus erythematosus
Intralesional triamcinolone acetonide 10 mg/ml every 4 weeks, in combination with
Oral hydroxychloroquine, first 4 weeks 2 × 200 mg daily, thereafter 200 mg daily
May be combined with 1,200 IU vitamin E and 500 mg vitamin C daily (in smokers)
Photoprotection
Folliculitis decalvans
Oral fusidic acid 3 × 500 mg daily for 3 weeks, in combination with
Oral zinc gluconate 30 mg daily for months (Fig. 3.24c, d)
or
Oral rifampicin 450 mg twice daily in combination with oral flucloxacillin 500 mg four times daily for 2 weeks and thereafter every 3 months for 5 days
or
Oral rifampicin 300 mg twice daily in combination with oral clindamycin 300 mg twice daily during 10 weeks
or
Oral levofloxacin 500 mg twice daily for 10 days
Daily antiseptic shampoo treatment with 0.2–2 % chlorhexidine gluconate
Surgical reduction of patches of scarring alopecia (Fig. 3.24e–g) or selective punch excision of hair tufts may be taken into consideration (during oral antibiotic treatment)
Dissecting cellulitis of the scalp
Oral isotretinoin 1 mg/kg body weight daily for at least 6 months, in combination with
Sustained, pathogen-specific, systemic antibiotic (according to antibiogram), and
Oral prednisone, 1 mg/kg body weight with subsequent tapering
or
Oral dapsone 100–200 mg daily, in combination with
Oral zinc gluconate 30 mg daily, and
Intralesional triamcinolone acetonide 5–10 mg/ml
In severe and refractory cases, large-scale surgical excision in combination with reconstructive surgery
or
Subcutaneous adalimumab 40 mg every 2 weeks (Fig. 3.24h, i)
Folliculitis keloidalis nuchae
Patient should refrain from shaving the nape of the neck
Early lesions may be treated with a combination of cryotherapy and intralesional triamcinolone acetonide 10–40 mg/ml
Daily topical antiseptics or antibiotics, such as povidone iodine shampoo, shampoo with 0.2–2 % chlorhexidine gluconate, or topical clindamycin solution
During inflammatory phases, oral doxycycline 200 mg daily, or minocycline 100 mg daily, or erythromycin 1–2 g daily
In case of keloid-like plaques may consider CO_2 laser evaporation
Tinea capitis (children)
Systemic antimycotic treatment, in case of endotrich infection with *Trichophyton* spp. with oral terbinafine 6 mg/kg body weight per day for 2–4 weeks, in case of exotrich infection with *Microsporum* spp. with oral itraconazole 5 mg/kg body weight per day for 4–6 weeks, in combination with
Topical antimycotic treatment, either as shampoo (selenium disulfide, ketoconazole, or povidone iodine) or topical antimycotic agent (ciclopiroxolamine, an imidazole, or terbinafine)
May combine oral prednisone 1 mg/kg body weight per day for 1–2 weeks in case of deep inflammatory tinea (Kerion)
Combine with oral antibiotic, preferably an oral macrolide antibiotic, if secondary pathogenic bacterial infection is present
Check for carrier status for sanitation of family members or pets, depending on anthropophilic or zoophilic fungal agent resp. detected in mycologic culture

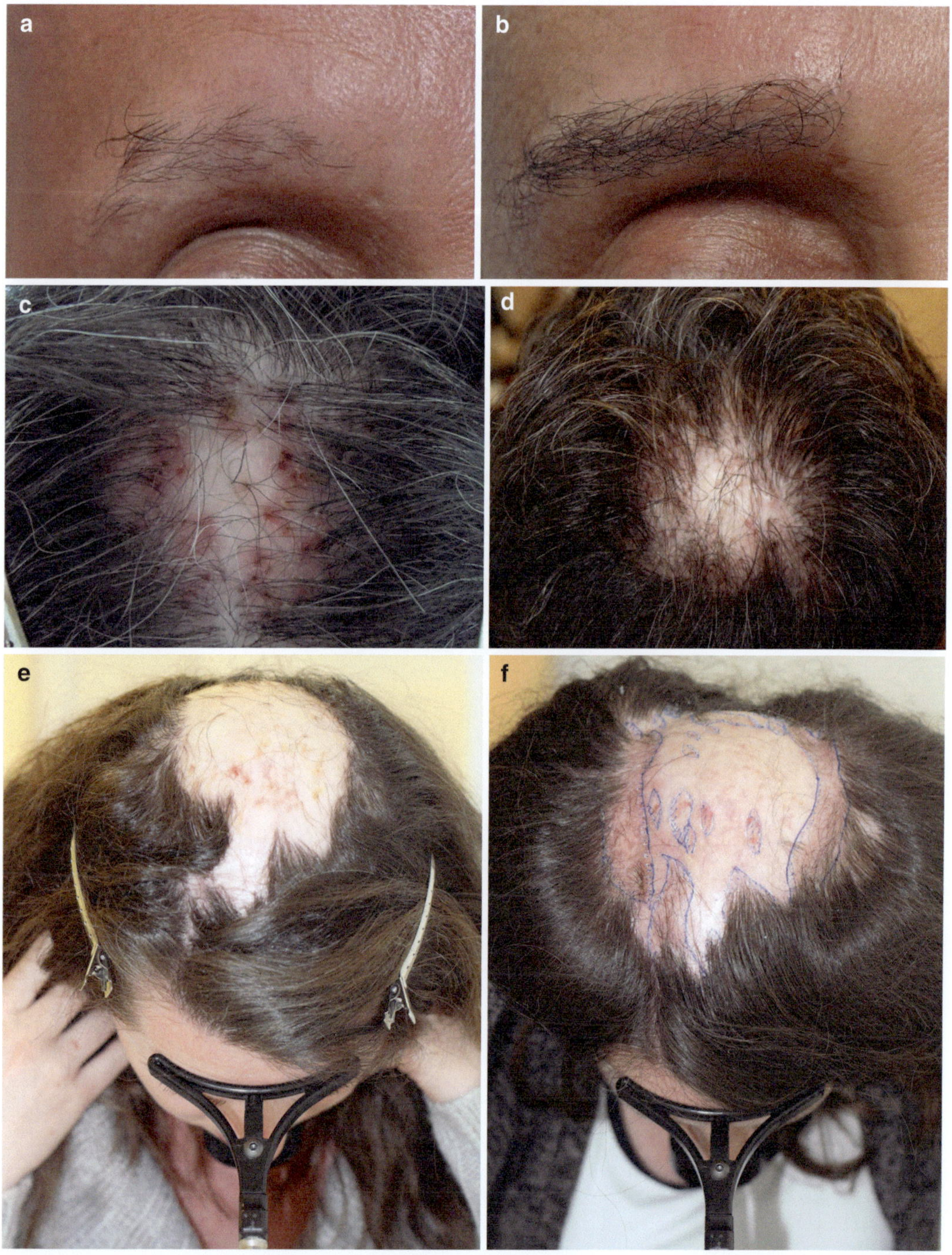

Fig. 3.24 (**a**–**i**) Successful treatment of scarring alopecias: (**a**, **b**) autologous hair transplantation of eyebrows in frontal fibrosing alopecia (Courtesy of Dr. B.Banholzer, MD); (**c**, **d**) folliculitis decalvans treated with oral fusidic acid, oral zinc gluconate, and daily antiseptic washing with a shampoo containing 2 % chlorhexidine gluconate; (**e**–**g**) surgical reduction of scarring alopecia due to folliculitis decalvans with use of expander; and (**h**, **i**) dissecting cellulitis of the scalp treated with subcutaneous adalimumab 40 mg every other week

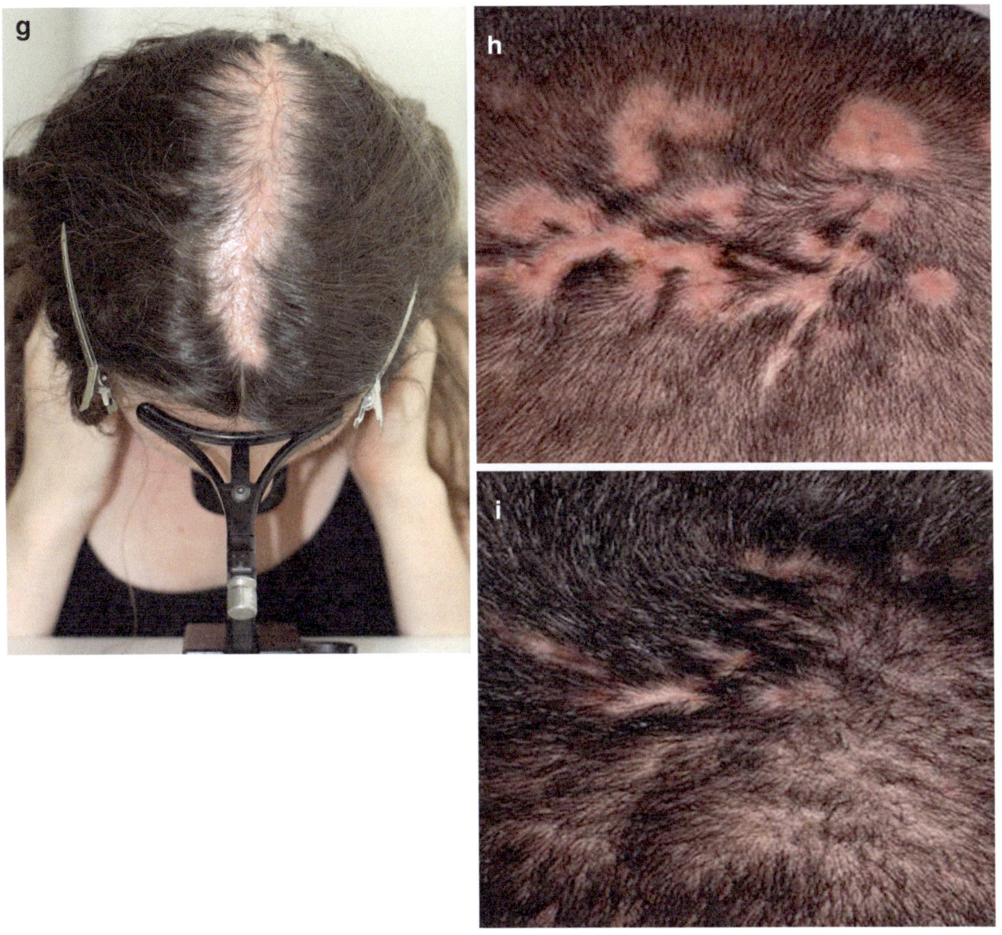

Fig. 3.24 (continued)

3.5.6 Alopecia Mucinosa

Follicular mucinosis is an uncommon condition affecting the pilosebaceous unit, presenting clinically as grouped follicular papules or plaques with associated hair loss (alopecia mucinosa), most commonly on the face, neck, and scalp (Fig. 3.25a). The term is used in pathology to describe mucinous infiltration with cystic mucinous changes in the epithelium of hair follicles. Follicular mucin can be viewed as follicular plugs of amorphous material in dilated follicular ostia by dermoscopy. Alopecia mucinosa may be primary (idiopathic) or secondary to cutaneous T-cell lymphoma (mycosis fungoides).

Since the original descriptions, evidence is accumulating that patient age, distribution of lesions, and duration or extent of disease do not reliably distinguish between benign primary follicular mucinosis and secondary follicular mucinosis, associated with cutaneous lymphoma. Finally, it has been suggested that individuals with follicular mucinosis demonstrating a clonal T-cell receptor gene rearrangement may be at higher risk for the development of lymphoma.

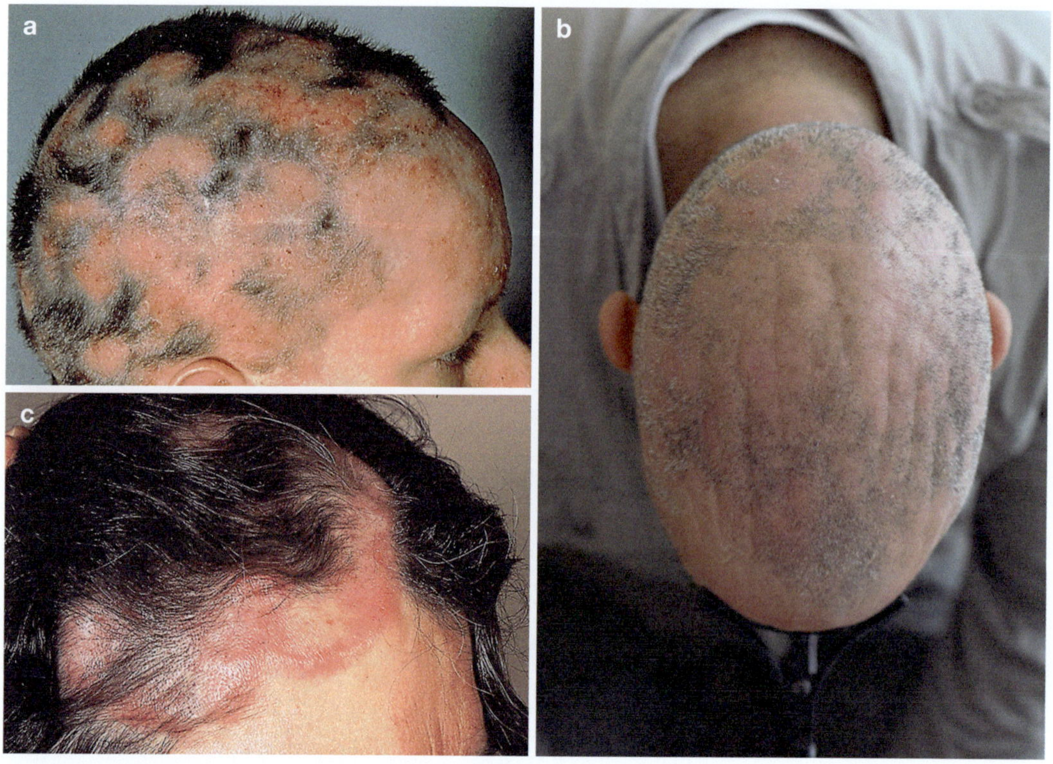

Fig. 3.25 (**a–c**) Lymphoproliferative diseases: (**a**) alopecia mucinosa, (**b**) folliculotropic mycosis fungoides, and (**c**) primary cutaneous follicle center cell lymphoma

Therefore, continued long-term follow-up of patients with clonal primary follicular mucinosis is necessary to determine the significance of infiltrates harboring a T-cell receptor gene rearrangement.

Folliculotropic mycosis fungoides represents another cutaneous lymphoproliferative disorder affecting the pilosebaceous unit. Histopathologic examination demonstrates an infiltration of atypical lymphocytes predominantly around the follicles, while alcian blue stain fails to show mucinosis. Southern blot analysis allows detection of monoclonal T-cell receptor gene rearrangement. The morphologic spectrum of clinical presentation is broad and distinct from conventional mycosis fungoides. This is at least partially due to the ability of the disease to simulate a variety of inflammatory conditions afflicting the follicular unit. In comparison to conventional mycosis fungoides, the disease course seems to be more aggressive, and many patients, including those with early disease, show a poorer outcome, particularly between 10 and 15 years after clinical onset of disease. The condition shows distinct clinical features, with predominant head and face involvement. The morphologic spectrum of lesions is broad and includes erythematous papules and plaques with follicular prominence with or without alopecic patches (Fig. 3.25b) and comedonal, acneiform, or cystic lesions that can be visualized by dermoscopy.

Of the lymphoproliferative diseases affecting the scalp, *primary cutaneous follicle center cell lymphoma* (follicular relates to the lymph follicle and not to the hair follicle) probably represents the most common. It is defined as a lymphoma of follicle center B cells (centrocytes and centroblasts), which has at least a partially follicular pattern. In immunohistopathology it is positive for the respective B-cell markers. It presents with indolent, erythematous nodules of the scalp (Fig. 3.25c). By definition, there is no evidence of extracutaneous disease at the time of diagnosis and after completion of an initial staging evaluation.

3.5.7 Alopecia Neoplastica

Alopecia neoplastica represents yet another condition that may present as a scarring alopecia, appearing anywhere on the scalp. In its original description, it has been defined as hair loss secondary to a visceral malignancy that has metastasized to the scalp. More recently a classification into primary and secondary alopecia neoplastica has been proposed. The clinical presentation may mimic alopecia areata (Fig. 3.26).

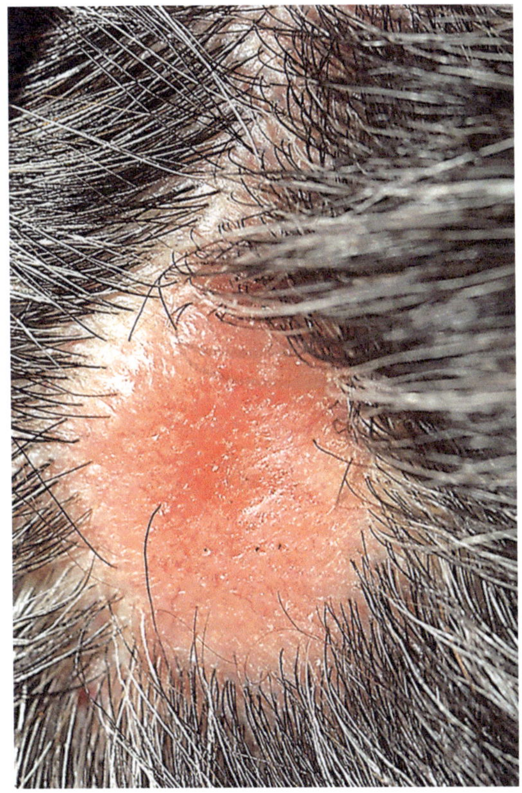

Fig. 3.26 Alopecia neoplastica (cutaneous metastasis to the scalp)

> At times, the diagnosis of alopecia neoplastica may antedate the diagnosis of the underlying malignancy. The suspicion must remain high, and a scalp biopsy will reveal the diagnosis.

In a study of 398 patients with malignant tumors of the scalp, basal (41 %) and squamous cell carcinoma (16.6 %) were the most frequent, followed my metastatic tumors to the scalp in 12.8 %, of which lung cancer was the most frequent primary tumor in both male and female patients. Another study of 197 scalp tumors in women identified basal cell carcinoma in 77 % and squamous cell carcinoma in 17 %, in stark contrast to a frequency of 54 % squamous cell carcinoma in men who were in average older.

Primary scalp tumors are infrequently associated with hair loss. Alopecia caused by primary skin neoplasias has been described most frequently in folliculotropic mycosis fungoides.

Secondary alopecia neoplastica seems to predominate in elderly women, in whom breast cancer accounts for over 80 % of primary tumors. Other primary tumors of which scalp metastases presented as neoplasm-related hair loss have been: gastric, colon, renal, pancreatic, and prostate carcinoma.

3.6 Dystrophic Anagen Effluvium

Dystrophic anagen effluvium is hair loss that results from the shedding of large numbers of hairs from the anagen phase of growth. It is a major characteristic of anagen that the epithelial hair follicle compartment undergoes proliferation, with the hair matrix keratinocytes showing the highest proliferative activity in building up the hair shaft.

The common pathogenesis which unites the different etiologies of dystrophic anagen effluvium is a direct insult to the rapidly dividing bulb matrix cells.

The abrupt cessation of mitotic activity leads to the weakening of the partially keratinized, proximal portion of the hair shaft, its narrowing and subsequent breakage within the hair canal and shedding. The morphologic consequence is the dystrophic anagen hair with a tapered proximal end and lack of root sheath.

Hair loss is usually dramatic, involving 90 % of affected scalp hair that is shed within days to few weeks of the inciting event. The hair loss may be diffuse (in chemotherapy and toxic alopecia) or focal (in radiation-induced alopecia and alopecia areata). Causes for dystrophic anagen effluvium are listed in Table 3.10.

Table 3.10 Causes for dystrophic anagen effluvium

Antineoplastic drugs (chemotherapy-induced alopecia)
X-ray (radiation-induced alopecia)
Environmental or occupational exposure to toxins (toxic alopecia)
Immunologic injury (alopecia areata)

3.6.1 Alopecia Areata

Alopecia areata represents the most frequent cause of dystrophic anagen effluvium, either localized or diffuse, occurring in the otherwise healthy child or adult. It is a common hair loss condition characterized by an acute onset of nonscarring hair loss in usually sharply defined areas. Any hair-bearing area can be affected, but the most noticeable are the scalp, the beard area, and the eyebrows. The characteristic patch of alopecia areata is usually round or oval and is completely bald and smooth. Trichoscopic examination reveals yellow dots, dystrophic hairs (cadaverized hairs, exclamation mark hairs), and/or short regrowing miniaturized hairs.

The progress of alopecia areata in an individual patient is unpredictable, though a large surface area, a long disease duration, and associated nail abnormalities have been connected with a poorer prognosis.

Some patients lose hair in only a small patch, while others may have more extensive or less frequently diffuse involvement. Alopecia totalis is the loss of all scalp hair; alopecia universalis is the loss of all scalp and body hair.

Alopecia areata is considered to be of autoimmune origin with an organ-specific, T-cell-mediated assault on the hair follicle at the level of the bulb. The hair bulb is an immune-protected site with deficient MHC expression. There is circumstantial evidence suggesting that alopecia areata results from loss of immune privilege with presentation of autoantigens. A peribulbar lymphocytic infiltrate induces hair follicle keratinocytes to undergo apoptosis resulting in inhibition of cell division in the hair matrix.

3.6.2 Thomas More Syndrome

Thomas More syndrome designates the condition in which scalp hair suddenly turns white in men (Fig. 3.27a, b). The name alludes to the English martyr Sir Thomas More (1478–1535), whose hair allegedly turned white overnight in the Tower

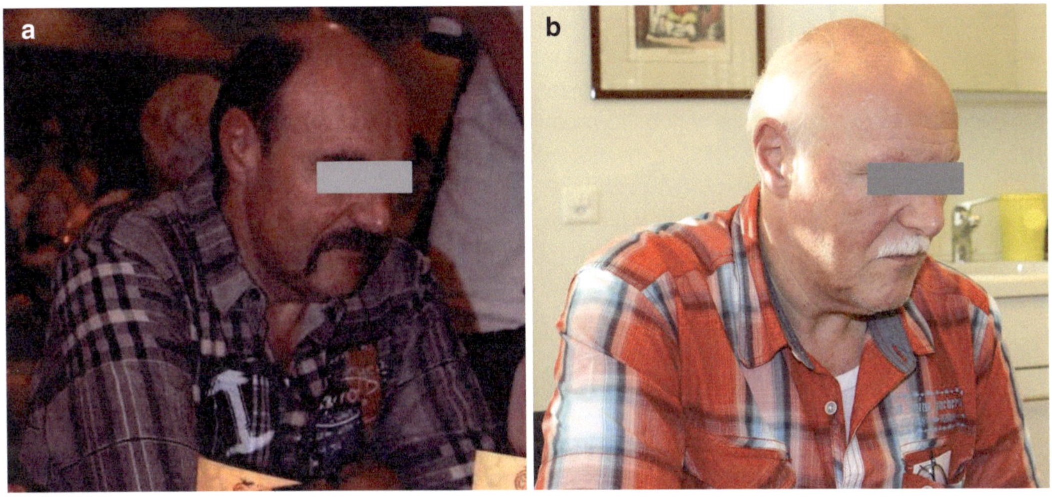

Fig. 3.27 (**a**, **b**) Thomas More syndrome

of London before his execution. Sir Thomas More, also known as Saint Thomas More, was an English lawyer, author, and statesman who in his lifetime gained a reputation as a leading Renaissance humanist scholar and occupied many public offices, including Lord Chancellor from 1529 to 1532. He was beheaded in 1535 after having refused to sign the Act of Supremacy that declared King Henry VIII Supreme Head of the Church of England over the Pope. In 1935, 400 years after More's death, Pope Pius XI canonized him in the Roman Catholic Church, and in 2000 Pope John Paul II officially declared More patron saint of politicians.

Although the actual incidence is rare, this stigmatizing phenomenon has captured storytellers' imagination like few other afflictions as a sign of grave sorrow. The first documented case of sudden hair whitening can be traced back to the Talmud (83 AD), which describes a scholar who was appointed chief of the main Israeli Talmudic academy at the young age of 17 years. Upon his wife's concern that he looked too youthful for the position, he developed 18 rows of white hair. The Jewish rabbi, physician, and philosopher Maimonides (1135–1204) suggested that this was the result of strenuous studying. History also records that the hair of the ill-fated French Queen Marie Antoinette (1755–1793) turned white the night before her last walk to the guillotine during the French Revolution. Hence the original term Marie Antoinette syndrome for the condition that has technically also been called *canities subita*. More modern accounts refer to the turning white of hair in survivors of bomb attacks during World War II.

> Although Marie Antoinette has originally been chosen as eponym for the syndrome, presumably out of dermatologic gallantry, Saint Thomas More, who turned white in 1535, ought to have the right of seniority over the Queen of France who succumbed to the same fate in 1793. Since there seems to be no other particular reason for favoring Marie Antoinette over Thomas More, out of fairness, it seems appropriate to use the term "Marie Antoinette syndrome" for the condition afflicting women and "Thomas More syndrome" for men.

Navarini and Trüeb reported a 56-year-old man with sudden total whitening of scalp hair and eyebrows within weeks. He was otherwise completely healthy and had not experienced any stressful event.

Today, the syndrome is interpreted as an acute episode of diffuse alopecia areata in which the very sudden "overnight" whitening of hair is caused by the preferential loss of pigmented hairs in this supposedly immune-mediated disorder. As early as 1901, immunology research pioneer and Nobel Prize Laureate (1908) in Medicine for his work on phagocytosis, Elie Metchnikoff (1845–1916), believed that whitening of hair was related to pigment absorbed and carried away by phagocytes he observed in the vicinity of dystrophic hair follicles and called "pigmentophages." In 1981, Guin et al. reported a lady whose hair turned white over 3 months with hair thinning but no patches of alopecia. Immunofluorescence studies demonstrated immune deposits along the follicular epithelium suggesting an underlying immunological mechanism. Finally, case reports of sudden canities in association with easily plucked hairs, exclamation mark hairs and patchy alopecia typical for alopecia areata, and in coexistence with other presumably autoimmune phenomena, such as vitiligo, supported the immune theory. Ultimately, these observations have led some authorities to speculate that the autoimmune target in alopecia areata may be related to the hair follicle melanin pigment system. McBride and Bergfeld described mosaic hair color changes in two patients with extensive alopecia areata and suggested that these processes may result from localized immunological reactions against hair follicle melanocytes in a multifocal pattern with subsequent changes in hair color. In contrast to total whitening of hair, this mechanism would account better for the pattern of "18 rows of white hair" originally described in the Talmud. In this case, we are rather dealing with the phenomenon of poliosis than canities subita, and *migratory poliosis* has indeed been described as yet another clinical presentation of alopecia areata.

> Although early accounts of overnight whitening of hair are substantiated by more recent case reports in the scientific literature, it may be suspected that the phenomenon has been used both as a literary stylistic means in fiction, with the aim of dramatizing, and in historical accounts with the claim of authenticity.

Scrutinizing the case of Henry III of Navarre (later King Henry IV of France), whose hair allegedly turned white overnight on the occasion of the horrors of St. Bartholomew's day massacre in 1572, Navarini and Trüeb found inconsistencies between Henry's biography and the current pathophysiological understanding of canities subita. According to the current pathogenetic understanding, a prerequisite for overnight whitening of hair would be that the individual in question has a salt-and-pepper pattern, with pigmented hairs interspersed with white hairs. Only if this is the case can the pigmented hairs be selectively shed, while the white hairs remain giving the impression of sudden whitening – otherwise total alopecia would result. Given that the current hypothesis of the syndrome's pathophysiology holds true, it seems quite improbable that Henry III of Navarre's hair should have turned white so rapidly, as he was only 19 years old at the time in question.

3.6.3 Treatment Algorithm for Alopecia Areata

A recent meta-analysis of published trials on treatment of alopecia areata states that only few treatments have been well evaluated in randomized trials. The authors found no randomized controlled trials on the use of diphenylcyclopropenone (DCP), intralesional corticosteroids, or dithranol, although commonly used in clinical practice. Although topical steroids and minoxidil are widely prescribed and appear to be safe, there is no convincing evidence that they are beneficial

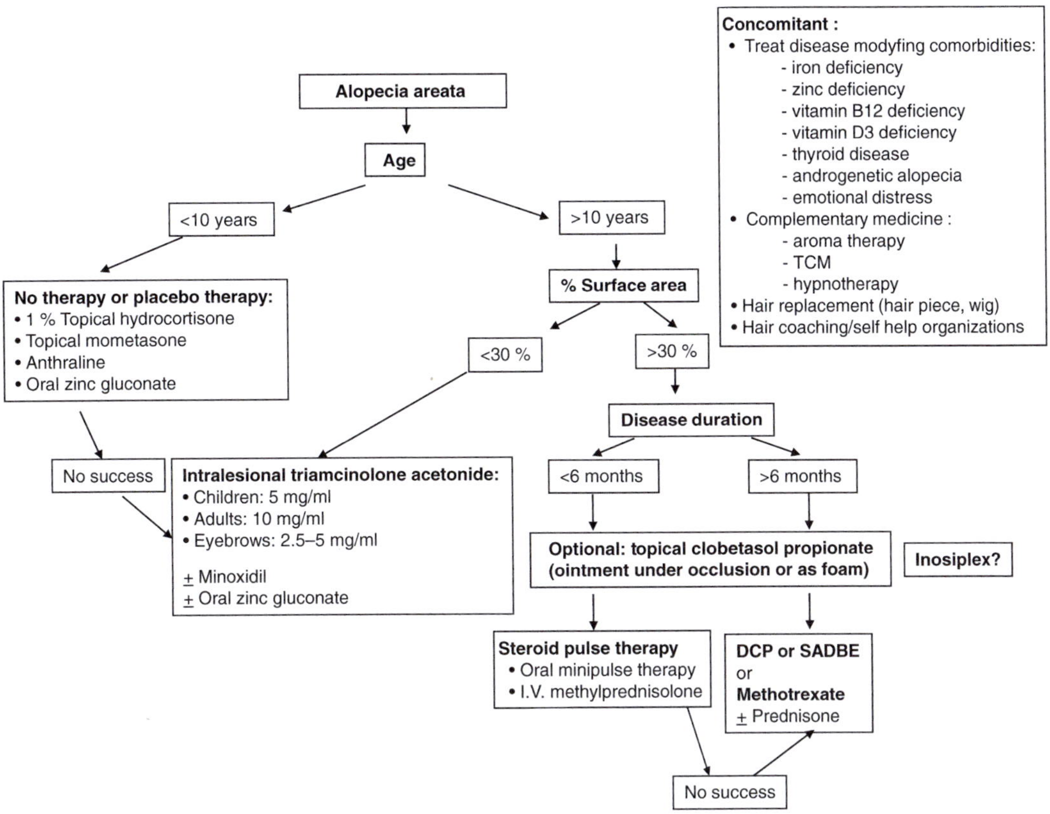

Fig. 3.28 Algorithm for treatment of alopecia areata

in the long term. Most trials have been reported poorly and are so small that any important clinical benefits are inconclusive. Of 17 trials including 6–85 participants with a total of 540 participants assessing a range of interventions that included topical and oral corticosteroids, topical ciclosporin, photodynamic therapy, and topical minoxidil, none showed significant treatment benefit in terms of hair growth when compared with placebo. The authors came to the conclusion that considering the possibility of spontaneous remission, especially for those in the early stages of the disease, the options of not being treated therapeutically or, depending on individual preference, of wearing a wig may be alternative ways of dealing with this condition.

Nonetheless, depending on patient age, surface area, and disease duration, a treatment algorithm can be designed (Fig. 3.28). Any treatment of alopecia areata should fulfill the following criteria:

- Remission rates superior to the spontaneous remission rates of alopecia areata
- Proof of efficacy in half-side treatment of alopecia totalis or universalis
- Good safety profile with minimal toxicity

The spontaneous remission rates for patchy alopecia areata are one-third within 6 months, half within 1 year, and two thirds within 5 years; thereafter, complete remissions are rare.

Recurrence rates within 5 years are 80 % and within 20 years 100 %. Total remission rates for alopecia totalis or universalis with a disease duration of 5 years or more are one percent in children and less than 10 % in adults.

Single patches of alopecia areata are best treated with intralesional triamcinolone acetonide 10 mg/ml by jet injector or insulin syringe on a monthly basis, for an average of 3 to a maximum of six consecutive treatments (in children 5 mg/ml, for eyebrows 2.5–5 mg/ml, and for beard 5 mg/ml by insulin syringe) (Fig. 3.29a, b).

With pulse corticosteroid therapy (500 mg IV methylprednisolone on three consecutive days, in three cycles 4 weeks apart) within 6 months of disease onset, remission rates are 88 % for multilocular alopecia areata with a surface area <50 %,

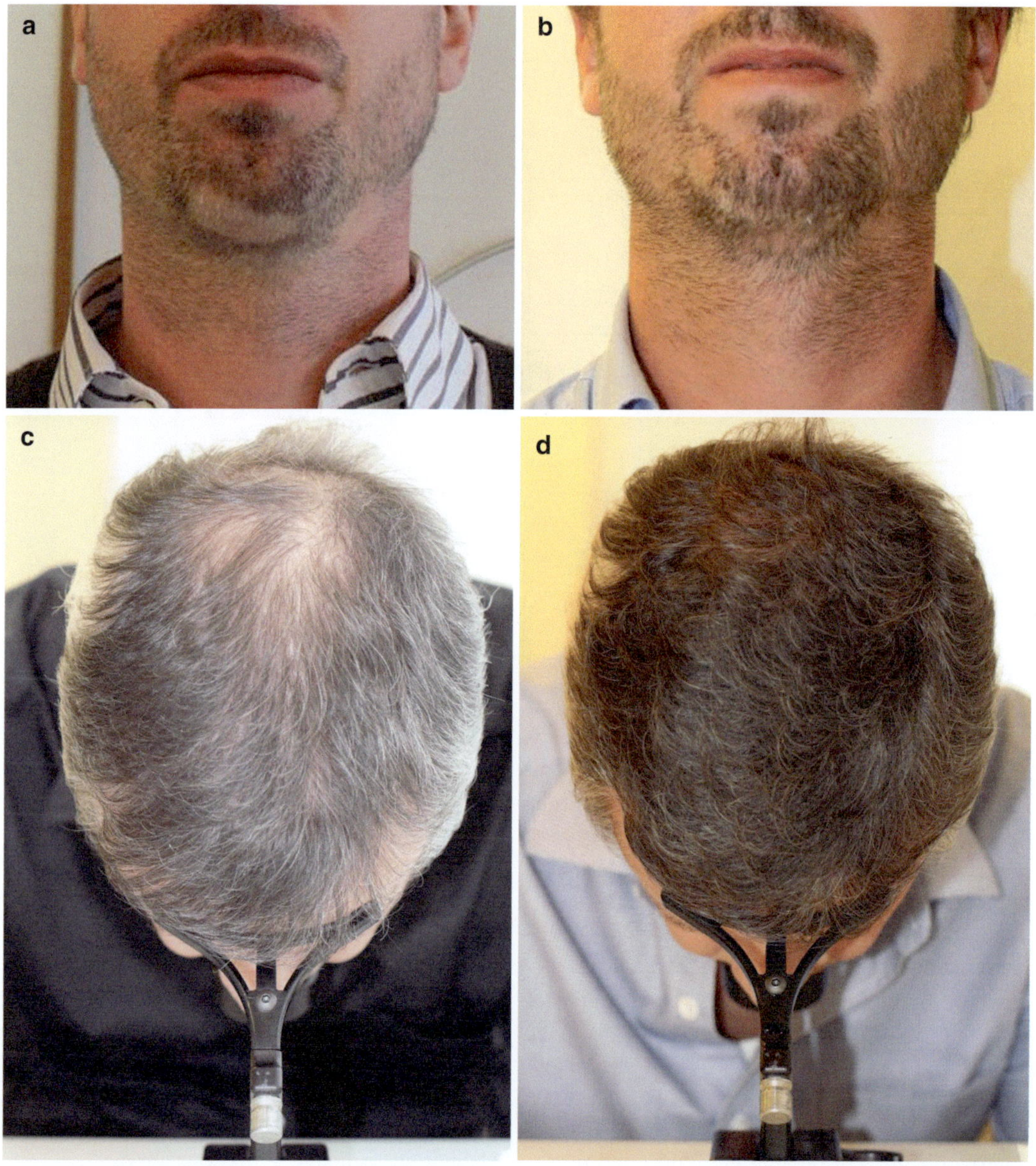

Fig. 3.29 (**a–j**) Successful treatments in alopecia areata: (**a**, **b**) of the beard area in a 31-year-old man with intralesional triamcinolone acetonide 10 mg/ml (**a**) before and (**b**) after 3 months of treatment; (**c**, **d**) in a 51-year-old man with compound of topical 5 % minoxidil and 0.2 % triamcinolone acetonide twice daily, (**c**) before and (**d**) after 3 months of treatment; (**e**, **f**) in a 10-year-old boy with IV methylprednisolone pulse therapy, (**e**) before and (**f**) 5 months after treatment; (**g**, **h**) in a 40-year-old man with clobetasol propionate ointment under occlusion, (**g**) before and (**h**) after 6 months treatment; and (**i**, **j**) in a 45-year-old man with topical immunotherapy (DCP) (**i**) before and (**j**) after 9 months treatment

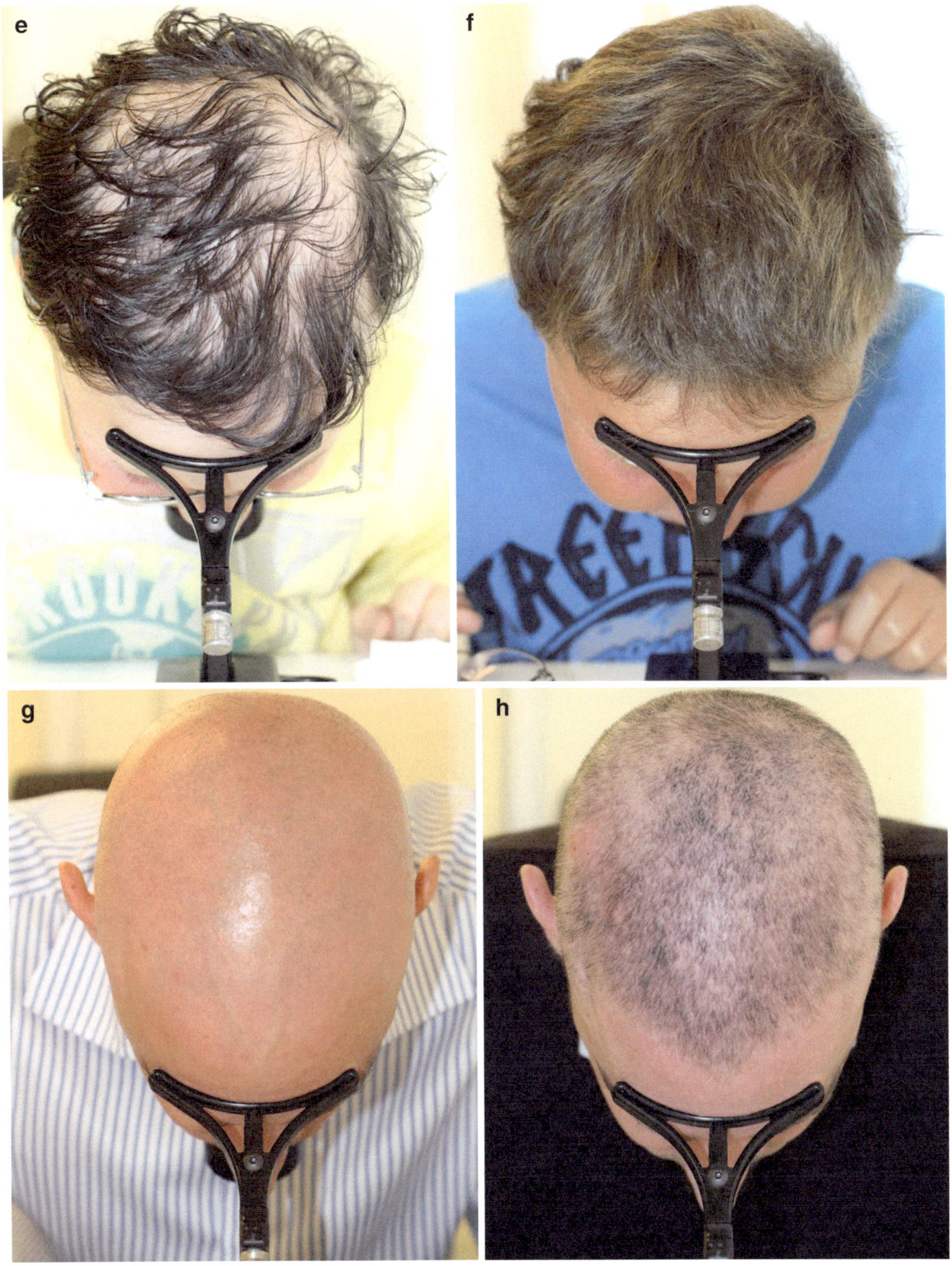

Fig. 3.29 (continued)

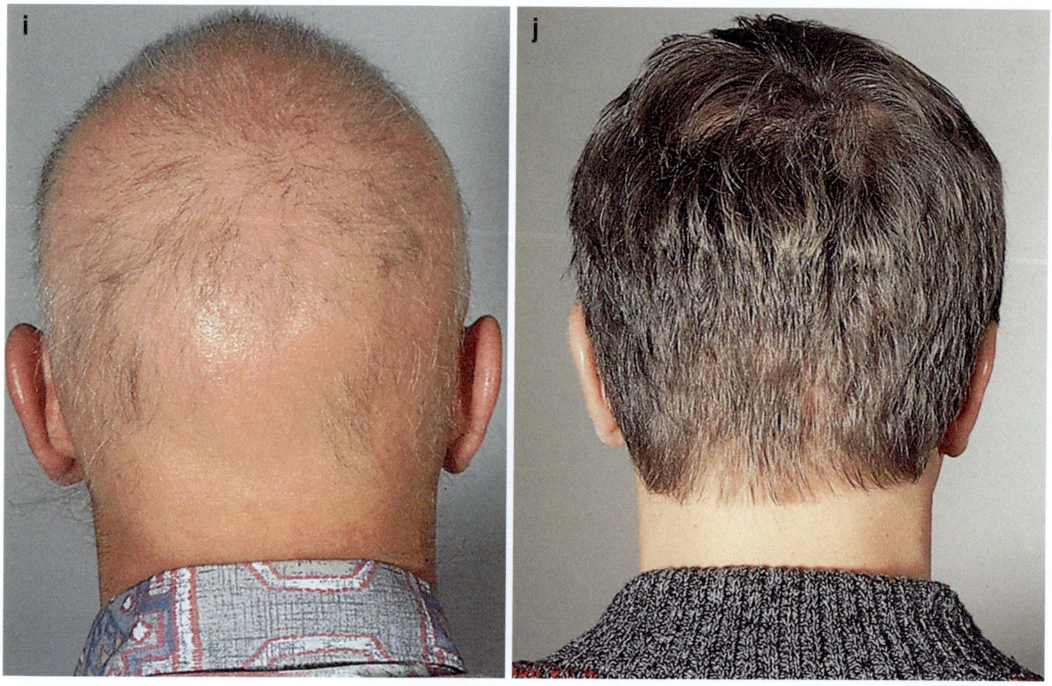

Fig. 3.29 (continued)

59.4 % with a surface area >50 %, and 21.4 % in alopecia totalis (Fig. 3.29e, f). After 6 months of disease onset, the remission rate is 15.8 %.

With 0.05 % topical clobetasol ointment under occlusion (Saran wrap) on six consecutive nights per week over 6 months, regrowth of hair is achieved in alopecia totalis or universalis in 17.8 %. Despite positive clinical results obtained using clobetasol ointment with occlusive dressing, this approach has a low patient compliance, especially in patients with residual hair (Fig. 3.29g, h). More recently, 0.05 % clobetasol foam applied twice daily on five consecutive days per week proved to also be an effective, safe, and well-tolerated treatment with good cosmetic acceptance and patient compliance.

In a retrospective study of 68 patients with severe alopecia areata (>40 % scalp hair loss) treated for at least 5 months with topical diphenylcyclopropenone (DCP), Pericin and Trüeb found an overall response rate of 70.6 % with 30.9 % complete remission and 39.7 % partial remission. Among the investigated prognostic factors for the outcome of DCP therapy, only the extent of alopecia areata at the time of initiation of treatment was found to be of significance. Total remission rates for multilocular alopecia areata was 43.8 %, for subtotal alopecia areata and ophiasis 33.3 %, and for alopecia totalis or universalis 21.4 %, irrespective of disease duration (Fig. 3.29i, j).

Joly proposed the use of methotrexate (MTX) alone or in combination with low doses of oral corticosteroids in the treatment of alopecia areata totalis and universalis with an overall success rate of 64 %. Best results are achieved with subcutaneous MTX in the maximal dosage of 30 mg weekly in combination with 20 mg oral prednisone daily with regrowth of hair beginning within 2–4 months of therapy. Drug toxicities are to be carefully weighed out against treatment benefit.

Potentially disease-modifying comorbidities are to be sought out and simultaneously treated such as deficiencies of iron, zinc, vitamin B12, and vitamin D3; thyroid dysfunction; androgenetic alopecia; and emotional distress.

Some authors advocate combination treatment with antidepressant agents in alopecia areata with comorbid depression. Others suggest that hypnotherapy may enhance the mental well-being of patients with alopecia areata, though no effect on hair regrowth could be shown. Ultimately, the options available for adapting to the disease rather than treating in an effort to cure are to be taken into consideration in selected long-standing widespread cases or recurrent small spot disease.

> New drug treatment opportunities based on the results of genome-wide association studies that implicate T cell and natural killer cell activation pathways are paving the way to new approaches in future clinical trials for alopecia areata.

Currently, there are ongoing studies with the CTLA4–Ig fusion protein abatacept (blocks costimulation of T cells), anti-IL15Rβ monoclonal antibodies (blocks activation of CD8+ T cells), and the Janus kinase (JAK) 3 inhibitor tofacitinib and JAK 1/3 inhibitor ruxolitinib (block signal transduction at the IL-15 receptor).

3.6.4 Postoperative Pressure Alopecia

Postoperative pressure alopecia represents another form of dystrophic anagen effluvium frequently mistaken for alopecia areata, but of traumatic origin and localized to the occipital scalp. Patients typically complain of occipital pain and tenderness within 24 h of surgery. Signs observed within the first week after surgery may be focal swelling, edema, crusting, and ulceration. The hair loss is set in between 2 and 3 weeks after surgery and is complete within 28 days (Fig. 3.30).

Postoperative pressure alopecia has been originally reported after open cardiac surgery and is now increasingly observed following lengthy plastic surgical procedures. It occurs after prolonged pressure on the scalp during general anesthesia with intubation, with the head fixed in one position, and understood to be due to pressure-induced ischemia.

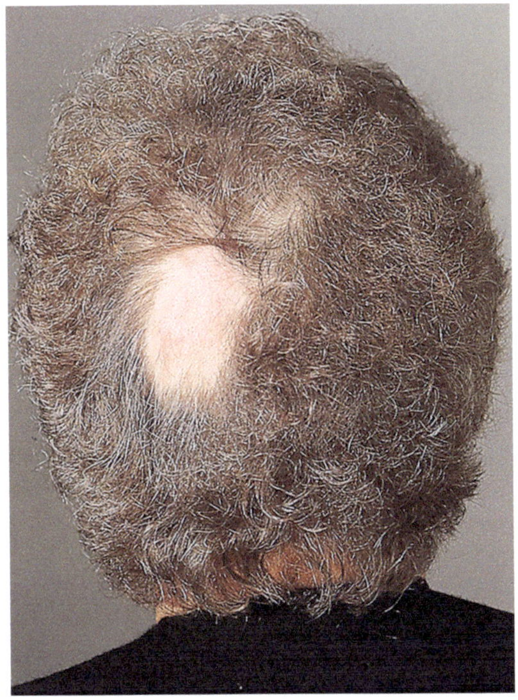

Fig. 3.30 Postoperative pressure alopecia

Risk factors for hair loss and scarring include length of the anesthesia, prolonged endotracheal intubation, prolonged head immobilization, intraoperative use of the Trendelenburg position, and additional factors potentially aggravating ischemia of the scalp, such as severe hypotension, massive blood loss, and use of vasoconstrictors.

The single most important aspect of prevention of this complication of surgery is knowledge of its existence and pathophysiology. A prospective study that incorporated head repositioning every 30 min in cardiac surgical patients significantly reduced the incidence of alopecia from a prospectively determined value of 14 to 1 %.

Fortunately, the condition is self-limiting in most cases with spontaneous regrowth of hair occurring within 3 months. In case of necrosis, ulceration, and scarring, the alopecia is permanent.

3.6.5 Temporary Radiation-Induced Epilation Following Neuroradiologically Guided Embolization Procedure

Temporary radiation-induced epilation following neuroradiologically guided embolization procedures represents yet another form of dystrophic anagen effluvium mistaken for alopecia areata. Since the anagen hair follicle is highly susceptible to x-ray exposure, loss of dystrophic hairs (dystrophic anagen effluvium) results from acute damage to the actively dividing matrix cells of anagen follicles. Hair loss occurs within the exposure area to x-rays (Fig. 3.31), and most patients notice hair loss two to 3 weeks following radiation exposure.

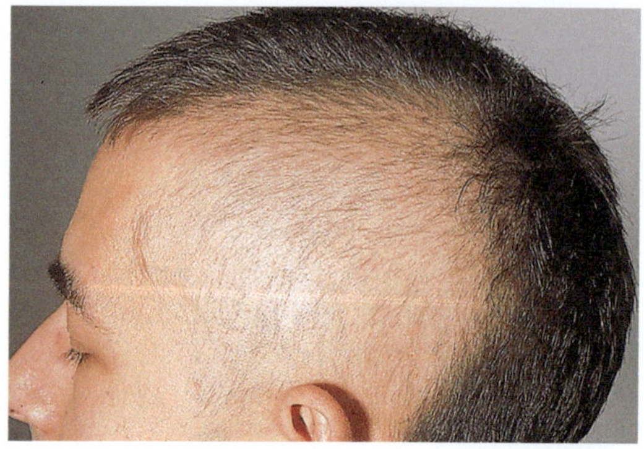

Fig. 3.31 Temporary radiation-induced epilation following neuroradiologically guided embolization procedure

> Radiation-induced alopecia may either be temporary or permanent, depending on the amount of radiation and other treatments received, such as concomitant chemotherapy. Hair loss occurs on hair-bearing skin with doses above 300–400 cGy and is permanent with a single dose above 1,200 cGy. If the dose is fractionated, permanent hair loss may not occur until the dose exceeds 4,500 cGy.

If the hair loss is temporary, complete hair regrowth occurs 2–4 months after x-ray exposure.

Krasovec and Trüeb originally reported temporary radiation-induced epilation following a neuroradiologically guided embolization procedure in the dermatologic literature. Endovascular procedures have become a widely used treatment of cerebral vascular malformation.

> Transient radiation-induced alopecia following neuroradiologically guided therapeutic embolization of cerebral vascular malformation is probably underreported, since it seems not to be an uncommon event.

It has been misinterpreted to be due to arterial occlusion; moreover, excluding the differential diagnosis of alopecia areata may be difficult, since the bald patch is devoid of inflammatory signs, and hair loss is characterized by dystrophic hair. The patient history, chronology of events, localization, and the geometry of the bald patch usually allow correct diagnosis.

3.6.6 Recommendations for Care to Minimize Scalp Reaction to Radiation

The scalp skin is sensitive to radiation and more so after hair loss. The skin may become erythematous, tender, or inflamed, much like a sunburn. After 2 or 3 weeks of radiation exposure, the scalp may become dry and itchy. If necessary, treatment can be prescribed to relieve discomfort and itching. Protection from UV radiation is mandatory. Recommendations for hair and scalp care are summarized in Table 3.11.

3.7 Chemotherapy-Induced Hair Loss

Chemotherapy-induced hair loss is considered a traumatic experience in cancer patient care, since hair loss negatively affects a patient's perception of appearance, body image, and self-esteem. Ultimately, patients feel deprived of their privacy

Table 3.11 Recommendations for patients to minimize scalp reaction to radiation treatment

Avoid frequent shampooing. Use a mild shampoo without any perfumes
Wash scalp with warm water only. Avoid rubbing or scratching. Pat dry with a soft towel
Avoid excessively combing or brushing hair
Avoid using hair spray, oils, or creams
Avoid using heat sources, including hair dryers, rollers, or curling irons
Do not perm or color hair until about 4 weeks after radiation treatment is complete
Protect head from sun, cold, and wind by wearing a head covering

Table 3.12 Cytotoxic agents and hair loss

Cytostatic agents which usually do cause hair loss	
Adriamycin	Docetaxel
Daunorubicin	Paclitaxel
Etoposide	Ifosfamide
Irinotecan	Vindesine
Cyclophosphamide	Vinorelbine
Epirubicin	Topotecan
Cytotoxic agents which sometimes cause hair loss	
Amsacrine	Vincristine
Cytarabine	Vinblastine
Bleomycin	Lomustine
Busulfan	Thiotepa
5-Fluorouracil	Gemcitabine
Melphalan	
Cytotoxic agents which unusually cause hair loss	
Methotrexate	Procarbazine
Carmustine	6-Mercaptopurine
Mitoxantrone	Streptozotocin
Mitomycin C	Fludarabine
Carboplatin	Raltritrexate
Cisplatin	Capecitabine

because the hair loss is readily interpreted by the lay public as associated with having cancer.

Chemotherapy-induced hair loss occurs with an estimated overall incidence of 65 %. The incidence and severity of the hair loss are variable and related to the particular chemotherapeutic agent and protocol: multiple classes of anticancer drugs induce alopecia (Table 3.12), with frequencies of chemotherapy-induced hair loss differing for the four major drug classes – more than 80 % for antimicrotubule agents (e.g., paclitaxel), 60–100 % for topoisomerase inhibitors (e.g., doxorubicin), more than 60 % for alkylators (e.g., cyclophosphamide), and 10–50 % for antimetabolites (e.g., 5-fluorouracil plus leucovorin). Combination therapy consisting of two or more agents usually produces greater incidences of more severe hair loss compared with single-agent therapy.

3.7.1 Patterns of Chemotherapy-Induced Hair Loss

Chemotherapy-induced hair loss is a consequence of direct toxic insult to the rapidly dividing cells of the hair follicle. It is a major characteristic of the anagen hair follicle that the epithelial compartment undergoes proliferation, with the bulb matrix cells showing the greatest proliferative activity in building up the hair shaft. The abrupt cessation of mitotic activity leads to the weakening of the partially keratinized, proximal portion of the hair shaft, a narrowing, and a subsequent breakage within the hair canal. The consequence is hair shedding that usually begins at 1–3 weeks after initiation of chemotherapy. Due to its long anagen phase, the scalp is the most common location for hair loss, while other terminal hairs are variably affected depending on the percentage of hairs in anagen. Since normally up to 90 % of scalp hair is in the anagen phase, hair loss is usually copious, and the resulting alopecia is quite obvious (Fig. 3.32). Nevertheless, chemotherapy given at high doses for a sufficiently long time and with multiple exposures may also affect the beard, eyebrows, eyelashes, and axillary and pubic hairs.

While chemotherapy-induced hair loss has traditionally been categorized as acute diffuse hair loss caused by dystrophic anagen effluvium, more recently it has been pointed out that, in fact, chemotherapy-induced hair loss may present with different pathomechanisms and clinical patterns.

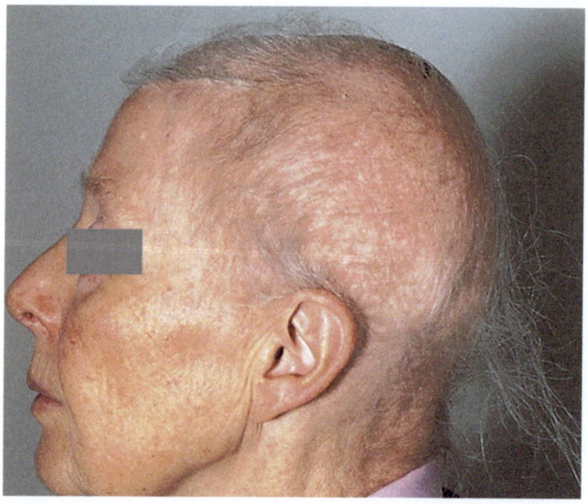

Fig. 3.32 Chemotherapy-induced alopecia

Evidence exists that the hair follicle may respond to the same insult capable of stopping mitosis with both shedding patterns, dystrophic anagen effluvium, and telogen effluvium. Accordingly, the hair may fall out very quickly in clumps or gradually. When mitotic activity is arrested, numerous and interacting factors may influence the shedding pattern. One of these factors is the mitotic activity of the hair follicle at the moment of the insult.

When the hair is in its late anagen phase, in which the mitotic rate is slowing down spontaneously, it simply accelerates its normal path to telogen, while mitotically inactive phases (catagen and telogen) are not affected. Since anagen duration is diminished in androgenetic alopecia, the probability is increased that the antimitotic insult strikes the hair close to the resting phase resulting in telogen effluvium. While synchronization of hair cycles also plays a role, and again in androgenetic alopecia, the hair cycles tend to synchronize due to the diminished duration of anagen, even a minor antimitotic insult may produce marked hair loss.

The hair loss generally is usually reversible, with hair regrowth typically occurring after a delay of 3–6 months. In some patients, the regrown hair shows changes in color and/or texture. It might be curlier than it was before, or it could be gray until the follicular melanocytes begin functioning again. But the difference is usually temporary.

Ultimately, permanent alopecia has been reported after chemotherapy with busulfan and cyclophosphamide after bone marrow transplantation and has been associated with certain risk factors, including chronic graft-versus-host reaction, previous exposure to x-ray, and patient age.

3.7.2 Possibilities for Prevention or Reversal of Chemotherapy-Induced Hair Loss

A number of preventive measures have been proposed and tried to reduce chemotherapy-induced hair loss. Nevertheless, no treatment exists that can guarantee to prevent chemotherapy-induced hair loss.

> Of the treatments so far investigated, scalp cooling (hypothermia) has been the most widely used and studied.

Of 53 multiple patient studies published between 1973 and 2003 on the results of scalp cooling for the prevention of chemotherapy-induced hair loss, seven trials were randomized. In six of the seven randomized studies, a significant advantage was observed with scalp cooling. The positive results were most evident when anthracyclines or taxanes were the chemotherapeutic agents.

In the most recent open-label, prospective, nonrandomized clinical trial, patients with solid tumors receiving docetaxel in a palliative setting were allocated according to patients' preference to short-term cooling (over 45 min postinfusion) with a Paxman® PSC-2 machine (PAX), with cold cap (CC), or with no cooling. The combined end point was alopecia World Health Organization (WHO) III or IV or the necessity to wear a wig. Two hundred thirty-eight patients were included in the trial (128 patients PAX, 71 CC, and 39 no cooling). The number of cycles (median 4) and median docetaxel doses were similar across the three groups (55–60 mg/day on weekly therapy, 135–140 mg/day on 3-week therapy). Alopecia occurred with PAX, CC, and no cooling under 3-week docetaxel in 23, 27, and 74 % and under weekly docetaxel in 7, 8, and 17 %, respectively. Overall, cooling (PAX and CC combined) reduced risk of alopecia by 78 % (hazard ratio 0.22; 95 % confidence interval 0.12–0.41). CC and PAX prophylaxis led to the same degree of prevention of alopecia. In this first comparison study published to date, both PAX and CC offered efficacious protection against hair loss, in particular when docetaxel was administered in a 3-week interval.

In several publications, authors have expressed their concerns about the risk of scalp skin metastases after cooling.

> Therefore, scalp cooling has remained contraindicated for those with hematological malignancies, and its use remains controversial in patients with non-hematological malignancies who undergo curative chemotherapy.

Patients undergoing scalp hypothermia commonly report feeling uncomfortably cold and suffering of headaches.

So far, no approved pharmacologic treatment exists for chemotherapy-induced hair loss. Among the agents that so far have been evaluated in cancer patients, the topical hair growth-promoting agent minoxidil was able to shorten the duration, albeit did not prevent chemotherapy-induced hair loss. Minoxidil also failed to induce significant regrowth of hair in busulfan- and cyclophosphamide-induced permanent alopecia.

Advances have been made in the understanding of the pathobiology of chemotherapy-induced hair loss, and several experimental approaches to the development of pharmacologic agents are under evaluation. Because the rapid cell proliferation of hair follicle keratinocytes during anagen renders the hair follicle susceptible to the toxicity of chemotherapy, a strategy to protect against chemotherapy-induced hair loss is arresting the cell cycle to reduce the sensitivity of the follicular epithelium to cell cycle-active antitumor agents. Inhibition of cyclin-dependent kinase 2 (CDK2), a positive regulator of the eukaryotic cell cycle, is believed to represent an approach for prevention of chemotherapy-induced hair loss by arresting the cell cycle. Potent small-molecule inhibitors of CDK2 are currently being developed using structure-based methods. Ultimately, the protection should be selective to the hair follicle, such that the anticancer efficacy of chemotherapy is not hampered. In view of the fact that cancer usually is treated with combinations of chemotherapeutics, an effective treatment of chemotherapy-induced hair loss would likely require agents that are effective for different chemotherapeutics with different action mechanisms. Moreover, variations in patient characteristics must be taken into account, since the pattern of chemotherapy-induced hair loss varies in individual patients.

Since chemotherapy-induced hair loss cannot be reliably prevented, the best way to deal with it is to plan ahead with a focus on making the patient as comfortable as possible with his appearance before, during, and after cancer treatment.

> The major approach to prevent or minimize chemotherapy-induced hair loss remains scalp cooling, while topical minoxidil may speed up hair regrowth.

Even if chemotherapy-induced hair loss cannot be prevented, it can be managed. Anticipating hair loss, coming to terms with the inevitability of hair loss, and taking control are the key steps in coping with chemotherapy-induced hair loss. Recommendations for hair care are summarized in Table 3.13.

3.7.3 Side Effects from Molecularly Targeted Therapies for Cancer

Molecularly targeted therapy for cancer is a type of medication that blocks the growth of cancer cells by interfering with specific targeted

Table 3.13 Chemotherapy-induced hair loss. Recommendations for hair care

Avoidance of physical or chemical trauma, such as bleaching, coloring, or perming of hair, curling irons, and hot rollers
Gentle hair strategies should be continued throughout chemotherapy, using a satin pillowcase, which is less likely to attract and catch fragile hair, using a soft brush, washing hair only as often as necessary and using a gentle shampoo
Cutting hair short or shaving hair. Short hair tends to look fuller than long hair, and when the hair is shed, it won't be as noticeable when it is short. Moreover, cut hair might help to make a better transition to total alopecia. Also, a shaved head may be easier for securing a wig or hairpiece
Appropriate head covering should be planned ahead. Head covering as the hair falls out is a very personal decision. For women in particular, chemotherapy-induced hair loss involves a confrontation with the nature of their disease, while for men it is a normal and inevitable consequence of treatment. Depending on individual preference, temporarily wearing a wig or another head covering until the hair regrows may be the most effective way of dealing with this condition, while protecting the scalp from sun and cold exposure at the same time

molecules needed for carcinogenesis and tumor growth, rather than by simply interfering with all rapidly dividing cells, as with traditional chemotherapy. Therefore, targeted cancer therapies are expected to be more effective than current treatments while being less harmful to normal cells.

Many are tyrosine kinase inhibitors. Among them are EGFR (epidermal growth factor receptor) inhibitors. Well-documented hair changes associated with EGFR inhibitors are transformation of the hair shaft property into curly, fine, and brittle texture; eyelash trichomegaly; and alopecia accompanied by a peculiar diffusely red, atrophic scalp studded with papulopustules, erosions, and crusting. Scarring alopecia may also occur and may represent a severe form of the condition.

3.8 Toxic Alopecia

Toxic alopecia is diffuse hair loss that occurs as a result of exposure to certain toxins. Following exposure, hair growth is abruptly interrupted, and dystrophic anagen hair is shed. Many heavy metals are capable of disrupting the formation of the hair shaft through covalent binding with the sulfhydryl groups in keratin: thallium, mercury, arsenic, copper, cadmium, and bismuth.

> Toxic alopecia from occupational exposure to hazardous chemicals has decreased over the years due to more stringent governmental regulations.

More recently, interest has focussed on mild aggressions from toxic metals of the environment. A study conducted in 1979 by Piérard in Belgium reported diffuse alopecia related to ingestion of toxic metals in 36 of 78 patients with diffuse alopecia.

> Toxic metals in abnormal amount in blood and urine were observed only when >10 % of hair bulbs were dystrophic.

Copper was involved in 17 alopecias, arsenic in 12, mercury in 5, and cadmium in 2. Copper intoxication was found to be related to ingestion of tap water containing a high concentration of copper salts, presumably from low pH, presence of chelating agents, or connection of electrical ground wires to copper water pipes, which caused sufficient flow of electrical current to ionize the metal.

The combination of rapid, diffuse alopecia, in combination with sudden abdominal pain and neurologic symptoms, such as painful polyneuropathy and acute muscle weakness ascending from the lower extremities, is pathognomonic for thallium toxicity. The hair mount, showing dystrophic anagen hair with black pigmentation at the base, may be diagnostic before the onset of alopecia. Thallium is an odorless, tasteless heavy metal formerly used in rodenticides and still used in some manufacturing processes, such as electronics, pharmaceuticals, and glass. Thallium also has been used for intentional poisonings.

Thallium remains a means of criminal poisoning and should be considered in any patient with acute onset of gastrointestinal symptoms, pain and paresthesias in the legs, and hair loss.

Finally, selenium is an essential element, which can result in significant toxicity if ingested in large amounts. Selenium is a micronutrient which represents an important constituent of the antioxidant enzyme glutathione peroxidase.

The potential health benefits of selenium in the prevention of cardiovascular disease and cancer motivate people to consume dietary compounds containing selenium. However, selenium at higher concentrations can cause multiple organ toxicity, a condition called selenosis.

Epidemiologic studies and case reports have shown that excess exposure to selenium is associated with several adverse health effects: an early toxic effect of selenium is on endocrine function, particularly on the synthesis of thyroid hormones following dietary exposure of around 300 μg selenium per day and on the metabolism of human growth hormone and insulin-like growth factor-1. At higher levels, other adverse effects can be hepatotoxicity, gastrointestinal disturbance, dermatitis, and hair and nail loss. In May 2008, US FDA reported 201 individuals with adverse reactions to liquid nutritional supplements containing excess selenium and chromium resulting in the largest epidemic of selenosis in the history of the USA.

3.8.1 Amalgam Illness

Adverse effects related to dental amalgam, including hair loss, have also been the subject of recent attention.

In one study, mercury levels in blood and urine correlated with the number of amalgam surfaces, indicating the release of mercury from dental amalgam restorations. Since the mercury levels were far below those where negative health effects would be expected and were similar in patients with complaints self-related to dental amalgam restorations and healthy control individuals, mercury was not found to be a likely cause of the impaired health reported by the patients.

In another study, assays of mercury in urine samples of patients with "amalgam illness" indicated that the exposure was far below the levels at which symptoms could be indicated by psychometric tests. Psychological investigation indicated that the symptoms were psychosomatic. All patients had experienced important psychic traumata in close correlation with the first appearance of symptoms.

Finally, in 2011 Sundström et al. compared 337 participants with amalgam-related complaints to 337 controls without such complaints. For 81 of the participants with amalgam-related complaints and their matched controls, data was also available approximately 5 years before the onset of complaints, making longitudinal analysis possible. All participants completed questionnaires assessing the occurrence of 55 life events. The results showed that many participants with amalgam-related complaints experienced negative life events before and at the onset of amalgam-related complaints. They also reported more unexpected and uncontrollable events difficult to adjust to in comparison with controls. Somatic illness or surgical operation was the most common life event; death of a very close family member and a major change in financial situation were also commonly reported. The authors concluded that adverse negative life events could play a vital role in understanding and explaining amalgam-related complaints.

In summary, a systematic relationship between increased mercury levels and the severity of reported symptoms of "amalgam illness" has so far not been demonstrated in any of several well-controlled multidisciplinary studies. These studies, however, have found a high prevalence of mental disorders among patients with self-diagnosed "amalgam illness."

3.9 Loose Anagen Hair and Short Anagen Hair of Childhood

Loose anagen hair and short anagen hair are conditions seen children with the chief complaint that the hair fails to grow long. While the hallmark of loose anagen hair is easily pluckable hairs in anagen, short anagen hair is characterized by a mild form of persistent telogen effluvium.

3.9.1 Loose Anagen Hair

Loose anagen hair, characterized by easily pluckable anagen hairs, is a disorder predominantly observed in children.

The diagnosis is based on the following criteria: on pull test, painless extraction of >10 anagen hairs (devoid of hair root sheaths), and in the trichogram >80 % of plucked hairs are anagen hairs devoid of sheaths.

Clinically the hair may show uneven ends. Additionally, there may be variations in hair texture, and the hair is often dry and lusterless (Fig. 3.33).

Histological studies of scalp biopsies have demonstrated abnormal clefting between the internal root sheath and the hair shaft, premature keratinization, and degeneration of the inner sheath. Also, poor cohesion of the cells of the outer sheath has been described.

Ultrastructural studies show longitudinal grooves of the hair shaft. The presence of these alterations supports the hypothesis of some abnormality of the root sheath adversely affecting anchoring of the anagen hair in the follicle.

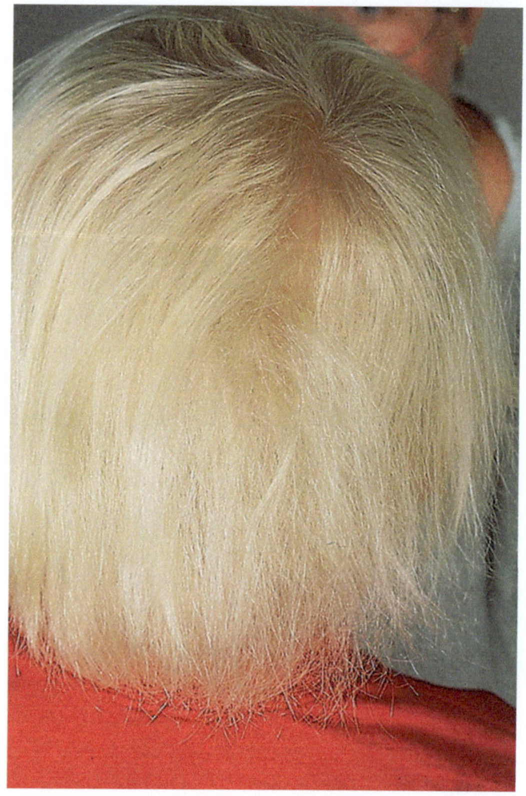

Fig. 3.33 Loose anagen hair of childhood

Loose anagen hair has originally been reported in girls, but may be underdiagnosed in males simply because of hairstyle differences between boys and girls.

The condition often recedes with age, but can be seen in adulthood, either as a continuation of the disorder that has lingered since childhood or as late-onset loose anagen hair. Patients with late-onset loose anagen hair state that their hair has increased shedding and does not grow as long as it used to.

There is no specific treatment for loose anagen hair, except for careful grooming of the hair to avoid extracting the loose anagen hairs. Oral biotin may be beneficial for the strength and texture of the hair.

3.9.2 Short Anagen Hair

In his classification proposal of telogen effluvium into five functional types on the basis of changes in the different phases of the follicular cycle, Headington suggested the existence of a mild form of persistent telogen effluvium in association with decreased hair length due to a short anagen phase.

Barraud-Klenovsek and Trüeb originally reported two children with a peculiar type of isolated congenital hypotrichosis. Both presented with persistent short, fine hair since birth (Fig. 3.34). Evidence was provided that the short hair observed in these patients was due to a short anagen phase of the hair cycle, with a normal rate of hair growth. Shortening of the anagen phase of the scalp hair cycle leads to a decrease in the maximal hair length and an increase in the number of hairs in telogen, resulting in an increase in hair shedding. Alternatively, Sinclair provided evidence of short anagen hair with a persistent synchronized pattern of scalp hair growth in a 4-year-old boy.

Scanning electron microscopy showed a widely spaced cuticular pattern, a finding typically seen in hair of thin caliber. One patient had affected family members with an apparently autosomal dominant mode of inheritance. The disorder appears to resolve spontaneously during puberty and adulthood.

The syndrome of short anagen hair was subsequently confirmed by Olsen who proposed methods for diagnosing this entity by clinical examination, trichogram, light microscopic examination of the hair shaft, scalp biopsy, and measurement of scalp hair growth rate.

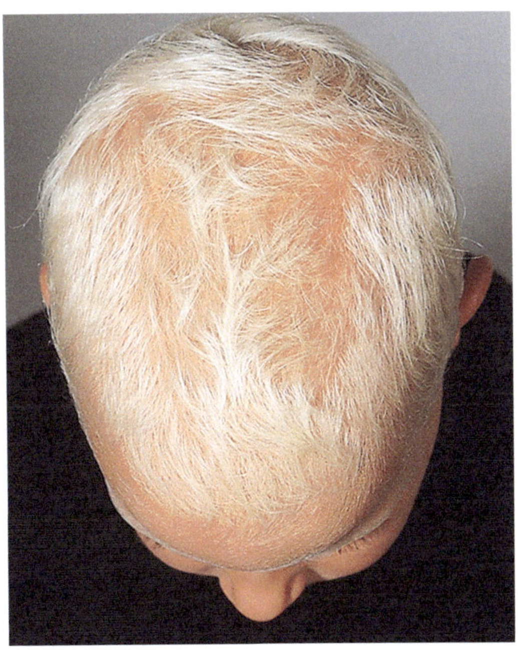

Fig. 3.34 Short anagen hair of childhood

> Short anagen hair appears to be an uncommon, though probably underreported condition, whose incidence is poorly documented in the medical literature.

The most important differential diagnosis includes short anagen hair in the trichodental syndrome, loose anagen hair, hereditary hypotrichosis simplex, and premature androgenetic alopecia.

Treatment is usually not necessary, though one would expect efficacy of topical minoxidil from reported successful treatment of a short anagen hair nevus.

3.10 Psychocutaneous Disorders of the Hair and Scalp

It is a common experience among dermatologists that significant numbers of their patients have psychological overlays to their chief complaints. This particularly holds true for complaints related to conditions of the hair and scalp. The exact incidence in any particular dermatologic practice most likely depends on the dermatologist's interest; however, even for those dermatologists who are not specially interested in the psychological aspects of dermatologic disease, some patients have such overt psychopathologic conditions, such as trichotillomania, factitial dermatitis, or delusions of parasitosis, that even the least psychologically minded dermatologist feels obliged somehow to address the psychological issues. Ideally, this would be accomplished simply through referral of the patient to a mental health professional. In reality, the majority of psychodermatologic patients are reluctant to be referred to a psychiatrist. Many lack the insight regarding the psychological contribution to their dermatologic complaints; others fear the social stigmatization of coming under the care of a psychiatrist.

The dermatologist is often the physician designated by the patient to handle their chief complaint, even if the main disorder is a psychological one. Therefore, it is essential for dermatologists dealing with such patients to expand their clinical acumen and therapeutic armamentarium to effectively handle the psychodermatologic cases in their practice. To accomplish this goal the following steps are required:

1. *Learn to classify and diagnose psychodermatologic disorders.* Because so many different types of conditions lie in between the fields of dermatology and psychiatry, it is paramount to have classification systems that will help clinicians understand what they are dealing with. There are two ways to classify psychocutaneous cases: first, by the category of the dermatologic presentation, e.g., neurotic excoriation, and, second, by the nature of the underlying psychopathologic condition, e.g., depressive disorder, generalized anxiety disorder, or obsessive–compulsive disorder.
2. *Become familiar with the various therapeutic options available*, both nonpharmacologic and psychopharmacologic.
3. *Recognize the limits of what can be accomplished in a dermatologic practice*: typically, a dermatologist does not have the time, training, or inclination necessary to administer most nonpharmacologic approaches. If a dermatologist seriously considers the challenge of treating these patients with psychopharmacologic agents, the selection of appropriate agents is dictated by the nature of the underlying psychopathologies that need to be treated. In order to prescribe effectively and safely for these patients, the dermatologist must have a basic understanding of the pharmacology of psychotropic agents.
4. *Optimize working relationships with psychiatrists*, since dermatologists and psychiatrists tend to have different perspectives when analyzing a clinical situation, different styles of communication, and different approaches to management.

3.10.1 Classification

Most psychocutaneous conditions of the hair and scalp can be grouped into the following four categories:

Psychophysiological disorders, in which the scalp disorder is exacerbated by emotional factors, e.g., hyperhidrosis, atopic dermatitis, psoriasis, and seborrheic dermatitis of the scalp.

Primary psychiatric disorders, in which there is no real skin condition, but all symptoms are either self-induced or delusional, e.g., trichotillomania, neurotic excoriations, factitial dermatitis, delusion of parasitosis, or psychogenic pseudoeffluvium.

Cutaneous sensory disorders, in which the patient has various abnormal sensations of the scalp with no primary dermatologic lesions and no diagnosable internal medical condition responsible for the sensations.

Secondary psychiatric disorders, in which patients develop emotional problems as a result of hair loss, usually as a consequence of disfigurement.

3.10.2 Psychophysiological Disorders

Psychophysiological disorders is the term used for psychocutaneous cases in which specific dermatologic skin disorders, such as psoriasis and eczema, are exacerbated by emotional stress in a significant proportion of patients. Examples affecting the scalp include hyperhidrosis, atopic dermatitis, psoriasis, and seborrheic dermatitis. In each of these conditions, one comes across two types of patients: those who experience a close chronologic association between stressful experiences and exacerbation of their dermatologic condition and those for whom the emotional state seems not to influence the natural course of their disease. These two groups are referred to as "stress responders" and "non-stress responders," respectively. The relative proportion of stress responders versus non-stress responders varies among the different psychophysiological conditions.

> A study involving a large number of subjects from the Harvard health care system in Boston, Massachusetts, determined the proportion with emotional trigger to be 100 % in patients with hyperhidrosis, 70 % in those with atopic dermatitis, 62 % with psoriasis, and 41 % with seborrheic dermatitis.

This category also includes the *psychosomatic disorders* – the physical symptomatic representation of unsolved emotional conflicts. For classification we may consider the different levels of psychosomatic disorder:

The *first level* is physiological and includes bodily sensations in response to emotional shifts, great or small. In health these bodily sensations make little or no impact on consciousness.

At the *second level*, the person becomes more or less constantly aware of the somatic sensations, which are of purely functional nature at this time point, attempts to analyze them, and becomes anxious that they might signify some serious organic disease.

The *third level* is the important one, at which internal somatic medicine and psychiatry meet. The organs and parts of the body have enormous elasticity and rebound, but if the underlying emotional distress is too prolonged, they supposedly lose their elasticity, no longer being able to cope, and finally protest in terms of the psychosomatic organ lesion or organ pathology.

It has long been recognized that psychosomatic factors play a role in dermatologic disease. It has been hypothesized that an organ system is vulnerable to psychosomatic ailments when several etiologic factors are operable. These factors include emotional factors mediated by the central nervous system; intrapsychic processes such as self-concept, identity, or eroticism; specific correlations between the emotional drive and the target organ, i.e., social values and standards linked with the organ system; and a constitutional vulnerability of the target organ.

3.10.3 Folliculitis Necrotica

Folliculitis necrotica is a peculiar dermatosis of the scalp that preferentially affects adult males, with chronic symptoms that wax and wane over time. Traditionally, the condition has been nosologically classified among the primary scarring alopecias. There is circumstantial evidence to also classify it among the psychophysiological disorders.

The disorder is characterized by minute and usually intensely pruritic follicular erythematous papules and pustules of the scalp that may become sore and crusted due to repeated scratching. The lesions may concentrate along the frontal hairline, but can appear anywhere on the scalp, varying in number from just a few to numerous lesions covering the scalp (Fig. 3.35). The disease has been classified into *acne necrotica miliaris* and *acne necrotica varioliformis*. The former affects the superficial portion of the hair follicle, allowing for hair regrowth after successful treatment. Miliaris refers to a millet, a term for a small seed. The latter represents

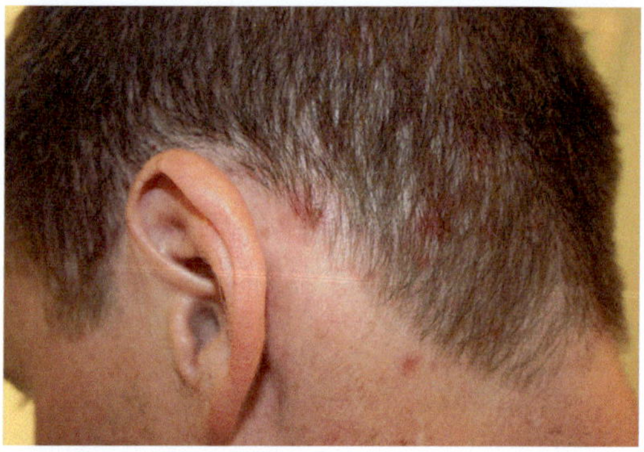

Fig. 3.35 Folliculitis necrotica

deeper lesions that progress to scabs that leave smallpox-like (varioliform) scars in their wake. Focal permanent alopecia may occur where the scalp has been scarred.

> Patients with folliculitis necrotica tend to be middle-aged executives, with lesions often triggered by stress. Many have jobs that place a lot of responsibility on them.

Histological studies of early lesions demonstrate lymphocytes centered around a hair follicle, with keratinocytes within the external hair root sheath and surrounding epidermis showing extensive cell necrosis.

The etiology is unknown; however, an abnormal inflammatory reaction to components of the hair follicle has been postulated, particularly to commensal or pathogenic microorganisms, such as *Propionibacterium acnes*, *Malassezia* spp., *Demodex folliculorum*, and in the more severe cases, *S. aureus*.

> Additionally extreme mechanical manipulation of the scalp due to scratching may be to blame.

The condition usually responds well to oral antibiotics, particularly long-term tetracyclines, in combination with a topical corticosteroid cream and a shampoo treatment alternating an antiseptic shampoo containing povidone iodine with an anti-dandruff shampoo containing ketoconazole. Mild cases may be treated with topical antibiotics such 0.5–1.0 g tetracycline in 70 % isopropyl alcohol (ad 100.0 g), 1 % clindamycin solution, or 4 % erythromycin gel. Refractory cases usually can be managed with long-term low-dose oral isotretinoin (start with 20 mg daily and taper to the individually required minimal dosage). In particularly tense patients, addition of oral doxepin hydrochloride 10–50 mg in the evening may be helpful in alleviating the itch–scratch cycle.

3.10.4 Primary Psychiatric Disorders

The term primary psychiatric disorders refers to cases in which there is no real skin condition. Everything that is seen on the scalp is self-induced, or there are no objective signs of complaints relating to the condition of the scalp and hair. This category includes conditions such as trichotillomania, neurotic excoriations, factitial dermatitis, delusions of parasitosis, and psychogenic pseudoeffluvium.

> Since the dermatologic presentations are quite stereotypic, but the underlying psychopathology varies, a critical step in psychodermatology is to try to ascertain the nature of the underlying psychopathologic condition.

Any one of the numerous psychopathologies listed in the *Diagnostic and Statistical Manual of Mental disorders*, 5th edition (DSM 5) and in the *International Statistical Classification of Diseases and Health-related Problems*, 10th edition (ICD-10) can be presented by these patients.

In general, one of the following four types of underlying psychopathology is present:

1. Generalized anxiety disorder
2. Depressive disorder
3. Delusional disorder
4. Obsessive–compulsive disorder

3.10.4.1 Generalized Anxiety Disorder

Generalized anxiety disorder is characterized by a sustained, increased free-floating anxiety, which is not orientated toward a certain object or situation. It expresses itself in the form of anxious expectations and enhanced alertness, combined with hypertension and, as a physiological correlate, vegetative hyperreactivity. Subjective symptoms include feelings of restlessness, irritability, feeling "on edge," tension, dizziness, agitation, and an inability to relax. These are frequently associated with physiological correlates such as muscle tension, sweating, shortness of breath, dry mouth, palpitations, abdominal complaints, and frequent urination.

When patients with psychophysiological disorders complain that they are "stressed," they are usually referring to an underlying sense of anxiety.

The uninhibited breakthroughs of tremendous anxiety show that the anxiety defense mechanisms have failed in the affected individuals. The causes of anxiety are repressed, but the ongoing arousal and fear are overwhelming. The patient's appearance is clinging and helpless. The patients signify a strong demand to be guided and assisted in their surroundings. The fixation toward fear of love deprivation may lead to attachments to strong "father figures," e.g., a physician, and strong emotional reactions on parting situations: a change of physician can cause severe separation anxiety and may therefore seem unbearable.

3.10.4.2 Depressive Disorder

In a depressive disorder the affected individual suffers from the symptoms of a depressive syndrome, which may be interspersed with shorter or longer periods of normal mood. Depression is characterized by subjective symptoms, such as depressed mood; crying spells; anhedonia (inability to experience pleasure); a sense of helplessness, hopelessness, and worthlessness; excessive guilt; and suicidal ideation. Frequently associated physiological correlates are psychomotor retardation or agitation, insomnia or hypersomnia, loss of appetite or hyperphagia, and, especially in older patients, complaints of constipation. In a depressive character disorder, affected individuals appear humble, unambitious, and sacrificing. They have high self-expectations and avoid close approaches from others; they would rather give up their own intentions and become subordinate to others. Usually there are coexisting wishes of dependency that others shall acknowledge the sacrifice and turn their attention and love to them. In others this may provoke an aggressive defense mechanism, which may appear as a hostile dissociation. These mismatched expectations mainly affect the patient's partnerships, when self-sacrifice and the excessive demand of love become overbearing.

3.10.4.3 Delusional Disorder

The presence of delusion defines psychosis. A delusion is a false idea on which the patient is absolutely fixed.

By definition, delusional patients have no insight, and others cannot talk them out of their belief system.

A delusion is deemed to be a basic psychotic phenomenon, in which the objective falseness and impossibility of the delusional content are usually easy to realize. Delusional convictions are not simple misbeliefs; they are constitutions of an abnormal mind that refer to the individual's cognitive experiences of his or her environment – their ego–environment relationship. Delusions are not voluntarily invented by the patients: they are caused by psychotic experiences. From the psychodynamic point of view, a delusional disorder is a special consequence of abnormal self-development. The delusion derives from the patient's desire to be in a safe place, away from the tension caused by the brittleness and contradictoriness of the patient's ego–environment relationship. The subjective certainty of the delusion's content causes its incorrectability: patients consistently keep their convictions, without considering their incompatibility with reality. Neither contrary experiences nor logical arguing can influence them.

> The type of psychotic patient most often seen by the dermatologist is not the schizophrenic, but the patient with monosymptomatic hypochondriacal psychosis.

Monosymptomatic hypochondriacal psychosis is characterized by a delusional ideation held by a patient that revolves around one particular hypochrondriacal concern, while with schizophrenia many other mental functions become compromised, besides the presence of delusional ideation.

3.10.4.4 Obsessive–Compulsive Disorder

Obsessive–compulsive symptoms may be seen across the whole spectrum of psychopathology. In early childhood they may occur as a temporary phenomenon in response to stress or anxiety, e.g., trichotillomania; they may occur as a psychoneurotic symptom in a person with an obsessive–compulsive personality configuration, e.g., onychophagia or acne excoriée; they may occur as a feature of the obsessive–compulsive disorder, or they may also occur in patients with psychosis. Individuals with an obsessive–compulsive personality configuration are rigid, perfectionistic, and indecisive for fear of making a mistake; they lack self-confidence, are sensitive to criticism, and are socially reserved. Perhaps most importantly, they have profound difficulty in handling anger and aggression, which sometimes is explosive and at other times is displaced into self-destructive picking of the skin rather than being expressed directly in a modulated fashion. The essential feature of obsessive–compulsive disorder required for diagnosis is recurrent obsessions or compulsions that are severe enough to be time-consuming or cause impairment in relationships, employment, school, or social activities. An obsession is a persistent idea, thought, impulse, or image that intrudes into a person's consciousness uncontrollably and causes distress, anxiety, and often feelings of shame.

> By definition, patients suffering from obsessive–compulsive disorder have insight into their condition, whereas delusional patients do not.

The individual with obsessive–compulsive disorder realizes that the obsession is inappropriate and irrational, but cannot resist. The obsessional concerns often lead to compulsive acts. Compulsions are repetitive, stereotyped motor acts, often ritualized and designed to reduce intolerable anxiety or distress. Obsessions may involve themes of aggression (harming the self or others), contamination (dirt, germs, body secretions), sex (forbidden thoughts or impulses), religion (concern with blasphemy or sacrilege), or somatic concerns.

The clinical manifestations on the hair and scalp of the respective psychopathologic conditions are listed in Table 3.14.

Table 3.14 Psychopathologic conditions and their clinical manifestations on the hair and scalp

Manifestations of generalized anxiety disorder
Neurotic excoriations of the scalp
Scalp dysesthesia
Manifestations of depressive disorder
Neurotic excoriations of the scalp
Scalp dysesthesia
Imaginary hair loss (psychogenic pseudoeffluvium)
Manifestations of delusional disorder
Delusions of parasitosis
Imaginary hair loss (psychogenic pseudoeffluvium)
Manifestations of obsessive–compulsive disorder
Trichotillomania
Neurotic excoriations of the scalp
Factitial dermatitis of the scalp

3.10.5 Neurotic Excoriations of the Scalp

The term neurotic excoriations refers to patients with self-inflicted excoriations of the scalp in the absence of an underlying specific dermatologic disease condition. The etiology is varied, and psychiatrically, patients with neurotic excoriations are not a homogenous group, each requiring an individual therapeutic approach.

The condition may occur at any time from childhood to old age, with the most severe and recalcitrant cases reportedly starting in the third to fifth decade.

Because the patients, by definition, can inflict lesions only on those areas of the body that can be reached, and because patients tend to excoriate areas that are easily accessible, the clinical distribution of lesions besides the scalp can give a clue to the diagnosis. The lesions may affect the scalp in an isolated manner or may be associated with excoriations of the face and/or of the upper trunk and extensor aspects of the arms. The excoriations may be initiated by minor irregularities of the skin surface, such as a keratin plug, insect bite, acne papule (acne excoriée), or irritated hair follicle, or may start de novo. There is a decreased threshold for itch with tendency to habitual or neurotic scratching. Picking activity may start inadvertently as the hand comes across on an irregularity of the skin, or it may occur in an organized and ritualistic manner, sometimes using an auxiliary instrument, such as the point of a knife. Tissue damage itself may again trigger itching, and the itch–scratch cycle may take on a life of its own. This activity typically takes place when the patient is unoccupied, and precipitating psychosocial stressors are usually present.

Neurotic excoriations occur across the spectrum of psychopathology. In mild and transient cases, it may be a response to stress, particularly in the younger patient, such as examination stress (thinker's itch), mainly in someone with obsessive–compulsive personality traits. In the more severe and sustained cases, psychiatric evaluation may diagnose a generalized anxiety disorder, depression, or obsessive–compulsive disorder.

The inflicted lesions are rather nonspecific. Varying in size from a few millimeters to several centimeters in the well-developed case, lesions are seen in all stages of evolution, from small superficial saucerized excoriations through deep scooped-out skin defects (Fig. 3.36a) to thickened hyperpigmented nodules and finally hypopigmented atrophic scars. Secondary bacterial infection may lead to regional lymphadenopathy. The histology is that of an excoriation with nonspecific inflammatory changes. Microbiological studies may reveal secondary bacterial infection, usually with *S. aureus*.

Since other dermatologic conditions can lead to similar lesions as neurotic excoriations of the scalp, clinicians must be careful not to make this diagnosis on the basis of the morphology of lesions alone. Specifically, pruritic skin conditions of dermatologic or other origin need to be excluded.

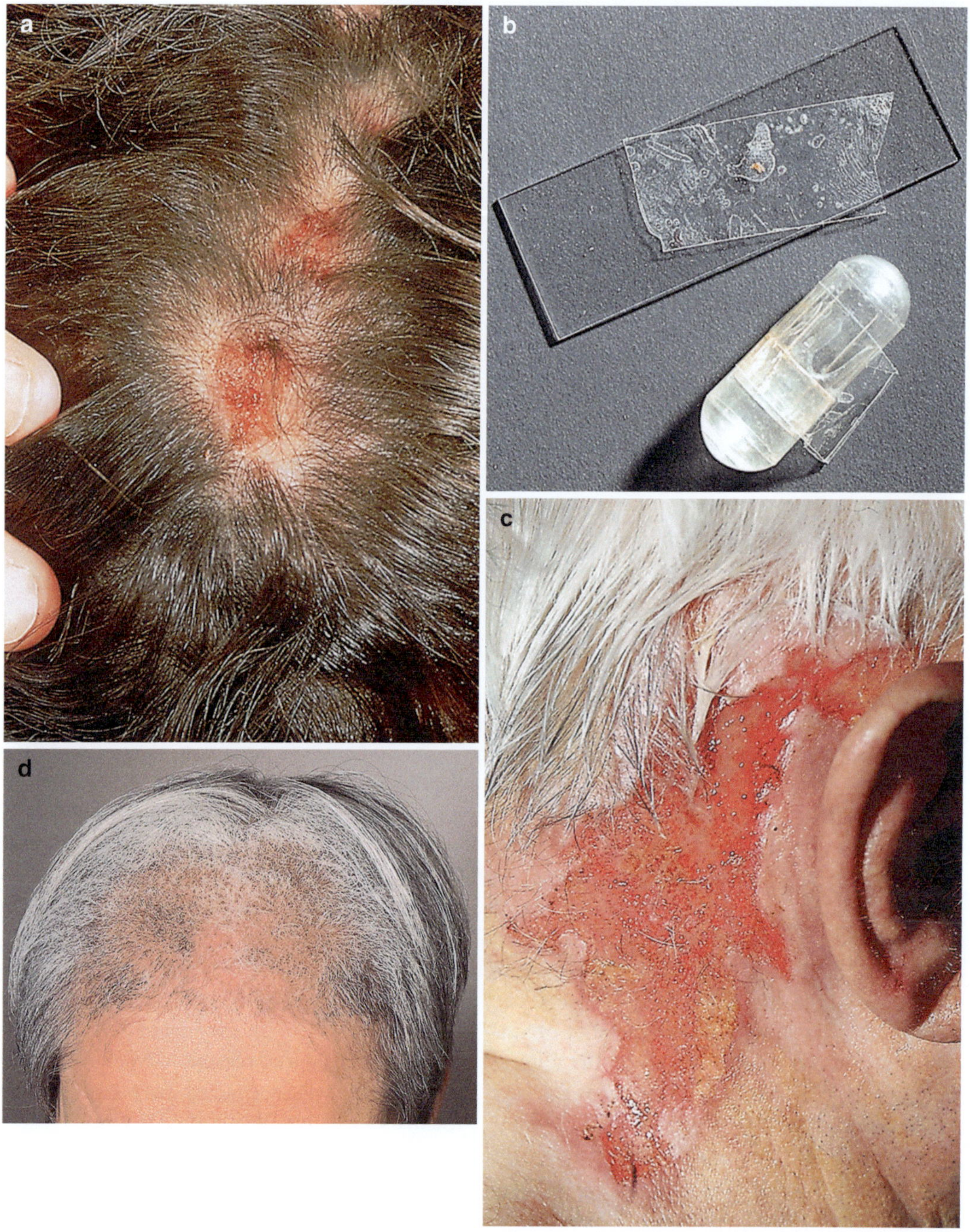

Fig. 3.36 (**a–d**) Psychodermatologic presentations on the scalp: (**a**) neurotic excoriations of the scalp, (**b**) patients with delusion of parasitosis often bring specimens to try to prove the existence of "parasites," (**c**) factitial dermatitis of the scalp, and (**d**) trichoteiromania

Examples are atopic dermatitis, folliculitis necrotica, chronic cutaneous lupus erythematosus, pemphigus vulgaris, pemphigoid, parasitic infestation, neurologic disorders, and other psychiatric disorders, such as cocaine intoxication, delusions of parasitosis, and factitial dermatitis.

Most importantly, one needs to confirm the diagnosis by ascertaining the presence of psychopathology through both clinical observation and direct patient questioning.

Dermatologic treatment includes the prescription of nonirritating or "sensitive" shampoos, topical glucocorticoid–antibiotic cream preparations, and sedative antihistamines, such as hydroxyzine or doxepin, preferably given at nighttime. Cool compresses are soothing, provide hydration, and facilitate debridement of crusts. When followed by the application of an emollient, they reduce any contribution that xerosis makes to itching. When present, secondary bacterial infection must be treated appropriately, usually with a short course of oral antibiotics.

Psychiatric treatment includes nonpharmacologic and pharmacologic therapeutic options. In both, the choice of the appropriate technique or pharmacologic agent depends on the underlying mental disorder.

Although behavioral modification, cognitive psychotherapy, psychodynamic psychotherapy, and an eclectic approach have met with variable success, many patients who present to the dermatologist are reluctant to agree to the psychiatric nature of their skin disorder and lack insight into the circumstances that trigger the drive to excoriate. Unless the patient is managed in a liaison clinic where dermatologists and psychiatrists can confer, it is the dermatologist who will take the responsibility for treatment.

If the patient is suffering from excessive stress, there are specific and nonspecific approaches. Those individuals who can find specific, real-life solutions to the difficulties they report are the more fortunate ones. Many patients experience stress from work or home relationships for which there is no easy way out. For these patients, a nonspecific solution to the stress can still be beneficial. Among the nonspecific solutions to stress, there are nonpharmacologic and pharmacologic means. The nonpharmacologic means include exercise, biofeedback, yoga, self-hypnosis, progressive relaxation, and other techniques learned in stress management courses. Some patients do not have time to take stress management courses, and others have special difficulty benefiting from this type of approach, for example, those who are not psychologically minded. For these patients, cautious use of antianxiety agents may be an alternative. In general, there are two types of anxiolytics: a quick-acting benzodiazepine type that can be sedating and produce dependency, such as alprazolam, and a slow-acting non-benzodiazepine type that is not sedating and does not produce dependency, such as buspirone. Alprazolam differs from the older benzodiazepines such as diazepam and chlordiazepoxide because its half-life is short and predictable. Another advantage is that it has an antidepressant effect, whereas most other benzodiazepines generally have a depressant effect. Because of the possible risk of addiction with long-term use, the most prudent way of using alprazolam would be to restrict its use to 2–3 weeks. If the patient requires long-term therapy for anxiety, buspirone may be considered. However, it must be kept in mind that the effect of buspirone is usually not experienced by the patient for the first 2–4 weeks of treatment. Also, buspirone cannot be used on an "as needed" basis. If buspirone does not work for a patient with chronic anxiety disorder, an alternative would be the use of low-dose doxepin. Even though doxepin is a tricyclic antidepressant, in low doses, it has been compared to benzodiazepines in terms of its anxiolytic effects. Sometimes, also a low dose of a low-potency antipsychotic agent such as thioridazine can be used.

Although there are a number of nonpharmacologic treatment options for depression, most dermatologists have neither the time nor the training to execute these treatment modalities. Nonetheless, it is advantageous to be conscious of these options, especially for those patients who agree to a referral to a mental health professional. Individual psychotherapy can be useful if there are definable psychological issues to be discussed, e.g., frustrations at work, a maladaptive style in interpersonal relationships, and the presence of maladaptive views of oneself, such as unrealistic expectations or fear of failure. Other patients have neurobiological predispositions to depression, and their depressive episodes may not be associated with any identifiable psychosocial difficulties. For these patients, the use of specific psychopharmacologic agents may in fact correct the primary cause of their depression. There are a number of antidepressants to choose from for treatment of depression pharmacologically. Among the tricyclic antidepressants, again doxepin is probably the most suitable for treatment of depressed patients with neurotic excoriations. If the patient cannot tolerate the sedative side effect of doxepin, desipramine or one of the newer, nontricyclic antidepressants such as fluoxetine, sertraline, and paroxetine are alternatives.

Finally, for the obsessive–compulsive patient with neurotic excoriations, there are, once again, nonpharmacologic and pharmacologic therapeutic options. However, if the dermatologist were to follow a nonpharmacologic approach for patients who reject referral to a mental health professional, it would have to be a technique that is simple enough to perform in a dermatologic setting. One such technique is the invocation of a "1- or 5-min rule," a simple behavioral technique to try to interrupt the progression from obsessive thoughts to compulsive behavior. The patient is asked to try to put an interval of 1–5 min between the occurrence of the obsessive thought and the execution of the compulsive behavior. Once the patient is successful in refraining for 1 min, the time is gradually increased to 5, 10, or even 15 min, and, eventually, with such a long interruption between the obsessive thought and the compulsive behavior, one anticipates to break the natural progression from one to the other. In a dermatologic setting, the pharmacologic approach may be most feasible for patients who refuse to be referred elsewhere. Moreover, the recognition that serotonin pathways are involved and that the SSRI group of antidepressant agents reduces compulsive activity has made it more likely that the dermatologist will meet with success. Frequent short visits should be scheduled for supervision of the dermatologic regimen and for emotional support, and either clomipramine (an older antidepressant with extensive documentation about its anti-obsessive–compulsive efficacy in the medical literature) or one of the newer SSRIs (fluoxetine or fluvoxamine maleate) should be prescribed.

3.10.6 Imaginary Hair Loss (Psychogenic Pseudoeffluvium)

Patients with imaginary hair loss or psychogenic pseudoeffluvium are frightened of the possibility of going bald or are convinced they are going bald without any objective findings of hair loss. Basically they suffer of what Cotterill has termed "dermatologic nondisease." Although dermatologists are used to seeing patients with minor skin and hair problems in significant body areas that cause disproportionate anxiety and cosmetic distress, with dermatologic nondisease there is no dermatologic pathology.

> It is important to realize that imaginary hair loss only makes up for a minority of patients complaining of hair loss and that patients with psychogenic pseudoeffluvium have varied underlying mental disorders.

The most common underlying psychiatric problems present are depressive disorder and body dysmorphic disorder. The clinical spectrum is wide, and the majority of patients are at the neurotic end of the spectrum and merely have overvalued ideas about their hair, whereas a minority of patients are truly deluded and suffer from delusional disorder. These patients lie at the psychotic end of the psychiatric spectrum. Those parts of the body that are important in body image are the focus of the preoccupation and concern.

True telogen effluvium resulting from androgenetic alopecia, telogen effluvium, or from involutional alopecia must carefully be excluded.

> Differential diagnosis of psychogenic pseudoeffluvium is particularly challenging, since there is considerable overlap between hair loss and psychological problems. Patients with hair loss have lower self-confidence, higher depression scores, greater introversion, as well as higher neuroticism and feelings of being unattractive.

A careful medical history, including medications, hormones, and crash diets; clinical examination of the hair and scalp (no alopecia, normal scalp); hair calendar (normal counts of hairs shed); trichogram (normal anagen and telogen rates); and laboratory workup should be performed to exclude real effluvium and if necessary repeated.

In addition to the relentless complaint of hair loss, patients suffering from body dysmorphic disorder adopt obsessional, repetitive ritualistic behavior and may come to spend the majority of the day in front of a mirror, repeatedly checking their hair. Another aspect of this behavior is a constant need for reassurance about the hair, not only from the immediate family, but also from the medical profession and from dermatologists in particular. These patients may become the most demanding types of patients to try to manage. The first step in treatment is to establish a good rapport with the patient.

It is important to recognize that patients with psychogenic pseudoeffluvium are expecting the clinician to treat them with respect as a trichologic patient and not as a psychiatric case. The most effective approach to psychogenic pseudoeffluvium is to take the chief complaint seriously and give the patient a complete trichologic examination.

Patients with overvalued ideas may respond to a sympathetic and unpatronizing dermatologist.

Psychotherapy is aimed at any associated symptomatology of depression, regardless of whether there is a causal relationship between the psychiatric findings and the imagined hair loss, because it is possible that patients who are depressed perceive even normal hair shedding in an exaggerated manner.

Patients with anxiety related to the fear of hair loss may also benefit from anxiolytic therapy with alprazolam or buspirone.

Many different treatments have been advocated to treat patients with body dysmorphic disorder: a wide variety of psychotropic agents (including tricyclic antidepressants and benzodiazepines) and antipsychotic drugs (including pimozide and thioridazine) have been tried in this condition, with poor results. Although there have been no controlled clinical trials of treatment of patients with body dysmorphic disorder, preliminary data indicate that SSRIs, such as fluoxetine and fluvoxamine maleate, may be effective, though the effective dosage of the SSRI drugs needs to be higher than the dosage conventionally employed to treat depression, and the duration of treatment is long term. Response to this group of drugs takes up to 3 months, and not all patients with body dysmorphic disorder will respond to treatment with SSRIs. In patients who fail to respond to SSRIs given for 3 months, it has been suggested either to add buspirone to the SSRIs or, if the patient has delusional body dysmorphic disorder, to add an antipsychotic agent such as pimozide.

Patients with body dysmorphic disorder expect the solutions to their problems in dermatologic (trichotropic agents) or surgical terms (hair transplantation).

Accordingly, following an initial consultation, it is common for a patient with body dysmorphic disorder to be given dermatologic treatment for alopecia. After repeated consultations with the patient, the dermatologist realizes that he or she is dealing with dermatologic nondisease. The result is often a frustrated dermatologist and a patient who eventually defaults from follow-up. The long and tough consultations, repeated telephone calls, and constant need for reassurance can put a significant strain on the dermatologist involved. Finally, a minority of patients with dysmorphic body disorder are angry, and these patients can direct this anger not only at themselves but also at the attending physician, with reproachful letters, threats, and even physical violence. It is important not to reject these patients and treat them mechanistically, but to adopt an empathetic approach.

The prognosis depends on the underlying psychopathology, its appropriate treatment, and the attending physician's capability to reassure and guide the patient.

3.10.7 Delusion of Parasitosis (Ekbom's Disease)

In delusions of parasitosis or Ekbom's disease, there is an unshakable conviction that the skin is infested by parasites. In the older literature, this condition is also described as "parasitophobia" or "acarophobia." However, the terms with "phobia" attached to them are misnomers and should be omitted, because in classic phobia, patients are aware of the fact that their fearful reactions are both excessive and irrational, while in the case of delusions of parasitosis, the patient is truly convinced of the validity of his or her perceptions.

In dermatologic practice the type of delusional patient most frequently seen is the patient with a delusional ideation that revolves around only one particular hypochondriacal concern. These patients are said to suffer from monosymptomatic hypochondriacal psychosis. These patients are different from other psychotic patients, such as schizophrenics or patients with a major depression, since the latter have many deficits in mental functioning, which is not the case in patients with monosymptomatic hypochondriacal psychosis. Moreover, a delusional disorder appears to run distinct from schizophrenia and mood disorders and does not appear to be a prodrome to either of these conditions. From a nosological point of view, delusions of parasitosis are classified as a delusional disorder of the somatic type with predominantly somatic delusions.

In the medical literature, the typical patient with delusions of parasitosis is reported to be a middle-aged woman, though there seems to be a bimodal distribution of age group.

> Delusion of parasitosis is frequently encountered in patients in their 20s and 30s of either sex who are at a lower socioeconomic status and who have a marginal existence in society, in work, and in interpersonal relationships.

Patients report cutaneous sensations such as crawling, biting, and stinging, which they relate to their unshakable conviction that their skin is infested by parasites. They often bring in bits of dry skin, debris, and other specimens to try to prove the existence of these "parasites" (Fig. 3.36b). Sometimes secondary injury to the skin or infection such as cellulitis may result from excessive scratching or the attempt to remove the "parasites" from the skin.

Though the patient with delusions of parasitosis presenting to the dermatologist more frequently suffers from monosymptomatic hypochondriacal psychosis, it must be remembered that the presence of a delusional ideation may be one particular manifestation of a more global psychiatric derangement, such as schizophrenia or major depression.

> Another subset of patients with delusions of parasitosis to consider are those who are substance abusers: drugs such as cocaine and amphetamine can induce formication and sometimes a delusional state that can be clinically identical to that of idiopathic delusions of parasitosis. Because the induction of formication is so well known among cocaine users, this phenomenon has been labeled cocaine bugs among substance abusers.

Also, neurologic disorders, such as multiple sclerosis, pernicious anemia, and especially in the elderly, brain dysfunction with manifest encephalomalacia due to cerebral arteriosclerosis should be considered in the differential diagnosis.

Chronic tactile hallucinosis describes those unusual cases in which patients develop chronic tactile sensations without delusions or other definable psychiatric disturbances and without associated medical or neurologic conditions.

Finally, the presence of inflammatory and pruritic skin disorders or real infestation, such as pediculosis capitis and furunculoid myiasis of the scalp, should not be overlooked.

Since trying to talk a patient out of a delusion is generally counterproductive, the most feasible way to have an impact on delusional ideation is to start the patient on an antipsychotic drug.

Traditionally, pimozide was prescribed. Newer agents include risperidone and olanzapine. The most challenging aspect of managing patients with delusions of parasitosis is to try to get their cooperation in taking one of these agents. This results from the discrepancy between the patient's belief system and the clinician's understanding of the situation. The first step is to establish a good rapport with the patient. In trying to do so, it is important to recognize that the patient with delusions of parasitosis is expecting the clinician to treat him with respect as a skin patient, not as a psychiatric case. Therefore, the most effective approach is to take the chief complaint seriously, give the patient a good skin examination, and pay attention to whatever "specimens" are brought in.

However, one should not make any comment that may reinforce the patient's delusional ideation.

Once the clinician senses that a reasonable working relationship is established with the patient, psychopharmacologic treatment is offered as an "empirical therapeutic trial," purposely avoiding any argument about the pathogenesis of the condition or the mechanism of action of the medication. No matter how skillful the clinician is, some delusional patients remain beyond reach. In this situation, the best the physician can do for the patient is simply to take on a supportive role and watch out for any secondary complication such as cellulitis, which may result from skin injury.

Untreated, the condition runs a chronic course. Many patients respond to pimozide, with symptomatic improvement occurring as early as 2 weeks after starting treatment, although several months of treatment may be needed for complete control. Most patients require ongoing maintenance therapy; some achieve remission; in a few, cure does occur. Remission is seldom associated with insight.

3.10.8 Trichotillomania

Trichotillomania involves the repetitive, uncontrollable pulling of one's hair, resulting in noticeable hair loss. It represents a disorder of impulse control. The disorder usually begins between early childhood and adolescence. It occurs six to seven times more frequently in children than in adults; before the age of 6, males predominate, females thereafter.

In the younger children, trichotillomania results from a mild form of frustration in a climate of psychosocial stress and soon becomes a habitual practice.

From puberty onward, trichotillomania is related to more severe pathologic psychodynamics, and prognosis is more guarded, particularly in female patients.

Most commonly, scalp hair is pulled, resulting in ill-defined areas of incomplete hair loss. In the affected areas, there are different lengths of hair, short, longer, and normal.

Associated features of trichotillomania may include excoriations of the scalp, nail biting (onychophagy), and eating hairs (trichophagy) with the risk of gastrointestinal obstruction by a mass of hair (trichobezoar), a complication that has been termed the *Rapunzel syndrome*.

Parents seldom notice their child's behavior, and most of them do not believe that their child would pull out his or her own hair. Once the diagnosis is suspected, it is confirmed in the following ways:

1. With the parents out of the room, in a friendly way ask the youngster to show you how this is done. This immediately tells the patient that you know what is going on and often initiates the disclosure or demonstration of how it is done.
2. If necessary, the next most simple way to prove the diagnosis is to perform a trichogram, which will typically show a significantly decreased telogen rate at the periphery of the area of hair loss (since the telogen hairs are more easily pulled out than the anagen hairs).
3. Finally, do a biopsy. This cannot rule out the diagnosis, but, if present, the following histopathologic findings will confirm it: wavy, wrinkled, corkscrew-shaped hair shaft (trichomalacia), the presence of many hairs in the catagen stage, and a lack of perifollicular inflammation (found in alopecia areata).

The most important differential diagnosis is alopecia areata.

Trichotillomania in connection with alopecia areata may pose a special diagnostic challenge. It may result from scratching at the site of alopecia areata that is symptomatic with pruritus, initiating a habit-forming behavior. Alternatively, patients with a mental predisposition may artificially prolong the disfigurement as the hair on the bald patches of alopecia areata regrows, with the aim to maintain gratification of dependency needs, which were being met during alopecia areata.

Children with trichophagy should be screened for iron deficiency as part of their evaluation, since the association of *pica* – an unusual craving for nonfood items – and iron deficiency has been reported. The compulsive oral behavior characteristically resolved with the oral administration of therapeutic doses of iron. It must be kept in mind though that iron deficiency may either be a cause of trichophagy or result from gastrointestinal bleeding in the case of trichobezoar.

The primary treatment approach for trichotillomania is habit reversal combined with stress management and behavioral contracting. Parents can help by recognizing the problem in its early stages and getting involved in its treatment. Treatment may involve self-monitoring of hair-pulling episodes as well as the feelings and situations that are most likely to lead to hair pulling. Youngsters are then systematically introduced to new behaviors, for example, squeezing a ball or tightening their fist whenever they feel the urge to pull at their hair. Relaxation training and other stress-reduction techniques may also be used, including reward charts that help track and monitor a child's progress with the added incentive of earning small rewards for continued progress. In addition, cognitive therapy is found to be effective.

The younger the patient, the smaller the percentage of cases referred to a psychiatrist; the rest are treated by the dermatologist who applies his or her own psychiatric knowledge (liaison psychiatry). A proper follow-up is required to establish whether improvement has actually occurred. When the symptom is present in adolescents or adults, competent help from a psychiatrist should be sought.

In a dermatologic setting, a pharmacologic approach may be most feasible for patients who refuse to be referred elsewhere. Basically, the same pharmacologic agents are used for the treatment of trichotillomania as for obsessive–compulsive disorder: the older tricyclic antidepressants imipramine and clomipramine and the newer selective serotonin reuptake inhibitors (SSRIs) fluoxetine, fluvoxamine, sertraline, and paroxetine. Physicians using SSRIs for treatment of patients with obsessive–compulsive disorders or trichotillomania are cautioned that the duration of treatment is critical in determining adequate treatment. Improvement continues to occur when the drugs are taken beyond 8- or 12-week trials. A patient showing a partial response after 4–6 weeks would be expected to continue to improve during the following weeks. Cessation of pharmacotherapy results in a relapse of the majority of patients. Despite success with SSRIs, patients with obsessive–compulsive disorders tend to respond to medication with only partial symptom reduction, suggesting that obsessive–compulsive disorders may be a neurobiological heterogeneous disorder that may require alternative treatment options in the individual patient. For example, successful treatment of five adult trichotillomania patients with a combination of the SSRI escitalopram with the anticonvulsant topiramate was originally reported. Subsequently, Lochner et al. performed an open-label pilot study to investigate the efficacy and safety of topiramate in 14 adults with trichotillomania. They found that topiramate may be useful in the treatment of trichotillomania and suggested that future studies should investigate the efficacy of topiramate in an appropriately powered, randomized, placebo-controlled trial.

An interesting new therapy is based on the glutamate modulator *N*-acetylcysteine. It is hypothesized that *N*-acetylcysteine, an amino acid, restores the extracellular glutamate concentration in the nucleus accumbens and, therefore, offers promise in the reduction of compulsive behavior. In a 12-week, double-blind, placebo-controlled study performed in 50 individuals with trichotillomania (45 women and 5 men with a mean age [SD] of 34.3 [12.1]), Grant et al. originally found that *N*-acetylcysteine (dosing range, 1,200–2,400 mg/day) demonstrated statistically significant reductions in trichotillomania symptoms. No adverse events occurred in the *N*-acetylcysteine group, and *N*-acetylcysteine was well tolerated.

To examine the efficacy of *N*-acetylcysteine for the treatment of trichotillomania in children, Bloch et al. again performed a double-blind, placebo-controlled (add-on) study with a total of 39 children and adolescents aged 8–17 years with trichotillomania randomly assigned to receive the active agent or matching placebo for 12 weeks. No significant difference between *N*-acetylcysteine and placebo was found on outcome measures. It is noteworthy that on several measures of hairpulling, subjects significantly improved with time regardless of treatment assignment: in the N-acetylcysteine group, 25 % of subjects were judged as treatment responders, compared to 21 % in the placebo group.

Dronabinol, a cannabinoid agonist, represents yet another novel pharmacologic approach, again studied by Grant et al. The authors hypothesized that dronabinol reduces the excitotoxic damage caused by glutamate release in the striatum again offering promise in reducing compulsive behavior. Fourteen female subjects with a mean age of 33.3 ± 8.9 diagnosed with trichotillomania were enrolled in a 12-week open-label treatment study of dronabinol (dose ranging from 2.5 to 15 mg/day). The authors found that dronabinol demonstrated statistically significant reductions in trichotillomania symptoms, in the absence of negative cognitive effects.

3.10.9 Factitial Dermatitis of the Scalp

Factitial dermatitis or factitious disorder with physical symptoms is a condition in which the patient creates lesions on the skin to satisfy a psychological need of which he or she is not consciously aware, usually a need to be taken care of by assuming the sick role. Patients with factitious disorder or factitial dermatitis create the lesions for psychological reasons and not for monetary or other discrete objectives as in the case of malingering. Patients knowingly fake symptoms, but will deny any part in the process. They desire the sick role and may move from physician to physician in order to receive care. They are usually loners with an early childhood background of trauma and deprivation. They are unable to establish close interpersonal relationships and generally have severe personality disorders. Unlike malingerers, they follow through with medical procedures and are at risk for drug addiction and for the complications of multiple operations. In the more severe form known as Münchausen syndrome or *laparotomophilia migrans*, a series of successive hospitalizations becomes a lifelong pattern.

Little is known about the etiology of factitious disorder. Besides the difficulties involved in making the diagnosis, the reluctance of these patients to undergo psychological testing and the heterogeneity in the details of cases published in the literature lie at the origin of this situation. Some clinicians have remarked that patients with factitious disorder often present traumatic events, particularly abuse and deprivation, and numerous hospitalizations in childhood, and as adults lack support from relatives and/or friends. The majority of patients suffer from borderline personality disorder. Because of emotional deficits in early life and a frequent history of physical or sexual abuse, patients have failed to develop a stable body image with clearly defined physical and emotional boundaries. For these patients, the factitial lesions serve many purposes: the excitement and stimulation ease the sense of emptiness and isolation, and skin sensation defines boundaries and helps establish personal and sexual identity, whereas the sick role gratifies dependency needs. In all reported series, females outnumber male patients from 3:1 to 20:1; onset is highest in adolescence and early adulthood, and a remarkably high number of patients work or have a close family member working in the health care field.

Factitial dermatitis of the scalp is only one aspect of the whole picture of factitious disease. The condition for which dermatologists are consulted often has already occasioned many visits to other physicians. The patient typically presents a bundle of normal investigative findings and a shopping bag filled with oral and topical medications. The lesions themselves are as varied as the different methods employed to create them; on the scalp there are usually ulcerations (Fig. 3.36c) or areas of cutoff hair (trichotemnomania). They are bizarre in shape and distribution and usually appear on normal skin. Though the possibilities are limitless, consistent is a "hollow" history – a term that refers to the patient's vagueness and inability to give details of how the lesions evolved. Consistent also are the affects of both the patient and their family. Although the patient seems astonishingly unmoved by the lesions, the family is angry, accusatory, and critical of what they interpret as medical incompetence.

A number of dermatologic, neurologic, and mental disorders may share similar symptoms. Clinically the differential diagnostic considerations are determined by the morphology and cover the scope of clinical dermatology. Among the most important disorders affecting the scalp that have to be taken into consideration are necrotizing herpes zoster (shingles), temporal arteritis, angiosarcoma, neurotrophic ulcerations of the scalp, and neurotic excoriations of the scalp.

With respect to treatment of factitial dermatitis, the essential and probably most difficult step is to secure an enduring and stable patient–physician relationship.

For achieving this goal most clinicians advocate a nonconfrontational strategy reframing the factitious manifestation as a "cry for help." An interesting approach is that of "contract conference." In this approach the psychiatrist emphasizes the need for the patient to express himself/herself in the common language of difficult relationships, feelings, and problems in living instead of the (factitious) language of illness. After that the patient and clinician can focus their efforts on resolving those real problems. Once a stable relationship is installed, the management of the disorder must be oriented to avoid unnecessary hospitalizations and medical procedures.

Another important issue in the management of this condition is recognition and adequate treatment of frequently associated disorders, such as personality disorders, depression, and drug and/or alcohol abuse and dependency.

Dermatologic treatment is symptomatic and determined by the clinical presentation. The uses of occlusive dressings are a diagnostic tool rather than an effective therapeutic intervention, since success is only of a temporary nature. Because of the patient's intense emotional investment in their skin, it may be helpful to prescribe positive measures such as wet dressings, emollients, and other bland topicals to replace the prior destructive activity.

Some case reports focus on the use of pharmacologic agents. A good response has been reported to the antipsychotic drug pimozide; other clinicians, because of the resemblance to the obsessive–compulsive disorder, advocate the use of clomipramine or the SSRIs fluoxetine and fluvoxamine maleate.

In the vast majority of patients, the condition remains chronic.

3.10.10 Chronic Cutaneous Sensory Disorders

Some patients only present with a cutaneous sensory complaint such as itching, burning, stinging, or other disagreeable sensations without any diagnosable dermatologic, neurologic, or medical diagnosis. Patients with chronic cutaneous sensory disturbance of unknown etiology can be divided into those with diagnosable psychiatric findings, such as a depression or anxiety, and those with no diagnosable psychiatric findings. The latter patients have been termed to be suffering from somatoform pain disorder.

> In dermatology the somatoform disorders consist of a heterogeneous pattern of differing clinical presentations based on a comparable emotional disorder, the characteristic of which is a repeated presentation of physical symptoms in combination with a stubborn demand for medical examination, despite repeated negative results, and the physician's assurance that the symptoms have no physical basis. The term *dermatologic nondisease* has also been coined for this disorder.

The somatoform disorders have been further classified into:

1. Conversion disorder, also known as hysteria
2. Hypochondriacal and body dysmorphic disorder
3. Somatization disorder (Briquet's syndrome)
4. Somatoform pain disorder

3.10.10.1 Conversion Disorder

Conversion disorder is characterized by the loss of a bodily function. It is involuntary, and diagnostic testing does not show a somatic cause for the dysfunction. The patient with conversion disorder confronts an acute stressor, which creates a psychic conflict, and the physical symptoms serve as the resolution of the conflict, while the patient may be unaware of the stressor. Conflicts or other stressors that precede the onset or worsening of the symptoms suggest that psychological factors are related to it. The disorder may be best thought of as disturbances of illness perception or need. They are paradigms of mind–body interactions and of the critical role that mental factors play in the production of illness. Again, the loss of function may symbolize the underlying conflict associated with it. Psychodynamic theory interprets the cause of the symptoms as a defense mechanism that absorbs and neutralizes the anxiety generated by an unacceptable impulse or wish. The patient doesn't consciously feign the symptoms for material gain or to occupy the sick role.

3.10.10.2 Hypochondriacal and Body Dysmorphic Disorder

Unlike conversion disorder, where the affected individual perceives a functional disorder and simply uses it to escape from uncomfortable situations, the patient with hypochondriacal disorder has no real illness, but is overly obsessed over normal bodily functions. They read into the sensations of these normal bodily functions the presence of a feared illness. Because of misinterpreting bodily symptoms, they become preoccupied with ideas or fears of having a serious illness, while appropriate medical investigation and reassurance do not relieve these ideas. These ideas cause distress that is clinically important or impairs work, social, or personal functioning. They are not delusional (as in delusional disorder) and are not restricted to concern about appearance (as in body dysmorphic disorder). Hypochondriacal disorder usually develops in middle age or later and tends to run a chronic course. Patients typically seek many tests and much reassurance from their doctor.

> Probably the more important group of problem patients for the dermatologist in practice is that with body dysmorphic disorder or "dysmorphophobia" (a term that is incorrect, since we are not dealing with a phobic disorder).

It is classified together with hypochondriacal disorder, though this classification will probably be abandoned in the future in favor of a new class of its own. This disorder tends to occur in younger adults. The patient becomes preoccupied with a nonexistent or minimal cosmetic defect and persistently seeks medical attention to correct it. Cases of body dysmorphic disorder can range from relatively mild to very severe. The patient is preoccupied with an imagined defect of appearance or is excessively concerned about a slight physical anomaly. This preoccupation causes clinically important distress or impairs work, social, or personal functioning. Another term used for body dysmorphic syndrome is *Thersites complex* (named after Thersites who was the ugliest soldier in Odysseus' army, according to Homer).

One of various theories attempting to make the onset of body dysmorphic disorder understandable is the "self-discrepancy theory," in which affected patients present conflicting self-beliefs with discrepancies between their actual and desired self. Patients have an unrealistic ideal as to how they should look. Media-induced factors are considered to predispose to body dysmorphic disorder by establishing role models for beauty and attractiveness.

3.10.10.3 Somatization Disorder

Somatization disorder presents with a pattern of recurrent, multiple somatic complaints that do not have an organic basis. Starting before the age of 30, the patient has usually had many physical complaints occurring over several years and sought treatment for them, or the complaints have materially impaired social, work, or personal functioning. Typically there is a combination of pain symptoms, related to different body sites or body functions, gastrointestinal symptoms, sexual dysfunction, and pseudoneurological symptoms. None of these are limited to pain (as in somatoform pain disorder). Physical or laboratory investigations determine that each of the symptoms cannot be fully explained by a general medical condition or by substance abuse, including medications and drugs of abuse, or if the patient does have a general medical condition, the impairment or complaint is greater than would be expected based on history, laboratory, and physical examinations.

In dermatology, environment-related physical complaints, the so-called *eco syndromes*, are noteworthy among the somatization disorders. The patients report multiple complaints in various organ systems, of which the purported cause is exposure to environmental toxins, without proof of any direct toxic causal relationship between exposure and symptomatology. Examples are the *multiple chemical sensitivity syndrome* and the *amalgam-related complaint syndrome*.

Occasionally, the complaint of hair loss is related to the amalgam in tooth fillings, and patients unnecessarily have all fillings removed and pay for expensive detoxification procedures.

3.10.10.4 Somatoform Pain Disorder

In somatoform pain disorder, by definition, pain is in the foreground. It is reported by the patient as clinically relevant, causes suffering and professional and/or social impairments, and cannot be adequately explained by either a somatic cause or another psychiatric disorder. In dermatology, mainly regional cutaneous or mucosal dysesthesias occur. Depending on their localization, specific names for the conditions are available, such as glossodynia (tongue) and penodynia (penis).

3.10.11 Trichodynia

The term "trichodynia" was proposed for discomfort, pain, or paresthesia of the scalp related to the complaint of hair loss. Rebora found that 34.2 % of female patients, who had their hair consultation because of hair loss, complained of this phenomenon. In a subsequent survey, Grimalt et al. claimed that 22.1 % of their female patients reported trichodynia.

The cause of trichodynia is not understood, though it has been proposed that it is probably polyetiologic.

> The most prevalent speculations with respect to the pathogenesis of trichodynia are perifollicular inflammation, increased expression of neuropeptide substance P localized in the vicinity of hair follicles, and underlying psychiatric disorders.

Originally, trichodynia was reported to be more prevalent in female patients with chronic telogen effluvium, and to a lesser extent in patients with androgenetic alopecia. Rebora et al. proposed the symptom to be distinctive for chronic telogen effluvium.

Willimann and Trüeb's study on 403 patients (311 female, 92 male) whose main complaint was hair loss confirms the previously published findings in the literature that trichodynia affects a significant proportion of patients complaining of hair loss. The aim of the study was to assess the frequency of trichodynia in patients complaining of hair loss and its correlation with gender, age, cause, and activity of hair loss. It was found that 17 % of patients complaining of hair loss, i.e., 20 % of female and 9 % of male patients, reported "hair pain," pain or discomfort of the scalp, not otherwise explained by presence of a specific dermatologic disease, such as psoriasis or eczema, or neurologic disorder, such as migraine equivalent.

> Statistical analysis failed to demonstrate any significant correlation between trichodynia, the extent of hair thinning, and hair loss activity, quantified by the hair pull, daily hair count, wash test, and trichogram. It is noteworthy though that trichodynia typically increases the anxiety related to the patient's preoccupation with hair loss or fear of hair loss.

As opposed to the suggestion of Rebora et al. that trichodynia would be typical for chronic telogen effluvium, the symptom did not allow any discrimination with respect to the cause of hair loss and was found with similar frequencies in association with androgenetic alopecia, chronic telogen effluvium, or a combination of both.

The cause of trichodynia remains obscure. Rebora et al. proposed a possible role of perifollicular microinflammation. Hoss and Segal interpreted scalp dysesthesia as a cutaneous dysesthesia syndrome related to underlying psychiatric disorders, with affected individuals either suffering of depressive, generalized anxiety, or somatoform disorder. Hordinsky and collaborators found localization of the neuropeptide substance P in the scalp skin of patients with painful scalp suggesting a causal relationship between the presence of substance P and trichodynia. Substance P represents a neuropeptide involved in nociception and neurogenic inflammation.

> Willimann and Trüeb proposed that trichodynia probably is polyetiologic. Though only a small number of patients with trichodynia in the studied patients showed telangiectasia of the scalp, this finding strongly correlated with presence of trichodynia.

An interesting analogy is the observation of Lonne-Rahm et al. who found that patients with the telangiectatic variant of rosacea respond more frequently with stinging sensations to the topical application of 5 % lactic acid on the cheeks than patients with the papulopustular type of rosacea or normal controls. On the basis of these findings, they concluded that the blood vessels are of importance in stinging sensations, and a connection exists between sensory or subjective irritation and cutaneous vascular reactivity. Also the observation of development of cutaneous allodynia during a migraine attack provides clinical evidence for the relation of vascular changes and pain.

In this context, it is interesting to note that substance P not only represents an important mediator of nociception and neurogenic inflammation, but also exerts a potent vasodilatatory effect. The role of substance P and related substances (neuropeptides) in the pathogenesis of trichodynia, and especially its relation to the nervous system and emotional stress, needs further elucidation.

By the virtue of their bidirectional effects on the neuroendocrine and immune systems, substance P and other neuropeptides may well represent key players in the interaction between the central nervous system and the skin immune and microvascular system.

Such mechanisms would explain the noxious effects not only of external stimuli (mechanical, thermal, chemical), but also of emotional distress on cutaneous nociception through the release of neuropeptides, such as substance P. Interestingly, Paus and collaborators have recently demonstrated that stress-induced immune changes of the hair follicles in mice could be mimicked by injection of substance P in non-stressed animals and were abrogated by selective substance P receptor antagonism in stressed animals.

A lower prevalence of male patients suffering of trichodynia might be connected to gender-related differences in pain perception, inasmuch as increase of pain perception in relation to anxiety scores has been found to be more pronounced in females.

Trichodynia tends to affect the centroparietal area of the scalp, seemingly surprising since the pain threshold of the centroparietal scalp is otherwise considered to be higher.

In the absence of any other specific morphologic changes of the scalp or correlation with quantitative parameters of hair loss, management of trichodynia remains empiric and empathetic, tailored to the individual patient's needs. The therapeutic choice includes nonirritating shampoos, topical antipruritic or anesthetic agents, topical capsaicin, corticosteroids, tricyclic antidepressants, gabapentin, and pregabalin. The efficacy of oral substance P (neurokinin 1 receptor) antagonists such as aprepitant in treatment of pain and depression has so far not been convincing.

As a general rule, topical overtreatment of the scalp is to be avoided. Most importantly, the patient needs to be reassured that trichodynia does not reflect hair loss activity, which may ease the patient's anxiety and in our experience also may beneficially influence cutaneous nociception.

Ultimately, treatment of trichodynia with botulinum toxin (BTX) seems a rational approach, since there is increasing evidence that BTX decreases the mechanical sensitivity of nociceptors and inhibits neurogenic vasodilation through inhibition of sensory neuropeptide release.

3.10.12 Trichoteiromania

Trichoteiromania is the term originally coined by Freyschmidt-Paul et al. in 2001 for breakage of hair by forcefully rubbing an area of the scalp. The typical clinical presentation is that of a bald patch with broken hairs (Fig. 3.36d). Subsequently, Reich and Trüeb reported four patients with trichoteiromania and further characterized them on the basis of clinical, morphologic, and psychopathologic criteria.

In contrast to trichotillomania, trichoteiromania has no diagnostic histopathologic features and a normal trichogram. Traumatic changes to the hair shaft are more conspicuous, with splitting at the ends of the hairs, giving the impression of white tips.

The underlying mental disorder in trichoteiromania varies among the patients, though an underlying cutaneous sensory disorder, not explained through any specific dermatologic disorder, is a common denominator in all cases.

While trichotillomania is considered to be an obsessive–compulsive disorder, the underlying mental disorder in trichoteiromania represents a more heterogeneous group, including anxiety, depression, or somatoform disorder.

Cooperation with the psychiatrist is indicated, as much as the management and prognosis of trichoteiromania again will depend on recognition of the underlying mental disorder and its specific psychotherapeutic and pharmacologic treatment.

3.10.13 Adjustment Disorders

Even though most patients with hair disorders experience significant psychological impact, it is usually not of an intensity to qualify as a mental illness. Nevertheless, the impact that hair disorders have on body image significantly contributes to the overall impact on the patient's quality of life. If one appreciates the psychosocial impact of hair disease, there is no doubt that appropriate treatment frequently has a huge bearing on the patients' quality of life. The clinician should keep in mind that the distress the patient feels from having a hair disease can be handled both dermatologically and psychologically.

Some patients have difficulties adjusting to hair loss. As a result, the individual may have difficulty with his or her mood and behavior. From a psychopathologic point of view, adjustment disorders may result from the stressful event of hair loss, depending on its acuity, extent, and prognosis. An adjustment disorder is a debilitating reaction to a stressful event or situation. These symptoms or behaviors are clinically significant as evidenced by either of the following: distress that is in excess of what would be expected or significant impairment in social, occupational, or educational functioning. Adjustment disorder subtypes include:

- Adjustment disorder with depressed mood
- Adjustment disorder with anxiety
- Adjustment disorder with mixed anxiety and depressed mood
- Adjustment disorder with disturbance of conduct
- Adjustment disorder with mixed disturbance of emotions and conduct

Associated features may be somatic and/or sexual dysfunction, feelings of guilt, and/or obsession.

The best way to alleviate the emotional distress caused by hair disease is to eliminate the hair disease that is causing the problem.

In other words, the intensity of the distress that the patient feels should be part of the clinician's formula in deciding how aggressively to treat the hair disease. For example, a decision to use or not to use topical minoxidil or oral finasteride in a patient with a borderline clinical state of androgenetic alopecia, or to recommend or not to recommend hair surgery to a patient with permanent alopecia, may hinge on the amount of distress the patient feels from the alopecia.

Besides being a sympathetic and concerned professional, a dermatologist may give a referral to a support organization, such as the National Alopecia Areata Foundation.

First, many of these support organizations specialize in providing educational materials to patients and their relatives, so they have an opportunity to inform themselves with respect to the nature and prognosis of their hair problem. Second, being part of such an organization breaks the sense of isolation patients often feel. Finally, by learning more about different treatment options, there is less risk that the patients will prematurely give up on treatment in despair and resign themselves to having uncontrolled alopecia. Keeping up hope is critical in not losing a positive outlook, in spite of having a chronic or recurrent condition.

3.11 Concept of Multitargeted Treatment

Besides an understanding of the pathologic dynamics of hair loss as they relate to the hair growth cycle and integrity of the hair follicle, insight into a multitude of cause relationships is prerequisite for delivering appropriate patient care. It must be borne in mind that hair loss often does not result from a single cause effect, but from a combination of internal and external factors that all need to be addressed simultaneously in an individualized manner for success, such as smoking and UV radiation, nutritional factors, medications, inflammatory phenomena and scarring, age-related phenomena, and ultimately the problems of comorbidities and multimorbidity in the elderly.

3.11.1 Value of Nutritional Supplementation Therapy

Since an important commercial interest lies in the nutritional value of various vitamin and amino acid supplements, an important question that arises is whether increasing the content of an already adequate diet with specific amino acids, vitamins, and/or trace elements may further promote hair growth.

Pharmacy aisles and Internet drugstores are full of nutritional supplements promising full, thick, luscious hair for prices that range from suspiciously cheap to dishearteningly exorbitant. Unless the hair is falling out due to a nutritional deficiency, there's only so much that nutrients can do to increase the size of individual hairs. This is because hair thickness is largely genetic.

> Nevertheless, there are external factors that influence hair health to a significant degree, and micronutrients can boost hair that's suffering from these problems. Specifically, there is growing evidence for the modes of action and efficacy of nutritional supplements on the basis of L-cystine and B vitamins.

The effects of nutrition on hair growth have been recognized from observations in inborn errors of metabolism, in deficiency disorders, and from supplementation studies in animals and humans.

In the 1960s, the role of L-cystine in the production of wool was investigated, and it was found that enrichment of even what appeared to be a normal diet with the sulfur-containing amino acids L-cystine and L-methionine increased wool production in sheep. When considering which dietary supplements could be used for improving hair growth in humans, L-cystine was therefore considered, and in the early 1990s studies on the effect of dietary supplements containing L-cystine, in combination with B-complex vitamins and medicinal yeast, a rich natural source of amino acids and B-complex vitamins, were performed, showing improvements in the trichogram, in hair swelling as a criterion for hair quality, and in the tensile strength of the hair fiber.

Interestingly, a more recent experiment demonstrated that C57BL/6 mice exposed to cigarette smoke developed hair loss, while no alopecia occurred in sham-exposed mice. Smoke-exposed mice had extensive atrophy of the epidermis, reduced thickness of the subcutaneous tissue, and scarcity of hair follicles with massive apoptosis in the hair bulbs at the edge of alopecic areas. This effect was prevented by the oral administration of *N*-acetylcysteine, an analogue and precursor of L-cysteine and reduced glutathione, as well as by L-cystine, the oxidized form of L-cysteine, which is a key hair component, in combination with vitamin B6, which plays a role in L-cystine incorporation in hair cells. The effect was interpreted as to be possibly related to the glutathione-related detoxification system.

Ultimately, combining with topical minoxidil in the treatment of androgenetic alopecia may prove to add extra benefit, since it has been shown in whole hair follicle cultures that minoxidil not only increases the incorporation of thymidine as marker of cell division, but also leads to increased uptake of cysteine by the hair follicle.

A role of the essential amino acid L-lysine in hair loss has also been suggested to be important. Double-blind data confirmed the findings of an open study in women with increased hair shedding, where a significant proportion responded to combination treatment with L-lysine and iron.

While nutritional factors affect the hair directly, one should not forget that they also may affect the skin. In the management of subjects with hair loss, evidence of associated scaling problems should draw the attention to the possibility of deficiency of vitamin A, biotin, zinc, or essential fatty acids.

Finally, excessive intake of certain nutritional supplements may actually cause hair loss and is not recommended in the absence of a proven deficiency. This applies particularly to vitamin A (>50,000 I.E. daily) and selenium, which in toxic doses cause hair loss. Also, a caveat should be spoken against uncritical iron supplementations, since there is the possibility that increased iron storage could enhance oxidative injury by inducing the Fenton reaction, with the prospective of increasing the risk of cardiovascular disease and cancer.

In an attempt to demonstrate the pro-oxidative capacity of oral iron supplementation, King et al. performed a study on women with low iron stores (plasma ferritin ≤20 μg/l) receiving a daily iron supplement for 8 weeks at a level commonly used to treat poor iron status. They measured increased lipid peroxidation by ethane exhalation rates and plasma malondialdehyde. The women served as their own control as pre- and post-supplementation periods were compared. After 6 weeks of iron supplementation, serum ferritin almost doubled and body iron more than doubled, hemoglobin levels increased slightly, and other indicators of iron status became normal. However, plasma malondialdehyde and breath ethane exhalation rates increased by more than 40 % between baseline and 6 weeks of supplementation. These increases correlated significantly with plasma iron and ferritin levels. The authors concluded that the increased indicators of lipid peroxidation with duration of supplementation and as iron status improved suggest that providing daily nearly 100 mg iron may not be a totally innocuous regimen for correcting iron depletion.

Micronutrients relevant to the hair and their recommended daily allowances are listed in Table 3.15.

Table 3.15 Micronutrients relevant to the hair and recommended daily allowances

Vitamins
B vitamins
Biotin (vitamin H) – 300 μg
Niacin (vitamin B3) – 20 mg
Folic acid – 300 μg
Riboflavin (vitamin B2) – 1.7 mg
Pantothenic acid (vitamin B5) – 5 mg
Pyridoxine (vitamin B6) – 1.5 mg
Cyanocobalamin (vitamin B12) – 3 mg
Antioxidants
Vitamin A/beta-carotene – 6 mg
Alpha-tocopherol (vitamin E) – 10 IU
Trace metals
Iron – depending on age and sex (in men – 8 to 10 mg)
Zinc – 15 mg
Selenium – 50 μg

3.11.2 Targeting the Inflammatory Component in Androgenetic Alopecia

The limited success rate of treatment of androgenetic alopecia with minoxidil and finasteride means that further pathogenic pathways may be taken into account. Clinical and investigative advances have helped us to understand some of the pathogenic steps leading to androgenetic alopecia: besides androgens and genetic imbalance, additional pathogenic factors are suspected, such as microbial flora, endogenous and exogenous stress, microinflammation, and others. While further suspects are likely to be exposed, individual diversity of causal agents, as well as of the sequence of events, or combined factors, must be kept in mind, when addressing the biological conditions contributing to androgenetic alopecia. Ultimately, dissecting the molecular controls of immune-mediated hair follicle degeneration by apoptosis-mediated organ deletion could provide insights into how progression to permanent hair loss due to follicular inflammatory phenomena and fibrosis might be halted.

So far, the inflammatory component has not been included in treatment protocols for androgenetic alopecia.

In an early study, Piérard-Franchimont et al. hypothesized on a microbial-driven inflammatory reaction abutting on the hair follicles and conducted a study to compare the effect of 2 % ketoconazole shampoo to that of an unmedicated shampoo used in combination with or without 2 % minoxidil therapy. They found that hair density and size and proportion of anagen follicles were improved almost similarly by both ketoconazole and minoxidil regimens and concluded that there may be a significant action of ketoconazole upon the course of androgenic alopecia and that *Malassezia* spp. may play a role in the inflammatory reaction. Later, Berger et al. performed a 6-month, randomized, investigator-blinded, parallel-group clinical study with healthy men between the ages of 18 and 49 years exhibiting Norwood–Hamilton type III vertex or type IV baldness to assess the hair growth benefits of a 1 % pyrithione zinc shampoo. The efficacy of a 1 % pyrithione zinc shampoo (used daily) was compared with that of 5 % minoxidil topical solution (applied twice daily), a placebo shampoo, and a combination of the 1 % pyrithione zinc shampoo and the 5 % minoxidil topical solution. Hair count results showed a significant net increase in total visible hair counts for the 1 % pyrithione zinc shampoo, the 5 % minoxidil topical solution, and the combination treatment groups relative to the placebo shampoo after 9 weeks of treatment. The relative increase in hair count for the 1 % pyrithione zinc shampoo was slightly less than half that for the minoxidil topical solution. However, no advantage was seen in using both the 5 % minoxidil topical solution and the 1 % pyrithione zinc shampoo.

Surprisingly, the use or addition of topical corticosteroids or of systemic anti-inflammatory agents such as oral hydroxychloroquine or oral doxycycline in the treatment plan of androgenetic alopecia (with microinflammation and fibrosis) has so far not been systematically studied. For now, we can only deduce a putative added benefit by analogy from their preliminary (successful) use in cicatricial pattern hair loss (Fig. 3.37a–e) or in central centrifugal cicatricial alopecia.

Proposed pathogenic mechanisms in androgenetic alopecia and respective therapeutic strategies are summarized in Fig. 3.38.

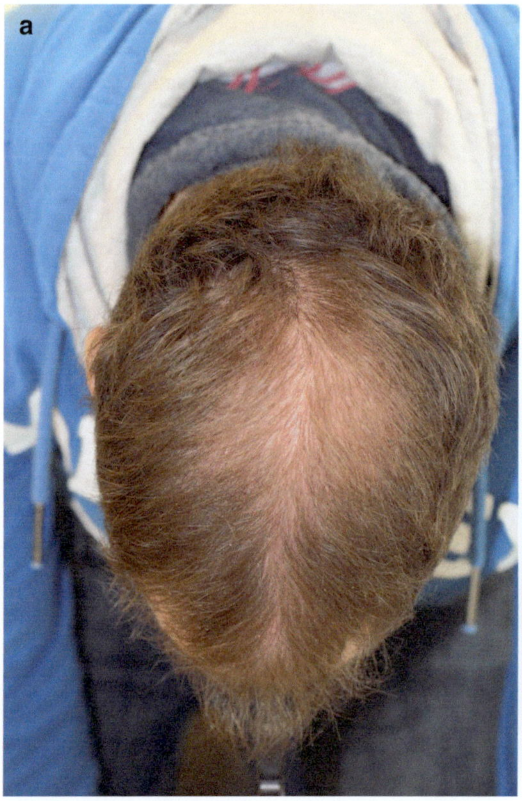

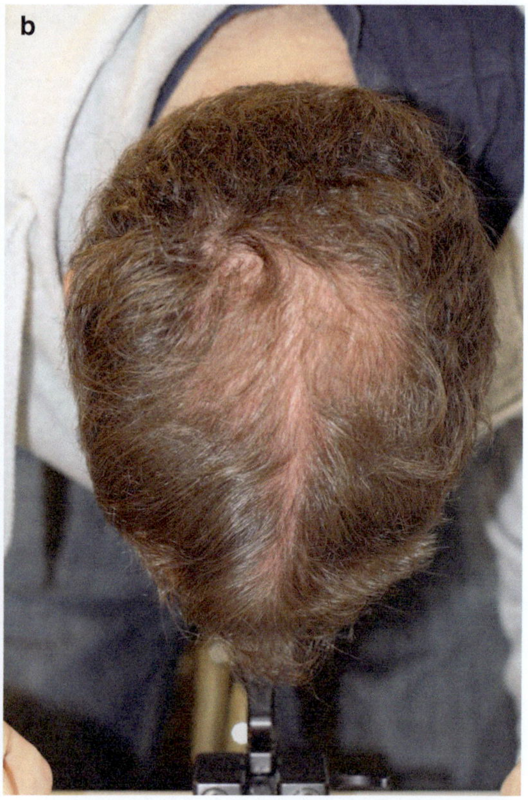

Fig. 3.37 (**a–e**) Successful treatment of fibrosing alopecia in a pattern distribution with a topical compound of 5 % minoxidil and 0.2 % triamcinolone acetonide in combination with 1 mg oral finasteride and oral hydroxychloroquine 200 mg daily, (**a**) before, (**b**) after 3, (**c**) 6, (**d**) 12, and (**e**) 24 months treatment

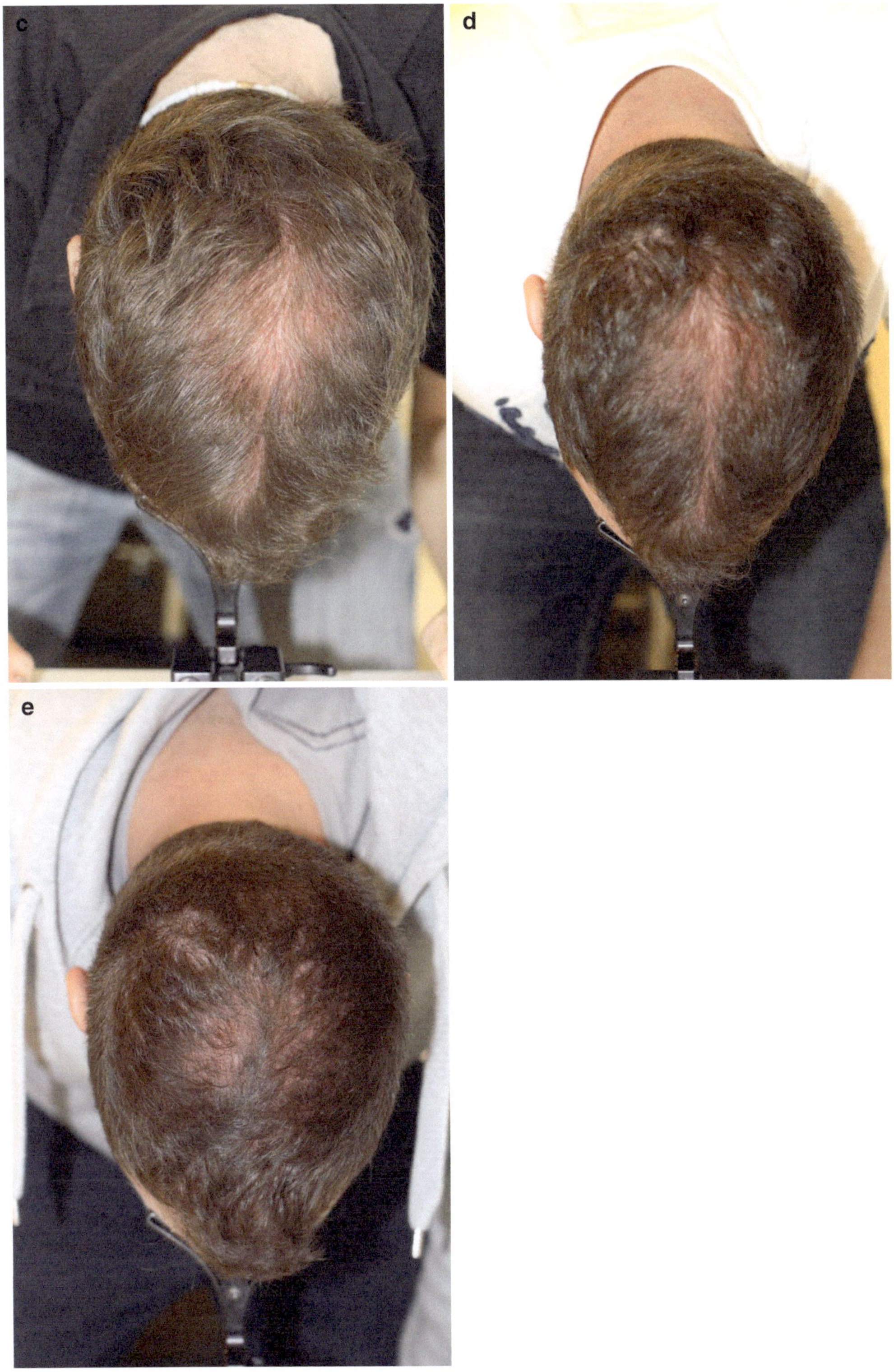

Fig. 3.37 (continued)

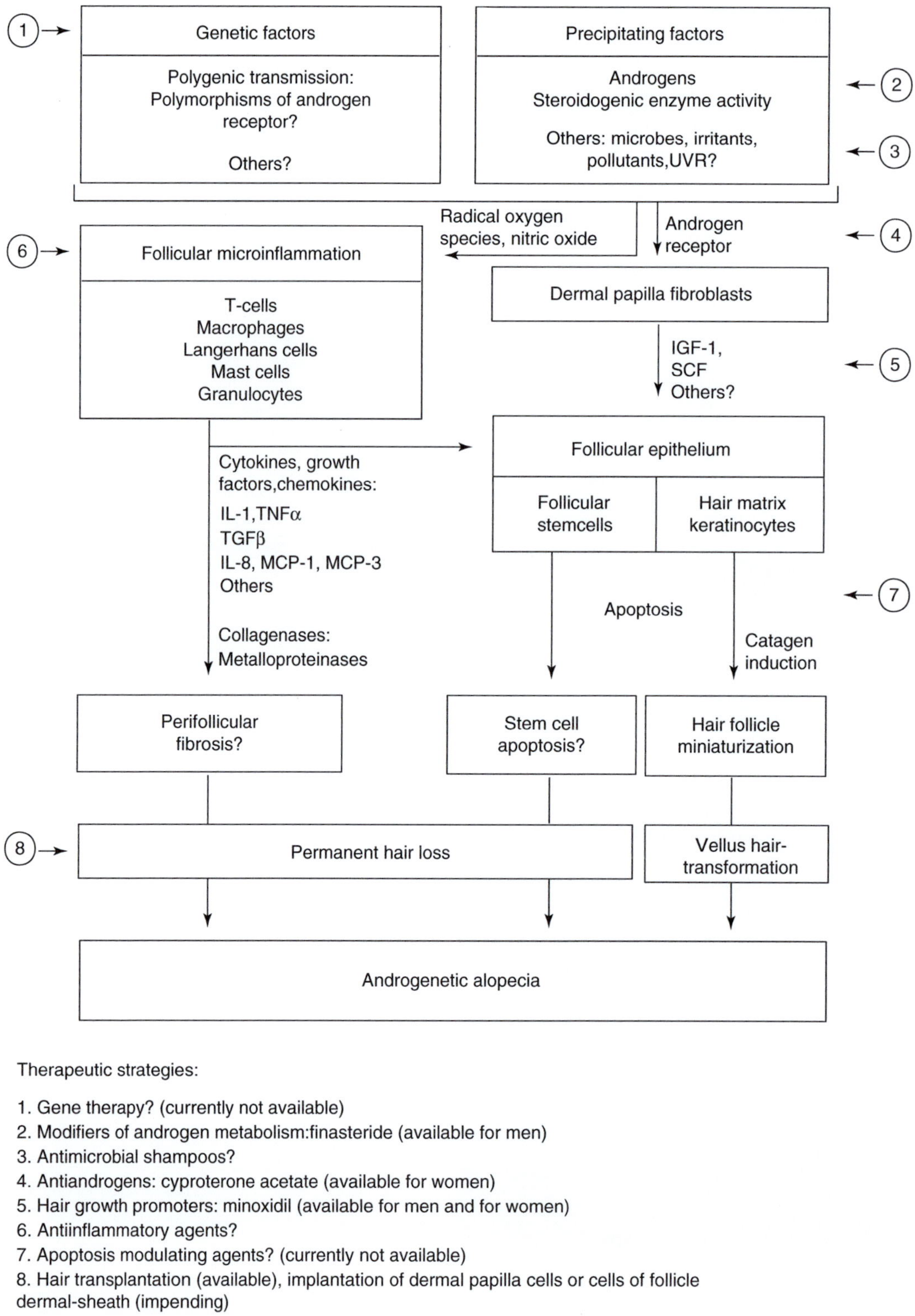

Fig. 3.38 Androgenetic alopecia: pathogenic mechanisms and therapeutic strategies (From: Trüeb RM (2002) Molecular mechanisms of androgenetic alopecia. Exp Gerontol 37:981–990)

3.11.3 Combination Treatments

While mainstream scientists are working on gene polymorphism diagnostics for prediction of risk, prevention, diagnosis, and targeted treatment development for male androgenetic alopecia, on stem cell technologies, and on bioengineering of the hair follicle, health care providers are becoming increasingly aware of a more holistic approach to the problem of hair loss.

Ultimately, combination treatments with oral finasteride, topical minoxidil, ketoconazole shampoo, LLLT, and appropriate nutritional supplementation may act synergistic to enhance hair growth and quality.

The scientific rationale for such an approach is given, but there is need for controlled studies to establish increase in efficacy of combination regimens for management of hair loss and new hair growth.

Examples of successful combination treatments in male androgenetic alopecia are illustrated in Fig. 3.39a–l.

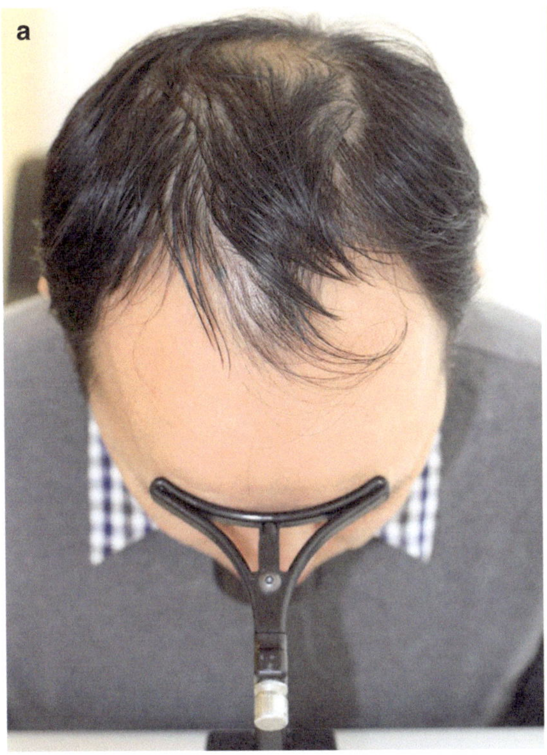

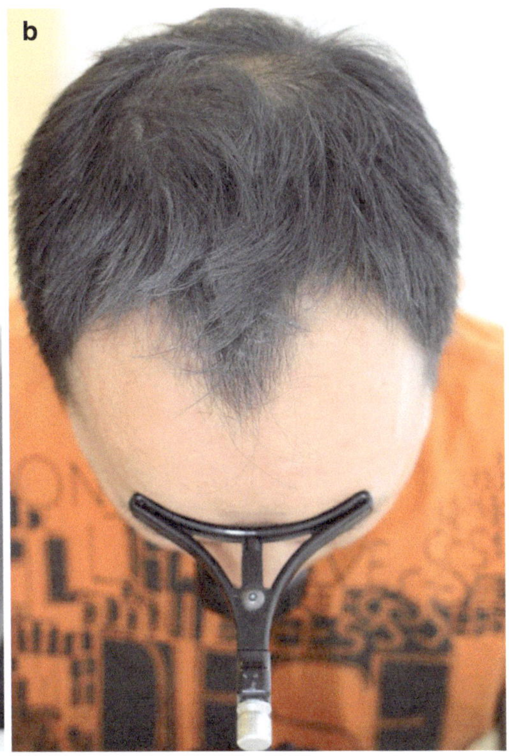

Fig. 3.39 (**a–l**) Successful combination treatments in male androgenetic alopecia. (**a–e**) In a 45-year-old male with 1 mg oral finasteride and topical 5 % minoxidil solution bid, (**a**) before, (**b**) after 3, (**c**) 6, (**d**) 12, and (**e**) 24 months treatment. (**f, g**) In a 54-year-old male adding on LLLT (HairMax LaserComb®) to 4 year pretreatment with topical 5 % minoxidil solution, (**f**) before and (**g**) after 3 months of LLLT. (**h, i**) In a 61-year-old male smoker with 1 mg oral finasteride in combination with oral supplementation with L-cystine and vitamin B6, (**h**) before and (**i**) after 3 months treatment. (**j-l**) In a 36-year-old male, (**j**) before, (**k**) after 9 months treatment with 1 mg oral finasteride and topical 5 % minoxidil solution bid, and (**l**) 3 months after adding on LLLT (HairMax LaserComb®)

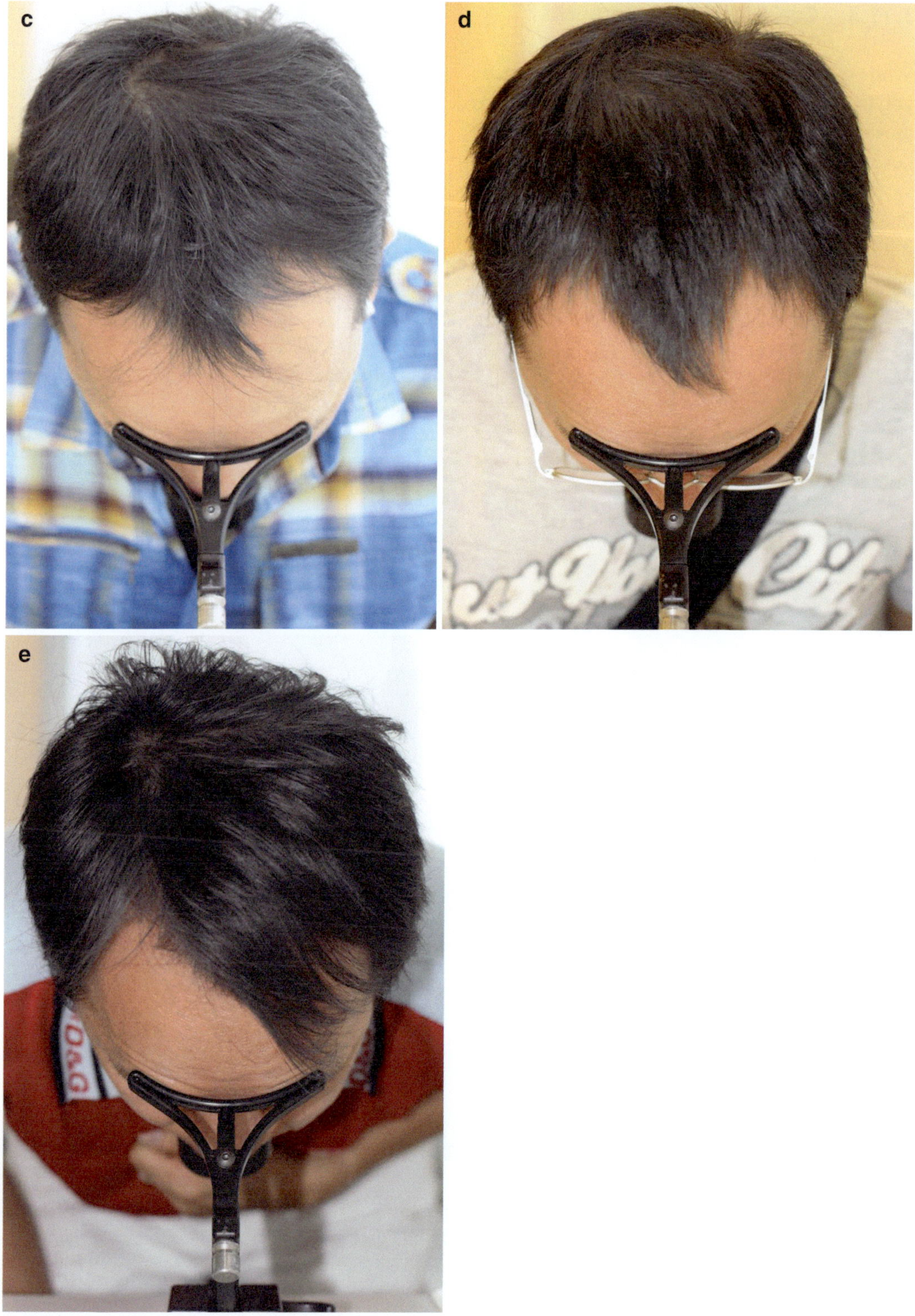

Fig. 3.39 (continued)

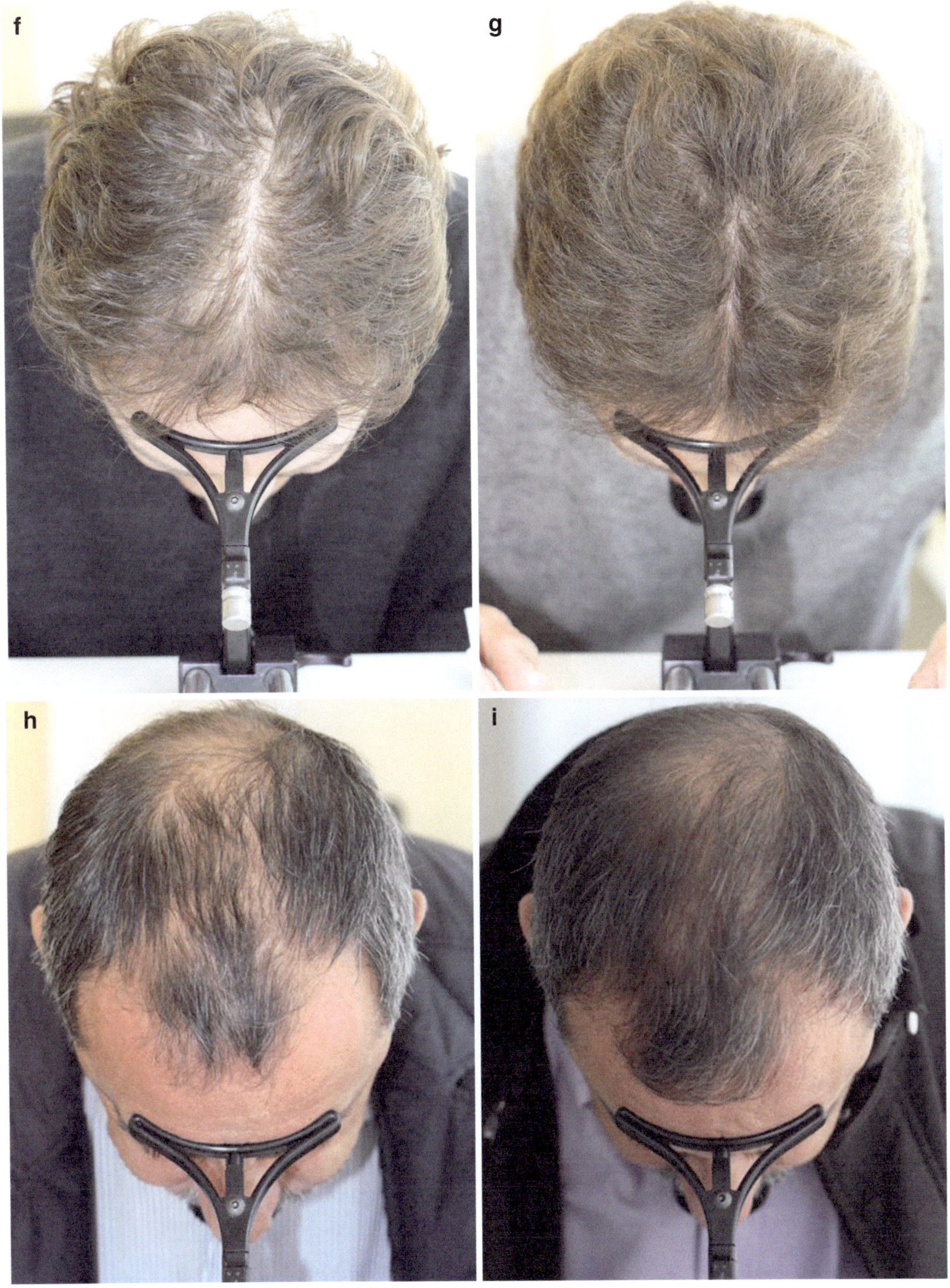

Fig. 3.39 (continued)

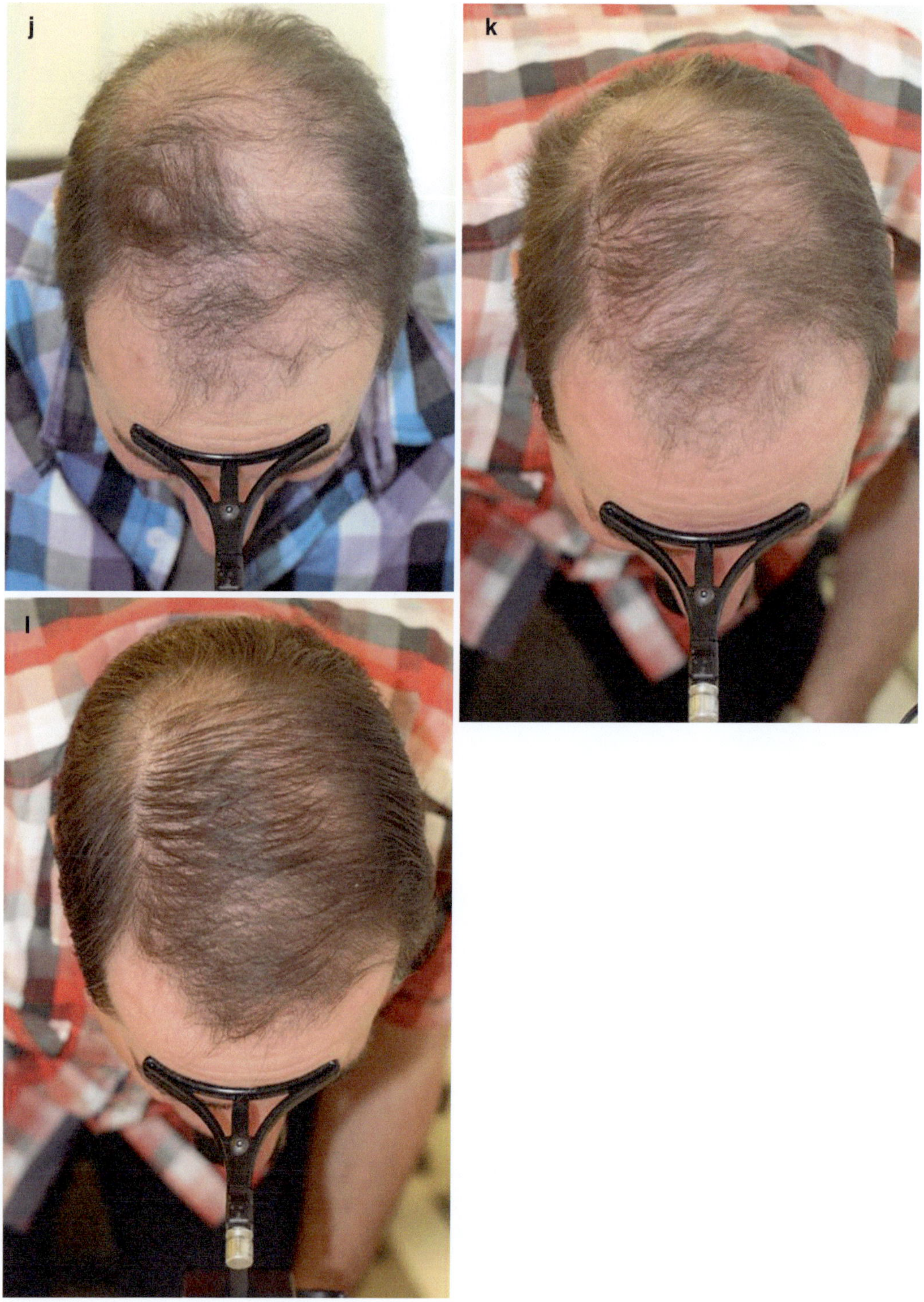

Fig. 3.39 (continued)

Further Reading

Male Androgenetic Alopecia: Pathobiology of Androgenetic Alopecia

Bayne EK, Flanagan J, Einstein M et al (1999) Immunohistochemical localization of types 1 and 2 5α-reductase in human scalp. Br J Dermatol 141:481–491

Cobb JE, White SJ, Harrap SB et al (2009) Androgen receptor copy number variation and androgenetic alopecia: a case-control study. PLoS One 4:e5081

Courtois M, Loussouarn G, Hourseau C (1995) Aging and hair cycles. Br J Dermatol 132:86–93

Fazekas AG, Lanthier A (1971) Metabolism of androgens by isolated human beard hair follicles. Steroids 18:367–379

Hair DX (2013) Available at: http://www.hairdx.com. Accessed 28 July

Hamada K, Randall VA (2006) Inhibitory autocrine factors produced by the mesenchyme-derived hair follicle dermal papilla may be a key to male pattern baldness. Br J Dermatol 154:609–618

Hamilton JB (1942) Male hormone stimulation is prerequisite and an incitant in common baldness. Am J Anat 71:451–480

Hibberts NA, Howell AE, Randall VA (1998) Balding hair follicle dermal papilla cells contain higher levels of androgen receptors than those from non-balding scalp. Endocrinology 156:59–65

Hillmer AM, Hanneken S, Ritzmann S et al (2005) Genetic variation in the human androgen receptor gene is the major determinant of common early-onset androgenetic alopecia. Am J Hum Genet 77:140–148

Hodgins MB, Murad S, Simpson NB (1985) A search for variation in hair follicle androgen metabolism which might be linked to male pattern baldness. Br J Dermatol 113:794 (abstract)

Hoffmann R, Happle R (2000) Current understanding of androgenetic alopecia. Part I: etiopathogenesis. Eur J Dermatol 10:319–326

Itami S, Kurata S, Takayasu S (1990) 5α-Reductase activity in cultured human dermal papilla cells from beard compared with reticular dermal fibroblasts. J Invest Dermatol 94:150–152

Itami S, Kurata S, Takayasu S (1995) Androgen induction of follicular epithelial cell growth is mediated via insulin-like growth factor I from dermal papilla cells. Biochem Biophys Res Commun 212:988–994

Kaufman KD (1996) Androgen metabolism as it affects hair growth in androgenetic alopecia. Dermatol Clin 14:697–711

Legro RS, Carmina E, Stanczyk FZ et al (1994) Alterations in androgen conjugate levels in women and men with alopecia. Fertil Steril 62:744–750

Ludwig E (1968) The role of sexual hormones in pattern alopecias. In: Baccaredda-Boy A, Moretti G, Frey JR (eds) Biopathology of pattern alopecia. Karger, New York, pp 50–60

Nyholt DR, Gillespie NA, Health AC et al (2003) Genetic basis of male pattern baldness. J Invest Dermatol 11:1561–1564

Paus R (1996) Control of the hair cycle and hair diseases as cycling disorders. Curr Opin Dermatol 3:248–258

Paus R, Cotsarelis G (1999) The biology of hair follicles. N Engl J Med 341:491–497

Trüeb RM (2002) Molecular mechanisms of androgenetic alopecia. Exp Gerontol 37:981–990

Trueb RM (2003) New and established methods in therapy of hair diseases. Hautarzt 54:732–740

Male Androgenetic Alopecia: Androgens, Androgen Metabolism, and the Androgen Receptor

Cobb JE, White SJ, Harrap SB et al (2009) Androgen receptor copy number variation and androgenetic alopecia: a case-control study. PLoS One 4:e5081

Fazekas AG, Lanthier A (1971) Metabolism of androgens by isolated human beard hair follicles. Steroids 18:367–379

Hamilton JB (1951) Patterned loss of hair in men; types and incidence. Ann N Y Acad Sci 53:708–728

Hibberts NA, Howell AE, Randall VA (1998) Balding hair follicle dermal papilla cells contain higher levels of androgen receptors than those from non-balding scalp. Endocrinology 156:59–65

Hillmer AM, Hanneken S, Ritzmann S et al (2005) Genetic variation in the human androgen receptor gene is the major determinant of common early-onset androgenetic alopecia. Am J Hum Genet 77:140–148

Hodgins MB, Murad S, Simpson NB (1985) A search for variation in hair follicle androgen metabolism which might be linked to male pattern baldness. Br J Dermatol 113:794 (abstract)

Kaufman KD (1996) Androgen metabolism as it affects hair growth in androgenetic alopecia. Dermatol Clin 14:697–711

Legro RS, Carmina E, Stanczyk FZ et al (1994) Alterations in androgen conjugate levels in women and men with alopecia. Fertil Steril 62:744–750

Quigley CA (1998) The androgen receptor: physiology and pathophysiology. In: Nieschlag E, Behre HM (eds) Testosterone: action, deficiency, substitution. Springer, Berlin, pp 33–106

Randall VA, Thornton MJ, Hamada K et al (1992a) Mechanism of androgen action in cultured dermal papilla cells derived from human hair follicles with varying responses to androgens in vivo. J Invest Dermatol 98:86S–91S

Randall VA, Thornton MJ, Messenger AG (1992b) Cultured dermal papilla cells from androgen-dependent human hair follicles (e.g. beard) contain more androgen receptors than those from non-balding areas of the scalp. J Endocrinol 133:141–147

Richards JB, Yuan X, Geller F et al (2008) Male-pattern baldness susceptibility locus at 20p11. Nat Genet 40:1282–1284

Sato A, Arima Y, Kojima Y et al (2008) Correlation between polymorphic CAG-repeats in the androgen receptor gene and therapeutic efficacy of Finasteride in androgenetic alopecia. Skin Surg 17:80–86

Sawaya ME, Honig LS, Garland LD et al (1988) Delta 5-3 beta-hydroxysteroid dehydrogenase activity in sebaceous glands of scalp in male-pattern baldness. J Invest Dermatol 91:101–105

Schmidt JB, Lindmaier A, Spona J (1991) Hormonal parameters in androgenetic hair loss in the male. Dermatologica 1832:214–217

Takashima I, Adachi K, Montagna W (1970) Studies of common baldness in the stumptailed macaque IV: in vitro metabolism of testosterone in the hair follicles. J Invest Dermatol 55:329–334

Trüeb RM (2002) Molecular mechanisms of androgenetic alopecia. Exp Gerontol 37:981–990

Genetic Involvement

Cobb JE, White SJ, Harrap SB et al (2009) Androgen receptor copy number variation and androgenetic alopecia: a case-control study. PLoS One 4:e5081

Ellis JA, Scurrah KJ, Cobb JE et al (2007) Baldness and the androgen receptor: the AR polyglycine repeat polymorphism does not confer susceptibility to androgenetic alopecia. Hum Genet 121:451–457

Heilmann S, Kiefer AK, Fricker N et al (2013) Androgenetic alopecia: identification of four genetic risk loci and evidence for the contribution of WNT signaling to its etiology. J Invest Dermatol 133: 1489–1496

Hillmer AM, Hanneken S, Ritzmann S et al (2005) Genetic variation in the human androgen receptor gene is the major determinant of common early-onset androgenetic alopecia. Am J Hum Genet 77: 140–148

Köonig A, Happle R, Tchitcherina E et al (2000) An X-linked gene involved in androgenetic alopecia: a lesson to be learned from adrenoleukodystrophy. Dermatology 200:213–218

Nyholt DR, Gillespie NA, Health AC et al (2003) Genetic basis of male pattern baldness. J Invest Dermatol 11:1561–1564

Paus R, Cotsarelis G (1999) The biology of hair follicles. N Engl J Med 341:491–497

Prodi DA, Pirastu N, Maninchedda G et al (2008) EDA2R is associated with androgenetic alopecia. J Invest Dermatol 128:2268–2270

Quigley CA (1998) The androgen receptor: physiology and pathophysiology. In: Nieschlag E, Behre HM (eds) Testosterone: action, deficiency, substitution. Springer, Berlin, pp 33–106

Randall VA, Thornton MJ, Hamada K et al (1992) Mechanism of androgen action in cultured dermal papilla cells derived from human hair follicles with varying responses to androgens in vivo. J Invest Dermatol 98:86S–91S

Richards JB, Yuan X, Geller F et al (2008) Male-pattern baldness susceptibility locus at 20p11. Nat Genet 40:1282–1284

Sato A, Arima Y, Kojima Y et al (2008) Correlation between polymorphic CAG-repeats in the androgen receptor gene and therapeutic efficacy of Finasteride in androgenetic alopecia. Skin Surg 17:80–86

Wakisaka N, Taira Y, Ishikawa M et al (2005) Effectiveness of finasteride on patients with male pattern baldness who have different androgen receptor gene polymorphism. J Investig Dermatol Symp Proc 10:293–294

Zhuo FL, Xu W, Wang Y et al (2011) Androgen receptor gene polymorphisms and risk for androgenetic alopecia: a meta-analysis. Clin Exp Dermatol 37:104–111

Male Androgenetic Alopecia: Gene Polymorphism Diagnostics in Androgenetic Alopecia

Cobb JE, White SJ, Harrap SB et al (2009) Androgen receptor copy number variation and androgenetic alopecia: a case-control study. PLoS One 4:e5081

Ellis JA, Scurrah KJ, Cobb JE et al (2007) Baldness and the androgen receptor: the AR polyglycine repeat polymorphism does not confer susceptibility to androgenetic alopecia. Hum Genet 121:451–457

Hair DX (2013) Available at: http://www.hairdx.com. Accessed 28 July

Heilmann S, Kiefer AK, Fricker N et al (2013) Androgenetic alopecia: identification of four genetic risk loci and evidence for the contribution of WNT signaling to its etiology. J Invest Dermatol 133:1489–1496

Hillmer AM, Hanneken S, Ritzmann S et al (2005) Genetic variation in the human androgen receptor gene is the major determinant of common early-onset androgenetic alopecia. Am J Hum Genet 77:140–148

Nyholt DR, Gillespie NA, Health AC et al (2003) Genetic basis of male pattern baldness. J Invest Dermatol 11:1561–1564

Quigley CA (1998) The androgen receptor: physiology and pathophysiology. In: Nieschlag E, Behre HM (eds) Testosterone: action, deficiency, substitution. Springer, Berlin, pp 33–106

Richards JB, Yuan X, Geller F et al (2008) Male-pattern baldness susceptibility locus at 20p11. Nat Genet 40:1282–1284

Sato A, Arima Y, Kojima Y et al (2008) Correlation between polymorphic CAG-repeats in the androgen receptor gene and therapeutic efficacy of Finasteride in androgenetic alopecia. Skin Surg 17:80–86

Wakisaka N, Taira Y, Ishikawa M et al (2005) Effectiveness of finasteride on patients with male pattern baldness who have different androgen receptor gene polymorphism. J Investig Dermatol Symp Proc 10:293–294

Zhuo FL, Xu W, Wang Y et al (2011) Androgen receptor gene polymorphisms and risk for androgenetic alopecia: a meta-analysis. Clin Exp Dermatol 37:104–111

Male Androgenetic Alopecia: Syndromatic Androgenetic Alopecia

Amorosi B, Giustini S, Rossi A, Giacanelli M, Calvieri S (1999) Myotonic dystrophy (Steinert disease): a morphologic and biochemical hair study. Int J Dermatol 38:434–438

Geh JL, Moss AL (1999) Multiple pilomatrixomata and myotonic dystrophy: a familial association. Br J Plast Surg 52:143–145

Lurie R, Ben-Amitai D, Laron Z (2004) Laron syndrome (primary growth hormone insensitivity): a unique model to explore the effect of insulin-like growth factor 1 deficiency on human hair. Dermatology 208:314–318

Sherrod QJ, Chiu MW, Gutierrez M (2008) Multiple pilomatricomas: cutaneous marker for myotonic dystrophy. Dermatol Online J 14:22

Male Androgenetic Alopecia: Premature Alopecia

Blume-Peytavi U, Blumeyer A, Tosti A, Finner A, Marmol V, Trakatelli M, Reygagne P, Messenger A, European Consensus Group (2001) S1 guideline for diagnostic evaluation in androgenetic alopecia in men, women and adolescents. Br J Dermatol 164:5–15

Georgala S, Befon A, Maniatopoulou E, Georgala C (2007) Topical use of minoxidil in children and systemic side effects. Dermatology 214:101–102

Tosti A, Iorizzo M, Piraccini BM (2005) Androgenetic alopecia in children: report of 20 cases. Br J Dermatol 152:556–559

Male Androgenetic Alopecia: Clinical Presentations and Classifications

Beek CH (1950) A study on extension and distribution of the human body hair. Dermatologica 101:317–331

Birch MP, Messenger JF, Messenger AG (2001) Hair density, hair diameter and the prevalence of female pattern hair loss. Br J Dermatol 144:297–304

Camacho-Martinez FM (2009) Hair loss in women. Semin Cutan Med Surg 28:19–32

Dinh QQ, Sinclair R (2007) Female pattern hair loss: current treatment concepts. Clin Interv Aging 2:189–199

Guarrera M, Cardo P, Arrigo P et al (2009) Reliability of hamilton-norwood classification. Int J Trichology 1:120–122

Hamilton JB (1951) Patterned loss of hair in men; types and incidence. Ann N Y Acad Sci 53:708–728

Hong H, Ji JH, Lee Y et al (2013) Reliability of the pattern hair loss classifications: a comparison of the basic and specific and Norwood-Hamilton classifications. J Dermatol 40:102–106

Jang WS, Son IP, Yeo IK et al (2013) The annual changes of clinical manifestation of androgenetic alopecia clinic in Korean males and females: a outpatient-based study. Ann Dermatol 25:181–188

Khumalo NP, Gumedze F (2012) The adapted classification of male pattern hair loss improves reliability. Dermatology 225:110–114

Koo SH, Chung HS, Yoon ES et al (2000) A new classification of male pattern baldness and a clinical study of the anterior hairline. Aesthetic Plast Surg 24:46–51

Lee WS, Lee HJ (2012) Characteristics of androgenetic alopecia in Asian. Ann Dermatol 24:243–252

Lee WS, Ro BI, Hong SP et al (2007) A new classification of pattern hair loss that is universal for men and women: basic and specific (BASP) classification. J Am Acad Dermatol 57(1):37–46

Lee WS, Oh Y, Ji JH et al (2011) Analysis of familial factors using the basic and specific (BASP) classification in Korean patients with androgenetic alopecia. J Am Acad Dermatol 65:40–47

Ludwig E (1977) Classification of the types of androgenetic alopecia (common baldness) occurring in the female sex. Br J Dermatol 97:247–254

Norwood OT (1975) Male pattern baldness: classification and incidence. South Med J 68:1359–1365

Olsen EA (2001) Female pattern hair loss. J Am Acad Dermatol 45:S70–S80

Olsen EA (2003) Current and novel methods for assessing efficacy of hair growth promoters in pattern hair loss. J Am Acad Dermatol 48:253–262

Olsen EA, Canfield D, Canfield W et al (2003) A novel method for assessing regional scalp hair density in male pattern hair loss. In: Van Neste D (ed) Hair science and technology. McGraw-Hill, New York, pp 251–254

Sehgal VN, Aggarwal AK, Srivastava G et al (2006) Male pattern androgenetic alopecia. Skin Med 5:128–135

Male Androgenetic Alopecia: Comorbidities of Male Androgenetic Alopecia

Abdel Fattah NS, Darwish YW (2011) Androgenetic alopecia and insulin resistance: are they truly associated? Int J Dermatol 50:417–422

Acibucu F, Kayatas M, Candan F (2010) The association of insulin resistance and metabolic syndrome in early androgenetic alopecia. Singapore Med J 51:931–936

Adams BB (2001) Water-slide alopecia. Cutis 67:399–400

Arias-Santiago S, Gutierrez-Salmeron MT, Buendia-Eisman A et al (2010a) Hypertension and aldosterone levels in women with early-onset androgenetic alopecia. Br J Dermatol 162:786–789

Arias-Santiago S, Gutierrez-Salmeron MT, Buendia-Eisman A et al (2010b) Lipid levels in women with androgenetic alopecia. Int J Dermatol 49:1340–1342

Arias-Santiago S, Gutierrez-Salmeron MT, Buendia-Eisman A et al (2010c) A comparative study of dyslipidaemia in men and woman with androgenic alopecia. Acta Derm Venereol 90:485–487

Arias-Santiago S, Gutierrez-Salmeron MT, Buendia-Eisman A et al (2011) Sex hormone-binding globulin and risk of hyperglycemia in patients with androgenetic alopecia. J Am Acad Dermatol 65:48–53
Cotton SG, Nixon JM, Carpenter RG et al (1972) Factors discriminating men with coronary heart disease from healthy controls. Br Heart J 34:458–464
Dogramaci AC, Balci DD, Balci A et al (2009) Is androgenetic alopecia a risk for atherosclerosis? J Eur Acad Dermatol Venereol 23:673–677
Duskova M, Hill M, Starka L (2010) Changes of metabolic profile in men treated for androgenetic alopecia with 1 mg finasteride. Endocr Regul 44:3–8
Gupta SN, Shaw JC (2002) Anterolateral leg alopecia revisited. Cutis 70:215–216
Hamilton JB (1951) Patterned loss of hair in man: types and incidence. Ann N Y Acad Sci 53:708–728
Kidd. Cited by: Danforth CH (1925) Studies on hair, with special reference to hypertrichosis, IV: regional characteristics of human hair. Arch Dermtol Syph 12:76
Kligman AM (1970) Is there a relation between leg hair loss and arteriosclerosis? JAMA 212:328
Lesko SM, Rosenberg L, Shapiro S (1993) A case-control study of baldness in relation to myocardial infarction in men. JAMA 269:998–1003
Mumcuoglu C, Ekmekci TR, Ucak S (2011) The investigation of insulin resistance and metabolic syndrome in male patients with early-onset androgenetic alopecia. Eur J Dermatol 21:79–82
Popkin RJ (1970) Relation of leg hair loss to arteriosclerosis. JAMA 213:130
Robertson PC (1938) Description and study of an area of atrophic skin occurring in men, with its relationship to the common type of diffuse alopecia of the scalp. Br J Dermatol Syph 50:581
Ronchese F, Chase RR (1939) Patterned alopecia about the calves and its apparent lack of significance. Arch Dermatol Syph 40:416–421
Su LH, Chen LS, Lin SC et al (2013) Association of androgenetic alopecia with mortality from diabetes mellitus and heart disease. JAMA Dermatol 149:601–606
Tommasi L (1940) Alopecia of the peroneal regions as a constitutional sign of neuro-arthritic diathesis. Br J Dermatol 52:1–9
Turpie ID (1983) Localized hair loss in an elderly man. Can Med Assoc J 129:536
Yi SM, Son SW, Lee KG et al (2012) Gender-specific association of androgenetic alopecia with metabolic syndrome in a middle-aged Korean population. Br J Dermatol 167:306–313

Male Androgenetic Alopecia: Evidence-Based Pharmacologic Treatments

Amory JK, Wang C, Swerdloff RS et al (2007) The effect of 5alpha-reductase inhibition with dutasteride and finasteride on semen parameters and serum hormones in healthy men. J Clin Endocrinol Metab 92:1659–1665
Beek CH (1950) A study on extension and distribution of the human body hair. Dermatologica 101:317–331
Blume-Peytavi U, Kunte C, Krisp A, Garcia Bartels N, Ellwanger U, Hoffmann R (2007) Comparison of the efficacy and safety of topical minoxidil and topical alfatradiol in the treatment of androgenetic alopecia in women. J Dtsch Dermatol Ges 5:391–395
Choi JW, Na SY, Park KC, Youn SW, Huh CH (2012) Relation between treatment efficacy and cumulative dose of 3% topical minoxidil in male pattern baldness. J Am Acad Dermatol 66(1):e10–e12
De Villez RL, Jacobs JP, Szpunar CA, Warner ML (1994) Androgenetic alopecia in the female. Treatment with 2% topical minoxidil solution. Arch Dermatol 3:303–307
Drake L, Hordinsky M, Fiedler V et al (1999) The effects of finasteride on scalp skin and serum androgen levels in men with androgenetic alopecia. J Am Acad Dermatol 41:550–554
Eun HC, Kwon OS, Yeon JH et al (2010) Efficacy, safety, and tolerability of dutasteride 0.5 mg once daily in male patients with male pattern hair loss: a randomized, double-blind, placebo-controlled, phase III study. J Am Acad Dermatol 63:252–258
Finasteride Male Pattern Hair Loss Study Group (2002) Long-term (5-year) multinational experience with finasteride 1 mg in the treatment of men with androgenetic alopecia. Eur J Dermatol 12:38–49
Gassmueller J, Hoffmann R, Webster A (2008) Topical fulvestrant solution has no effect on male and postmenopausal female androgenetic alopecia: results from two randomized, proof-of-concept studies. Br J Dermatol 158:109–115
Hajheydari Z, Akbari J, Saeedi M, Shokoohi L (2009) Comparing the therapeutic effects of finasteride gel and tablet in treatment of the androgenetic alopecia. Indian J Dermatol Venereol Leprol 75:47–51
Kaufman KD, Olsen EA, Whiting D et al (1998) Finasteride in the treatment of men with androgenetic alopecia. Finasteride Male Pattern Hair Loss Study Group. J Am Acad Dermatol 39:578–589
Kaufman KD, Rotonda J, Shah AK et al (2008) Long-term treatment with finasteride 1 mg decreases the likelihood of developing further visible hair loss in men with androgenetic alopecia (male pattern hair loss). Eur J Dermatol 18:400–406
Kawashima M, Hayashi N, Igarashi A et al (2004) Finasteride in the treatment of Japanese men with male pattern hair loss. Eur J Dermatol 14:247–254
Kumar R, Singh B, Bakshi G, Katare OP (2007) Development of liposomal systems of finasteride for topical applications: design, characterization, and in vitro evaluation. Pharm Dev Technol 12:591–601
Lachgar S, Charveron M, Gall Y et al (1998) Minoxidil upregulates the expression of vascular endothelial growth factor in human hair dermal papilla cells. Br J Dermatol 138:407–411

Leyden J, Dunlap F, Miller B et al (1999) Finasteride in the treatment of men with frontal male pattern hair loss. J Am Acad Dermatol 40:930–937

Li M, Marubayashi A, Nakaya Y, Fukui K, Arase S (2001) Minoxidil-induced hair growth is mediated by adenosine in cultured dermal papilla cells: possible involvement of sulfonylurea receptor 2B as a target of minoxidil. J Invest Dermatol 117:1594–1600

Madheswaran T, Baskaran R, Thapa RK, Rhyu JY, Choi HY, Kim JO, Yong CS, Yoo BK (2013) Design and in vitro evaluation of finasteride-loaded liquid crystalline nanoparticles for topical delivery. AAPS PharmSciTech 14:45–52

Matzkin H, Barak M, Braf Z (1996) Effect of finasteride on free and total serum prostate-specific antigen in men with benign prostatic hyperplasia. Br J Urol 78:405–408

Mazzarrella F, Loconsole F, Cammisa F et al (1997) Topical finasteride in the treatment of androgenetic alopecia. J Dermatolog Treat 8:189–192

Murugusundram S (2009) Serenoa repens: does it have any role in the management of androgenetic alopecia? J Cutan Aesthet Surg 2:31–32

Olsen EA, Weiner MS, Delong ER et al (1985) Topical minoxidil in early male pattern baldness. J Am Acad Dermatol 13:185–192

Olsen EA, DeLong ER, Weiner MS (1987) Long-term follow-up of men with male pattern baldness treated with topical minoxidil. J Am Acad Dermatol 16:688–695

Olsen EA, Weiner MS, Amara IA, DeLong ER (1990) Five-year follow-up of men with androgenetic alopecia treated with topical minoxidil. J Am Acad Dermatol 22:643–646

Olsen EA, Dunlap FE, Funicella T et al (2002) A randomized clinical trial of 5% topical minoxidil versus 2% topical minoxidil and placebo in the treatment of androgenetic alopecia in men. J Am Acad Dermatol 47:377–385

Olsen EA, Hordinsky M, Whiting D et al (2006) The importance of dual 5alpha-reductase inhibition in the treatment of male pattern hair loss: results of a randomized placebo-controlled study of dutasteride versus finasteride. J Am Acad Dermatol 55:1014–1023

Prager N, Bickett K, French N, Marcovici G (2002) A randomized, double-blind, placebo-controlled trial to determine the effectiveness of botanically derived inhibitors of 5-alpha-reductase in the treatment of androgenetic alopecia. J Altern Complement Med 8:143–152

Price VH, Menefee E, Sanchez M et al (2006) Changes in hair weight in men with androgenetic alopecia after treatment with finasteride (1 mg daily): three- and 4-year results. J Am Acad Dermatol 55:71–74

Rossi A, Mari E, Scarno M, Garelli V, Maxia C, Scali E, Iorio A, Carlesimo M (2012) Comparative effectiveness of finasteride vs serenoa repens in male androgenetic alopecia: a two-year study. Int J Immunopathol Pharmacol 25:1167–1173

Rundegren J (2004) Pattern alopecia: what clinical features determine the response to topical minoxidil treatment? IHRS2004 abstract B2.4. JDDG 2:500

Sovak M, Seligson AL, Kucerova R et al (2002) Fluridil, a rationally designed topical agent for androgenetic alopecia: first clinical experience. Dermatol Surg 28:678–685

Stough D (2007) Dutasteride improves male pattern hair loss in a randomized study in identical twins. J Cosmet Dermatol 6:9–13

Tanglertsampan C (2013) Efficacy and safety of 3% minoxidil versus combined 3% minoxidil / 0.1% finasteride in male pattern hair loss: a randomized, double-blind, comparative study. J Med Assoc Thai 95:1312–1316

Trueb RM (2003) New and established methods in therapy of hair diseases. Hautarzt 54:732–740

Van Neste D, Fuh V, Sanchez-Pedreno P et al (2000) Finasteride increases anagen hair in men with androgenetic alopecia. Br J Dermatol 143:804–810

Wester RC, Maibach HI, Guy RH et al (1984) Minoxidil stimulates cutaneous blood flow in human balding scalps: pharmacodynamics measured by laser Doppler velocimetry and photopulse plethysmography. J Invest Dermatol 82:515–517

Whiting DA, Waldstreicher J, Sanchez M et al (1999) Measuring reversal of hair miniaturization in androgenetic alopecia by follicular counts in horizontal sections of serial scalp biopsies: results of finasteride 1 mg treatment of men and postmenopausal women. J Investig Dermatol Symp Proc 4:282–284

Male Androgenetic Alopecia: Autologous Hair Transplantation

Avram MR (2005) Laser-assisted hair transplantation – a status report in the 21st century. J Cosmet Dermatol 4:135–139

Avram MR (2006) Hair transplantation for men and women. Semin Cutan Med Surg 25:60–64

Bernstein RM, Rassman WR (1998) Dissecting microscope versus magnifying loupes with transillumination in the preparation of follicular unit grafts. A bilateral controlled study. Dermatol Surg 24(8):875–880

Bunagan MJ, Banka N, Shapiro J (2013) Hair transplantation update: procedural techniques, innovations, and applications. Dermatol Clin 31:141–153

Chiang YZ, Tosti A, Chaudhry IH et al (2012) Lichen planopilaris following hair transplantation and face-lift surgery. Br J Dermatol 166:666–670

Kim JC, Unger W, Shapiro R et al (2011) Hair transplantation, 5th edn. Marcel Dekker, New York, pp 404–406

Marc RA (2012) Hair transplantation. Cutis 90:317–320

Pathomvanich D (2000) Donor harvesting: a new approach to minimize transaction of hair follicles. Dermatol Surg 26:345–348

Ross EK, Shapiro J (2005) Management of hair loss. Dermatol Clin 23:227–243

Salanitri S, Gonçalves AJ, Helene A Jr et al (2009) Surgical complications in hair transplantation: a series of 533 procedures. Aesthet Surg J 29:72–76

Unger W, Unger R, Wesley C (2008) The surgical treatment of cicatricial alopecia. Dermatol Ther 21: 295–311

Male Androgenetic Alopecia: Miscellaneous Treatments

Avram MR, Rogers NE (2009) The use of low-level light for hair growth: part I. J Cosmet Laser Ther 11:110–117

Avram MR, Leonard RT Jr, Epstein ES, Williams JL, Bauman AJ (2007) The current role of laser/light sources in the treatment of male and female pattern hair loss. J Cosmet Laser Ther 9:27–28

Bernstein EF (2005) Hair growth induced by diode laser treatment. Dermatol Surg 31:584–586

Blume-Peytavi U, Lönnfors S, Hillmann K et al (2012) A randomized double-blind placebo-controlled pilot study to assess the efficacy of a 24-week topical treatment by latanoprost 0.1% on hair growth and pigmentation in healthy volunteers with androgenetic alopecia. J Am Acad Dermatol 66:794–800

Blumeyer A, Tosti A, Messenger A et al (2011) Evidence-based (S3) guideline for the treatment of androgenetic alopecia in women and in men. J Dtsch Dermatol Ges 9(Suppl 6):S1–S57

Drake LA, Dinehart SM, Farmer ER et al (1996) Guidelines of care for androgenetic alopecia. American Academy of Dermatology. J Am Acad Dermatol 35:465–469

Duque-Estrada B, Vincenzi C, Misciali C, Tosti A (2009) Alopecia secondary to mesotherapy. J Am Acad Dermatol 61:707–709

Ellis JA, Sinclair RD (2008) Male pattern baldness: current treatments, future prospects. Drug Discov Today 13:791–797

Ferry JJ, Forbes KK, Vander Lugt JT et al (1990) Influence of tretinoin on the percutaneous absorption of minoxidil from an aqueous topical solution. Clin Pharmacol Ther 47:439–446

Fischer TW, Trüeb RM, Hänggi G et al (2012) Topical melatonin for treatment of androgenetic alopecia. Int J Trichology 4:236–245

Ghanaat M (2010) Types of hair loss and treatment options, including the novel low-level light therapy and its proposed mechanism. South Med J 103:917–921

Hugo Perez BS (2004) Ketoconazole as an adjunct to finasteride in the treatment of androgenetic alopecia in men. Med Hypotheses 62:112–115

Kadry R, Hamadah I, Al-Issa A, Field L, Alrabiah F (2008) Multifocal scalp abscess with subcutaneous fat necrosis and scarring alopecia as a complication of scalp mesotherapy. J Drugs Dermatol 7:72–73

Khandpur S, Suman M, Reddy BS (2002) Comparative efficacy of various treatment regimens for androgenetic alopecia in men. J Dermatol 8:489–498

Khidhir KG, Woodward DF, Farjo NP et al (2013) The prostamide-related glaucoma therapy, bimatoprost, offers a novel approach for treating scalp alopecias. FASEB J 27:557–567

Kim JH, Lee SY, Lee HJ et al (2012) The efficacy and safety of 17alpha-Estradiol (Ell-Cranell(R) alpha 0.025%) solution on female pattern hair loss: single center, open-label, Non-comparative, phase IV study. Ann Dermatol 24:295–305

Kim H, Choi JW, Kim JY et al (2013) Low-level light therapy for androgenetic alopecia: a 24-week, randomized, double-blind, sham device-controlled multicenter trial. Dermatol Surg 39:8

Leavitt M, Perez-Meza D, Rao NA et al (2003) Effects of finasteride (1 mg) on hair transplant. Dermatol Surg 31:1268–1276

Leavitt M, Charles G, Heyman E, Michaels D (2009) HairMax LaserComb laser phototherapy device in the treatment of male androgenetic alopecia: a randomized, double-blind, sham device-controlled, multicentre trial. Clin Drug Investig 29:283–292

Lee WS, Lee HJ, Choi GS et al (2013) Guidelines for management of androgenetic alopecia based on BASP classification-the Asian consensus committee guideline. J Eur Acad Dermatol Venereol 27: 1026–1034

Mester E, Szende B, Gärtner P (1968) The effect of laser beams on the growth of hair in mice. Radiobiol Radiother (Berl) 9:621–626 [Article in German]

Moreno-Arias G, Castelo-Branco C, Ferrando J (2002) Paradoxical effect after IPL photoepilation. Dermatol Surg 28:1013–1016

Olsen EA, Messenger AG, Shapiro J et al (2005) Evaluation and treatment of male and female pattern hair loss. J Am Acad Dermatol 52:301–311

Price VH (1999) Treatment of hair loss. N Engl J Med 341:964–973

Sasaki S, Hozumi Y, Kondo S (2005) Influence of prostaglandin F2 alpha and its analogues on hair regrowth and follicular melanogenesis in a murine model. Exp Dermatol 14:323–328

Shapiro J, Wiseman M, Lui H (2000) Practical management of hair loss. Can Fam Physician 46:1469–1477

Shin HS, Won CH, Lee SH et al (2007) Efficacy of 5% minoxidil versus combined 5% minoxidil and 0.01% tretinoin for male pattern hair loss: a randomized, double- blind, comparative clinical trial. Am J Clin Dermatol 8:285–290

Trueb RM (2003) New and established methods in therapy of hair diseases. Hautarzt 54:732–740

Trink A, Sorbellini E, Bezzola P, Rodella L, Rezzani R, Ramot Y, Rinaldi F (2013) A randomized, double-blind, placebo- and active-controlled, half-head study to evaluate the effects of platelet-rich plasma on alopecia areata. Br J Dermatol 2013169:690–694

Tsuboi R, Itami S, Inui S et al (2012) Guidelines for the management of androgenetic alopecia. J Dermatol 39:113–120

Effect of Cigarette Smoking and UV Radiation: Effect of Cigarette Smoking on Hair Growth

Arck PC, Handjiski B, Hagen E et al (2001) Indications for a 'brain-hair follicle axis (BHA)': inhibition of keratinocyte proliferation and up-regulation of keratinocyte apoptosis in telogen hair follicles by stress and substance P. FASEB J 15:2536–2538

Boyd AS, Stasko T, King LE et al (1999) Cigarette smoking-associated elastotic changes in the skin. J Am Acad Dermatol 41:23–26

Cash TF (1992) The psychological effects of androgenetic alopecia in men. J Am Acad Dermatol 26:926–931

Cash TF, Price VH, Savin RC (1993) Psychological effects of androgenetic alopecia on women: comparisons with balding men and with female control subjects. J Am Acad Dermatol 29:568–575

Daniell HW (1971) Smoker's wrinkles: a study in the epidemiology of "crow's feet". Ann Intern Med 75: 873–880

Dardour JC, Pugash E, Aziza R (1988) The one-stage preauricular flap for male pattern baldness: long-term results and risk factors. Plast Reconstr Surg 81:907–912

Davis BE, Koh HK (1992) Faces going up in smoke. Arch Dermatol 128:1106–1107

Demierre MF, Brooks D, Koh HK, Geller AC (1999) Public knowledge, awareness, and perceptions of the association between skin aging and smoking. J Am Acad Dermatol 41:27–30

Ernster VL, Grady D, Milke R et al (1995) Facial wrinkling in men and women, by smoking status. Am J Public Health 85:78–82

Frances C (1992) Smoking and the skin. Int J Dermatol 31:779–780

Frances C, Boisnic S, Hartmann DJ (1991) Changes in elastic tissue of the non-sun-exposed skin of cigarette smokers. Br J Dermatol 125:43–47

Grandy D, Ernster V (1992) Does cigarette smoking make you ugly and old? Am J Epidemiol 135:839–842

Haley NJ, Hoffmann D (1985) Analysis for nicotine and cotinine in hair to determine cigarette smoker status. Clin Chem 31:1598–1600

Hayakawa K, Shimizu T, Ohba Y et al (1992) Intrapair differences of physical aging and longevity in identical twins. Acta Genet Med Gemellol (Roma) 141: 177–185

Ippen M, Ippen H (1965) Approaches to a prophylaxis of skin ageing. J Soc Cosmet Chem 16:305–308

Joffe I (1991) Cigarette smoking and facial wrinkling. Ann Intern Med 115:659

Kadunce DP, Burr R, Gress R et al (1991) Cigarette smoking: risk factor for premature facial wrinkling. Ann Intern Med 114:840–844

Lahmann C, Bergemann J, Harrison G, Young AR (2001) Matrix metalloproteinase-1 and skin ageing in smokers. Lancet 357:935–936

Laurent P, Janoff A, Kagan HM (1983) Cigarette smoke blocks cross-linking of elastin in vitro. Am Rev Respir Dis 127:189–194

Liu CS, Kao SH, Wei YH (1997) Smoking-associated mitochondrial DNA mutations in human hair follicles. Environ Mol Mutagen 30:47–55

Mahé YF, Michelet JF, Billoni N et al (2000) Androgenetic alopecia and microinflammation. Int J Dermatol 39:576–584

Model D (1985) Smokers face: an underrated clinical sign? BMJ 291:1760–1762

Mosley JG, Gibbs CC (1996) Premature grey hair and hair loss among smokers: a new opportunity for health education? BMJ 313:1616

Osawa Y, Tochigi B, Tochigi M et al (1990) Aromatase inhibitors in cigarette smoke, tobacco leaves and other plants. J Enzyme Inhib 4:187–200

Paus R, Krejci-Papa N, Li L et al (1994) Correlation of proteolytic activities of organ cultured intact mouse skin with defined hair cycle stages. J Dermatol Sci 7:202–209

Philpott MP, Sander DA, Bowen J, Kealey T (1996) Effects of interleukins, colony stimulating factor and tumour necrosis factor on human hair follicle growth in vitro: a possible role for interleukin-1 and tumour necrosis factor-a in alopecia areata. Br J Dermatol 135:942–948

Raitio A, Risteli J, Väjäkangas K, Oikarinen A (2000) Evidence of disturbed collagen metabolism in smokers – a possible etiologic factor for accelerated skin aging. J Invest Dermatol 114:822

Severi G, Sinclair R, Hopper JL et al (2003) Androgenetic alopecia in men aged 40-69 years: prevalence and risk factors. Br J Dermatol 149:1207–1213

Smith JB, Fenske NA (1996) Cutaneous manifestations and consequences of smoking. J Am Acad Dermatol 34:717–732

Solly S (1856) Clinical lectures on paralysis. Lancet ii:641–643

Su L-S, Chen TH-H (2007) Association of androgenetic alopecia with smoking and its prevalence among Asian men. Arch Dermatol 143:1401–1406

Trüeb RM (2003) Association between smoking and hair loss: another opportunity for health education against smoking? Dermatology 206:189–191

Trüeb RM (2005) Aging of hair. J Cosmet Dermatol 4:60–72

Tur E, Yosipovitch G, Oren-Vulfs S (1992) Chronic and acute effects of cigarette smoking on skin blood flow. Angiology 43:328–335

Weber C, Erl W, Weber K, Weber PC (1996) Increased adhesiveness of isolated monocytes to endothelium is prevented by vitamin C intake in smokers. Circulation 93:1488–1492

Weiss W (1973) Smoker's wrinkles. JAMA 226:788

Weitz JL, Crowley KA, Landman SL et al (1987) Increased neutrophil elastase activity in cigarette smokers. Ann Intern Med 107:680–682

Wolf R, Lo Schiavo A, Ruocco V (1995) Smoking out the skin. J Appl Cosmetol 13:1–14
Yin L, Morita A, Tsuji T (2000) Alterations of extracellular matrix induced by tobacco smoke extract. Arch Dermatol Res 292:188–194
UV-associated activation of telomerase in human skin. Cancer Res 57:370–374
Wissing SA, Muller RH (2001) Solid lipid nanoparticles (SLN) – a novel carrier for UV blockers. Pharmazie 56:783–786

Effect of Cigarette Smoking and UV Radiation: Effect of UV Radiation on Hair Growth and Scalp Condition

Bangha E, Elsner P, Kistler GS (1996) Suppression of UV-induced erythema by topical treatment with melatonin (N-acetyl-5-methoxytryptamine). Arch Dermatol Res 288:522–526
Camacho F, Moreno JC, Garcia-Hernández MJ (1996) Telogen alopecia from UV rays. Arch Dermatol 132:1398–1399
Dourmishev L, Meffert H, Piazena H (2004) Dermatomyositis: comparative studies of cutaneous photosensitivity in lupus erythematosus and normal subjects. Photodermatol Photoimmunol Photomed 20:230–234
Fischer TW, Scholz G, Knoll B et al (2001) Melatonin reduces UV-induced reactive oxygen species in a dose-dependent manner in IL-3-stimulated leukocytes. J Pineal Res 31:39–45
Gao T, Bedell A (2001) Ultraviolet damage on natural gray hair and its photoprotection. J Cosmet Sci 52:103–118
Iyengar B (1998) The hair follicle: a specialized UV receptor in the human skin? Biol Signals Recept 7:188–194
Kasteler JS, Callen JP (1994) Scalp involvement in dermatomyositis. Often overlooked or misdiagnosed. JAMA 272:1939–1941
Kligman AM (1979) Perspectives and problems in cutaneous gerontology. J Invest Dermatol 73:39–46
Lehmann P, Holzle E, Kind P, Goerz G, Plewig G (1990) Experimental reproduction of skin lesions in lupus erythematosus by UVA and UVB radiation. J Am Acad Dermatol 22:181–187
Moehrle M, Dennenmoser B, Schlagenhauff B et al (2000) High prevalence of seborrhoeic dermatitis on the face and scalp in mountain guides. Dermatology 201:146–147
Pande CM, Albrecht L, Yang B (2001) Hair photoprotection by dyes. J Cosmet Sci 52:377–389
Piérard-Franchimont C, Uhoda I, Saint-Léger D, Piérard GE (2002) Androgenetic alopecia and stress-induced premature senescence by cumulative ultraviolet light exposure. Exog Dermatol 1:203–206
Starcher B, Pierce R, Hinek A (1999) UVB irradiation stimulates deposition of new elastic fibers by modified epithelial cells surrounding the hair follicles and sebaceous glands in mice. J Invest Dermatol 112:450–455
Sulica VI, Kao GF (1988) Squamous cell carcinoma of the scalp arising in lesions of discoid lupus erythematosus. Am J Dermatopathol 10:137–141
Trüeb RM (2003) Is androgenetic alopecia a photoaggravated dermatosis? Dermatology 207:343–348
Ueda M, Ouhtit A, Bito T, Nakazawa K, Lübbe J, Ichihashi M, Yamasaki H, Nakazawa H (1997) Evidence for

Effect of Cigarette Smoking and UV Radiation: Diffuse Red Scalp Disease

Ayres S Jr (1987) Extrafacial rosacea is rare but does exist. J Am Acad Dermatol 16:391–392
Baima B, Sticherling M (2002) Demodicidosis revisited. Acta Derm Venereol 82:3–6
Dupont C (1986) How common is extrafacial rosacea? J Am Acad Dermatol 14:839
Gajewska M (1975) Rosacea of common male baldness. Br J Dermatol 93:63–66
Grimalt R, Lacueva L, Hasmann G, Ferrando J (2000) Red scalp syndrome. Annual Meeting of the European Hair Research Society (EHRS) Abstract F11: 22
Karaman U, Celik T, Calik S, Sener S, Aydin NE, Daldal UN (2008) Demodex spp. In hairy skin biopsy specimens. Turkiye Parazitol Derg 32:343–345
Marks R, Jones EW (1969) Disseminated rosacea. Br J Dermatol 81:16–28
Miskjian HG (1951) Demodicidosis (demodex infestation of the scalp). AMA Arch Derm Syphilol 63:282–283
Moschella SL (1994) Written personal communication. August 14, 1992. In: Bernhard JD. Itch. Mechanisms and management of pruritus. McGraw-Hill, New York, p 51
Oberholzer PA, Nobbe S, Kolm I et al (2009) Red scalp disease–a rosacea-like dermatosis of the scalp? Successful therapy with oral tetracycline. Dermatology 219:179–181
Pereira TM, Vieira AP, Basto AS (2008) Rosacea with extensive extrafacial lesions. Int J Dermatol 47:52–55
Thestrup-Pedersen K, Hjorth N (1987) Rod skalp. En ikke tidligere beskrevet harbundssygdom? Ugeskr Laeger 149:2141–2142
Wilkin JK (1980) Epigastric rosacea. Arch Dermatol 116:584
Wilkin J, Dahl M, Detmar M et al (2002) Standard classification of rosacea: report of the national rosacea society expert committee on the classification and staging of rosacea. J Am Acad Dermatol 46:584–587
Wong CS, Kirby B (2004) Demodicidosis in scalp rosacea? Clin Exp Dermatol 29:318–319

Effect of Cigarette Smoking and UV Radiation: Erosive Pustular Dermatosis of the Scalp

Burton JL, Peachey RDG, Pye RJ (1988) Erosive pustular dermatosis of the scalp – a definition. Br J Dermatol 119:411
Caputo R, Veraldi S (1993) Erosive pustular dermatosis of the scalp. J Am Acad Dermatol 28:96–98

Ena P, Lissia M, Doneddu GME, Campus GV (1997) Erosive pustular dermatosis of the scalp in skin grafts: report of three cases. Dermatology 194:80–84

Grattan CEH, Peachu RD, Boon A (1988) Evidence for a role of local trauma in the pathogenesis of erosive pustular dermatosis of the scalp. Clin Exp Dermatol 13:7–10

Laffitte E, Kaya G, Piguet V, Saurat JH (2003) Erosive pustular dermatosis of the scalp: treatment with topical tacrolimus. Arch Dermatol 139:712–714

Laffitte E, Panizzon RG, Saurat JH (2004) Delayed wound healing on the scalp following treatment of actinic keratoses: erosive pustular dermatosis of the scalp. Dermatol Surg 30:1610

Lovell CR, Harmann RM, Bradfield JW (1980) Cutaneous carcinoma arising in erosive pustular dermatosis of the scalp. Br J Dermatol 102:325–328

Pye RJ, Peachey RDG, Burton JL (1979) Erosive pustular dermatosis of the scalp. Br J Dermatol 100:559–566

Rongioletti F, Delmonte S et al (1999) Erosive pustular dermatosis of the scalp following cryotherapy and topical tretinoin for actinic keratoses. Clin Exp Dermatol 24:499–500

Trüeb RM, Krasovec M (1999) Erosive pustular dermatosis of the scalp following radiation therapy for solar keratoses. Br J Dermatol 141:763–765

Effect of Cigarette Smoking and UV Radiation: Actinic Field Cancerization of the Bald Scalp

Cantisani C, De Gado F, Ulrich M, Bottoni U, Iacobellis F, Richetta AG, Calvieri S (2013) Actinic keratosis: review of the literature and new patents. Recent Pat Inflamm Allergy Drug Discov 7:168–175

Quatresooz P, Xhauflaire-Uhoda E, Piérard-Franchimont C, Piérard GE (2009) Epidermal field carcinogenesis in bald-headed: an attempt at finetuning early non-invasive detection. Oncol Rep 21:1313–1316

Stockfleth E (2012) The paradigm shift in treating actinic keratosis: a comprehensive strategy. J Drugs Dermatol 11:1462–1467

Tsatsou F, Trakatelli M, Patsatsi A, Kalokasidis K, Sotiriadis D (2012) Extrinsic aging: UV-mediated skin carcinogenesis. Dermatoendocrinol 4:285–297

Ueda M, Ouhtit A, Bito T, Nakazawa K, Lübbe J, Ichihashi M, Yamasaki H, Nakazawa H (1997) Evidence for UV-associated activation of telomerase in human skin. Cancer Res 57:370–374

Vatve M, Ortonne JP, Birch-Machin MA, Gupta G (2007) Management of field change in actinic keratosis. Br J Dermatol 157(Suppl 2):21–24

Effect of Cigarette Smoking and UV Radiation: Hair Photoaging

Borges CR, Roberts JC, Wilkins DG et al (2001) Relationship of melanin degradation products to actual melanin content: application to human hair. Anal Biochem 290:116–125

Braida D, Dubief C, Lang G (1994) Photoageing of hair fiber and photoprotection. Skin Pharmacol 7:73–77

Dean RT, Fu S, Stocker R et al (1997) Biochemistry and pathology of radical-mediated protein oxidation. Biochem J 324:1–18

Draelos ZD (2000) The biology of hair care. Dermatol Clin 18:651–658

Engelkamp D, Schafer BW, Mattei MG et al (1993) Six S100 genes are clustered on human chromosome 1q21: identification of two genes coding for the two previously unreported calcium-binding proteins S100D and S100E. Proc Natl Acad Sci U S A 90: 6547–6551

Hoting E, Zimmermann M (1995) Photochemical alterations in human hair 1. Artificial irradiation and investigations of hair proteins. J Soc Cosmet Chem 46: 85–99

Hoting E, Zimmermann M, Hocker H (1995) Photochemical alterations in human hair 2. Analysis of melanin. J Soc Cosmet Chem 46:181–190

Inoue T, Sasaki I, Yamaguchi M et al (2000) Elution of S100A3 from hair fiber: new model for hair damage emphasizing the loss of S100A3 from cuticle. J Cosmet Sci 51:15–25

Inoue T, Ito M, Kizawa K (2002) Labile proteins accumulated in damaged hair upon permanent waving and bleaching treatments. J Cosmet Sci 53:337–344

Jeon SY, Pi LQ, Lee WS (2008) Comparison of hair shaft damage after UVA and UVB irradiation. J Cosmet Sci 59:151–156

Jones LN, Rivett DE (1997) The role of 18-methyleicosanoic acid in the structure and formation of mammalian hair fibers. Micron 28:469–485

Kizawa K, Uchiwa H, Murakami U (1996) Highly-expressed S100A3, a calcium-binding protein, in human hair cuticle. Biochim Biophys Acta 1312:94–98

Lee WS (2009) Photoaggravation of hair aging. Int J Trichology 1:94–99

Lee WS (2011) Integral hair lipid in human hair follicle. J Dermatol Sci 64:153–158

Lee WS, Oh TH, Chun SH et al (2005) Integral lipid in human hair follicle. J Investig Dermatol Symp Proc 10:234–237

Marsh JM, Iveson R, Flagler MJ et al (2013) Role of copper in photochemical damage to hair. Int J Cosmet Sci [Epub ahead of print]

Menon IA, Persad S, Haberman HF et al (1983) A comparative study of the physical and chemical properties of melanins isolated from human black and red hair. J Invest Dermatol 80(3):202–206

Nicolaides N, Rothman S (1953) Studies on the chemical composition of human hair fat. II. The overall composition with regard to age, sex and race. J Invest Dermatol 21:9–14

Robbins CR, Bahl M (1984) Analysis of hair by electron spectroscopy for chemical analysis. J Soc Cosmetic Chem 35:379–390

Robbins CR, Crawford RJ (1991) Cuticle damage and the tensile properties of human hair. J Soc Cosmet Chem 42:59–67

Signori V (2004) Review of the current understanding of the effect of ultraviolet and visible radiation on hair structure and options for photoprotection. J Cosmet Sci 55:95–113

Takahashi T, Nakamura K (2005) A study of the photo-lightening mechanism of red hair with visible and ultraviolet light: comparison with blond hair. J Cosmet Sci 56:47–56

Takizawa T, Takizawa T, Arai S et al (1999) Ultrastructural localization of S100A3, a cysteine-rich, calcium binding protein, in human scalp hair shafts revealed by rapid-freezing immunocytochemistry. J Histochem Cytochem 47:525–532

Wertz PW (1997) Integral lipids of hair and stratum corneum. EXS 78:227–237

Wertz PW, Downing DT (1988) Integral lipids of human hair. Lipids 23:878–881

Telogen Effluvium: Pathologic Dynamics of Telogen Effluvium

Barraud-Klenovsek MM, Trüeb RM (2000) Congenital hypotrichosis due to short anagen. Br J Dermatol 143:612–617

Guarrera M, Rebora A (1996) Anagen hairs may fail to replace telogen hairs in early androgenic female alopecia. Dermatology 192:28–31

Guarrera M, Rebora A (2005) Kenogen in female androgenetic alopecia. A longitudinal study. Dermatology 210:18–20

Headington JT (1993) Telogen effluvium. New concepts and review. Arch Dermatol 129:356–363

Kligman AM (1961) Pathologic dynamics of human hair loss, I. Telogen effluvium. Arch Dermatol 83: 175–198

Paus R (1996) Control of the hair cycle and hair diseases as cycling disorders. Curr Opin Dermatol 3:248–258

Paus R, Cotsarelis G (1999) The biology of hair follicles. N Engl J Med 341:491–497

Piérard-Franchimont C, Piérard GE (2001) Teloptosis, a turning point in hair shedding biorhythms. Dermatology 203:115–117

Rathman-Josserand M, Genty G, Lecardonnel J, Chabane S, Cousson A, François Michelet J, Bernard BA (2013) Human hair follicle stem/progenitor cells express hypoxia markers. J Invest Dermatol 133: 2094–2097

Rebora A (1997) Telogen effluvium. Dermatology 195:209–212

Rebora A, Guarrera M (2002) Kenogen. A new phase of the hair cycle? Dermatology 205:108–110

Rebora A, Guarrera M (2004) Teloptosis and kenogen: two new concepts in human trichology. Arch Dermatol 140:619–620

Stenn K (2005) Exogen is an active, separately controlled phase of the hair growth cycle. J Am Acad Dermatol 52:374–375

Telogen Effluvium: Seasonal Hair Shedding

Courtois M, Loussouarn G, Hourseau S, Grollier JF (1996) Periodicity in the growth and shedding of hair. Br J Dermatol 134:47–54

Kunz M, Seifert B, Trüeb RM (2009) Seasonality of hair shedding in healthy women complaining of hair loss. Dermatology 219:105–110

Orentreich N (1969) Scalp replacement in man. In: Montagna W, Bobson RL (eds) Advances in biology of skin, vol IX, Hair growth. Pergamon, Oxford, pp 99–108

Randall VA, Ebling FJG (1991) Seasonal changes in human hair growth. Br J Dermatol 124:146–151

Telogen Effluvium: General Medical Problems Affecting the Condition of Hair

Billoni N, Buan B, Gautier B, Gaillard O, Mahé YF, Bernard BA (2000) Thyroid hormone receptor beta1 is expressed in the human hair follicle. Br J Dermatol 142:645–652

Comaisch S (1985) The thyroid and hair growth. Sem Dermatol 4:4–8

Gummer CL (1985) Diet and hair loss. Semin Dermatol 4:35–39

Schell H, Kiesewetter F, Seidel C, von Hintzenstern J (1991) Cell cycle kinetics of human anagen scalp hair bulbs in thyroid disorders determined by DNA flow cytometry. Dermatologica 182:23–26

Sinclair R (1999) Diffuse hair loss. Int J Dermatol 38(Suppl 1):8–18

Spencer LV, Callen JP (1987) Hair loss in systemic disease. Dermatol Clin 5:565–570

Stroud JP (1987) Diagnosis and management of the hair loss patient. Cutis 40:272–276

Wysenbeek AI, Leibovici L, Amit M, Weinberger A (1991) Alopecia in systemic lupus erythematosus. Relation to disease manifestations. J Rheumatol 18:1185–1186

York J, Nicholson T, Minors P, Duncan DF (1998) Stressful life events and loss of hair among adult women, a case-control study. Psychol Rep 82:1044–1046

Telogen Effluvium: Drug-Induced Hair Loss

Reeves JRT, Maibach HI (1977) Drug and chemical induced hair loss. In: Marzulli FN, Maibach HI (eds) Advances in modern toxicology, vol 4. Hemisphere Publishing Corp, Washington, DC/London, pp 487–500

Tosti A, Misciali C, Piraccini BM et al (1994) Drug-induced hair loss and hair growth. Incidence, management and avoidance. Drug Saf 10:310–317

Telogen Effluvium: Antitumor Necrosis Alpha Therapy-Induced Alopecia

Chaves Y, Duarte G, Ben-Said B, Tebib J, Berard F, Nicolas JF (2008) Alopecia areata universalis during treatment of rheumatoid arthritis with anti-TNF-alpha antibody (adalimumab). Dermatology 217:380

Doyle LA, Sperling LC, Baksh S, Lackey J, Thomas B, Vleugels RA, Qureshi AA, Velazquez EF (2011) Psoriatic alopecia/alopecia areata-like reactions secondary to anti-tumor necrosis factor-α therapy: a novel cause of noncicatricial alopecia. Am J Dermatopathol 33:161–166

El Shabrawi-Caelen L, La Placa M, Vincenzi C, Haidn T, Muellegger R, Tosti A (2010) Adalimumab-induced psoriasis of the scalp with diffuse alopecia: a severe potentially irreversible cutaneous side effect of TNF-alpha blockers. Inflamm Bowel Dis 16:182–183

Ettefagh L, Nedorost S, Mirmirani P (2004) Alopecia areata in a patient using infliximab: new insights into the role of tumor necrosis factor on human hair follicles. Arch Dermatol 140:1012

Ettler J, Wetter DA, Pittelkow MR (2012) Pityriasis amiantacea: a distinctive presentation of psoriasis associated with tumour necrosis factor-α inhibitor therapy. Clin Exp Dermatol 37:639–641

Fabre C, Dereure O (2008) Worsening alopecia areata and de novo occurrence of multiple halo nevi in a patient receiving infliximab. Dermatology 216:185–186

Garcia Bartels N, Lee HH, Worm M, Burmester GR, Sterry W, Blume-Peytavi U (2006) Development of alopecia areata universalis in a patient receiving adalimumab. Arch Dermatol 142:1654–1655

Hernández MV, Nogués S, Ruiz-Esquide V, Alsina M, Cañete JD, Sanmartí R (2009) Development of alopecia areata after biological therapy with TNF-alpha blockers: description of a case and review of the literature. Clin Exp Rheumatol 27:892–893

Joyau C, Veyrac G, Dixneuf V, Jolliet P (2012) Anti-tumour necrosis factor alpha therapy and increased risk of de novo psoriasis: is it really a paradoxical side effect? Clin Exp Rheumatol 30:700–706

Kirshen C, Kanigsberg N (2009) Alopecia areata following adalimumab. J Cutan Med Surg 13:48–50

Nakagomi D, Harada K, Yagasaki A, Kawamura T, Shibagaki N, Shimada S (2009) Psoriasiform eruption associated with alopecia areata during infliximab therapy. Clin Exp Dermatol 34:923–924

Osório F, Magro F, Lisboa C, Lopes S, Macedo G, Bettencourt H, Azevedo F, Magina S (2012) Anti-TNF-alpha induced psoriasiform eruptions with severe scalp involvement and alopecia: report of five cases and review of the literature. Dermatology 225:163–167

Pan Y, Rao NA (2009) Alopecia areata during etanercept therapy. Ocul Immunol Inflamm 17:127–129

Pelivani N, Hassan AS, Braathen LR, Hunger RE, Yawalkar N (2008) Alopecia areata universalis elicited during treatment with adalimumab. Dermatology 216:320–323

Hair Aging

Courtois M, Loussouarn G, Hourseau C (1995) Aging and hair cycles. Br J Dermatol 132:86–93

Flagler MJ, Schwartz JR, Robbins C, Dawson TL (2012) The effects of aging oh hair – more than just amount. In: Evans T, Wickett RR (eds) Practical modern hair science. Alluredbooks, Carol Stream

Harman D (1956) Aging: a theory based on free radical and radiation chemistry. J Gerontol 11:298–300

Nagase S, Tsuchiya M, Matsui T, Shibuichi S, Tsujimura H, Masukawa Y, Satoh N, Itou T, Koike K, Tsujii K (2008) Characterization of curved hair of Japanese women with reference to internal structures and amino acid composition. J Cosmet Sci 59:317–332

Otsukoa H, Nemoto T (1988) Study on Japanese hair. Koshokaishi 12:192–197

Sadighha A, Zahed GM (2008) Hair darkening after treatment with cyclosporin in a patient with psoriasis. J Eur Acad Dermatol Venereol 22:1239–1241

Tobin DJ, Paus R (2001) Graying: gerontobiology of the hair follicle pigmentary unit. Exp Gerontol 36:29–54

Trotter M, Dawson HL (1934) The hair of French Canadians. Am J Phys Anthrop 18:443–445

Trüeb RM (2005a) Aging of hair. J Cosmet Dermatol 4:60–72

Trüeb RM (2005b) Dermocosmetic aspects of hair and scalp. J Investig Dermatol Symp Proc 10:289–292

Trüeb RM (2006) Pharmacologic interventions in aging hair. Clin Interv Aging 1:121–129

Trüeb RM (2009) Oxidative stress in ageing of hair. Int J Trichology 1(1):6–14

Hair Aging: Rare Premature Aging Syndromes

Amorosi B, Giustini S, Rossi A, Giacanelli M, Calvieri S (1999) Myotonic dystrophy (Steinert disease): a morphologic and biochemical hair study. Int J Dermatol 38:434–438

Brown WT, Kieras FJ, Houck GE Jr, Dutkowski R, Jenins EC (1985) A comparison of adult and childhood progerias: Werner syndrome and Hutchinson-Gilford progeria syndrome. In: Salk D, Fujwara Y, Martin GM

(eds) Werner's syndrome and human aging. Plenum Press, New York, pp 229–244
Cooper SM, Dawber RP, Hilton-Jones D (2003) Three cases of androgen-dependent disease associated with myotonic dystrophy. J Eur Acad Dermatol Venereol 17:56–58
Finsterer J, Fellinger J (2011) Alopecia as a prominent feature of myotonic dystrophy type 1. Rev Invest Clin 63:322–324
Macieira-Coelho A (2003) Biology of aging. Progress in molecular and subcellular biology. Springer, Heidelberg, pp 50–52

Hair Aging: Graying

Arck PC, Overall R, Spatz K et al (2006) Towards a "free radical theory of graying": melanocyte apoptosis in the aging human hair follicle is an indicator of oxidative stress induced tissue damage. FASEB J 20:1567–1569
Commo S, Gaillard O, Bernard BA (2004) Human hair greying is linked to a specific depletion of hair follicle melanocytes affecting both the bulb and the outer root sheath. Br J Dermatol 150:435–443
Hollfelder B, Blankenburg G, Wolfram LJ, Höcker H (1995) Chemical and physical properties of pigmented and non-pigmented hair ('grey hair'). Int J Cosmet Sci 17:87–89
Jeon SY, Pi LQ, Lee WS (2008) Comparison of hair shaft damage after UVA and UVB irradiation. J Cosmet Sci 59:151–156
Macieira-Coelho A (2003) Biology of aging. Progress in molecular and subcellular biology. Springer, Heidelberg, pp 50–52
Mosley JG, Gibbs CC (1996) Premature grey hair and hair loss among smokers: a new opportunity for health education? BMJ 313:1616
Nagl W (1995) Different growth rates of pigmented and white hair in the beard: differentiation vs. proliferation? Br J Dermatol 132:94–97
Nishimura EK, Jordan SA, Oshima H et al (2002) Dominant role of the niche in melanocyte stem-cell fate determination. Nature 416:854–860
Nishimura EK, Granter SR, Fisher DE (2005) Mechanisms of hair graying: incomplete melanocyte stem cell maintenance in the niche. Science 307:720–724
Nogueira AC, Dicelio LE, Joekes I (2006) About photodamage of human hair. Photochem Photobiol Sci 5:165–169
Santos Nogueira AC, Joekes I (2004) Hair color changes and protein damage caused by ultraviolet radiation. J Photochem Photobiol B 74:109–117
Schallreuter KU, Wood JM, Pittelkow MR et al (1994) Regulation of melanin biosynthesis in the human epidermis by tetrahydrobiopterin. Science 263:1444–1446
Spencer JD, Gibbons NC, Rokos H et al (2007) Oxidative stress via hydrogen peroxide affects propriomelanocortin peptides directly in the epidermis of patients with vitiligo. J Invest Dermatol 127:411–420
Spencer JD, Gibbons NC, Böhm M, Schallreuter KU (2008) The Ca2+-binding capacity of epidermal furin is disrupted by H2O2-mediated oxidation in vitiligo. Endocrinology 149:163–1645
Tobin DJ (2008) Biology of hair follicle pigmentation. In: Blume-Peytavi U, Tosti A, Whiting DA, Trüeb R (eds) Hair growth and disorders. Springer, Berlin/Heidelberg, p 51
Tobin DJ, Paus R (2001) Graying: gerontobiology of the hair follicle pigmentary unit. Exp Gerontol 36:29–54
van Neste D (2004) Thickness, medullation and growth rate of female scalp hair are subject to significant variation according to pigmentation of scalp location during aging. Eur J Dermatol 14:28–32
van Neste D, Tobin DJ (2004) Hair cycle and hair pigmentation: dynamic interactions and changes associated with aging. Micron 35:193–200
Wood JM, Decker H, Hartmann H et al (2009) Senile hair graying: H2O2-mediated oxidative stress affects human hair color by blunting methionine sulfoxide repair. FASEB J 23:2065–2075

Hair Aging: Senescent Alopecia

Courtois M, Loussouarn G, Hourseau C (1995) Aging and hair cycles. Br J Dermatol 132:86–93
Eichmüller S, van der Veen C, Mill I et al (1998) Clusters of perifollicular macrophages in normal murine skin: physiological degeneration of selected hair follicles by programmed organ deletion. J Histochem Cytochem 46:361–370
Kligman AM (1988) The comparative histopathology of male-pattern baldness and senescent baldness. Clin Dermatol 16:108–118
Paradi M, Shahee O, Shaza D et al (2007) Comparison of senescent and androgenetic alopecia using microarray analysis. 5th International Hair Research Societies Meeting, Vancouver: Abstract O-10-3
Price V, Sawaya M, Headington J, Kibarian M (2001) Histology and hormonal activity in senescent thinning in males (abstract 266). J Invest Dermatol 117:434

Hair Aging: Age-Related General Medical Problems Affecting the Condition of Hair

Bodenheimer T (1999) Disease management: promises and pitfalls. N Engl J Med 340:1202–1205
Daveluy C, Pica L, Audet N et al (1998) Enquête sociale et de santé, 2nd edn. Institut de la statistique du Québec, Quebec City

Fischer TW, Slominski A, Tobin DJ, Paus R (2008) Melatonin and the hair follicle. J Pineal Res 44:1–15

Fischer TW, Trüeb RM, Hänggi G et al (2012) Topical melatonin for treatment of androgenetic alopecia. Int J Trichology 4:236–245

Holman H, Lorig K (2000) Patients as partners in managing chronic disease. Partnership is a prerequisite for effective and efficient health care. BMJ 320: 526–527

Johnson KA, Bernard MA, Funderberg K (2002) Vitamin nutrition in older adults. Clin Geriatr Med 18:773–799

Trüeb RM (2010) Hormones and hair growth. Hautarzt 61:487–495

Wolff JL, Starfield B, Anderson G (2002) Prevalence, expenditures, and complications of multiple chronic conditions in the elderly. Arch Intern Med 162:2269–2276

Hair Aging: Possibilities and Limitations for Reversal of Age-Related Pigment Loss

Comaish S (1972) White scalp hairs turning black – an unusual reversal of the aging process. Br J Dermatol 86:513–514

Dawber RPR (1997) Hair colour. In: Camacho F, Montagna W (eds) Trichology. Diseases of the pilosebaceous follicle. Libros Princeps, Biblioteca Aula Medica, Madrid, p 169

Dawber R, van Neste D (1995) Hair and scalp disorders. Common presenting signs, differential diagnosis and treatment. Martin Dunitz, London

Hoffman RM (1998) Topical liposome targeting of dyes, melanins, genes, and proteins electively to hair follicles. J Drug Target 5:67–74

Pattier P (2001) Spontaneous repigmentation of white hair. Ann Dermatol Venereol 128:1082–1083

Rook AJ, Dawber RPR (1991) The colour of the hair. In: Rook A, Dawber R (eds) Diseases of the hair and scalp, 2nd edn. Blackwell Scientific Publications, London, p 370

Saha B, Singh SK, Mallick S et al (2009) Sphingolipid-mediated restoration of Mitf expression and repigmentation in vivo in a mouse model of hair graying. Pigment Cell Melanoma Res 222:205–218

Sieve B (1941) Darkening of gray hair following para-aminobenzoic acid. Science 94:257–258

Tobin DJ, Cargnello JA (1993) Partial reversal of canities in a 22-year-old normal Chinese male. Arch Dermatol 129:789–791

Tobin DJ, Paus R (2001) Graying: gerontobiology of the hair follicle pigmentary unit. Exp Gerontol 36:29–54

Vanscheidt W, Hunziker T (2009) Repigmentation by outer-root-sheath-derived melanocytes: proof of concept in vitiligo and leucoderma. Dermatology 218:342–343

Wood JM, Decker H, Hartmann H et al (2009) Senile hair graying: H2O2-mediated oxidative stress affects human hair color by blunting methionine sulfoxide repair. FASEB J 23:2065–2075

Yonetani S, Moriyama M, Nishigori C et al (2008) In vitro expansion of immature melanoblasts and their ability to repopulate melanocyte stem cells in the hair follicle. J Invest Dermatol 128:408–420

Zarafonetis C (1950) Darkening of gray hair during para-aminobenzoic acid therapy. J Invest Dermatol 15:399–491

Hair Aging: Possibilities and Limitations for Reversal of Age-Related Hair Loss

Brenner S, Matz H (1999) Improvement in androgenetic alopecia in 53-76-year-old men using oral finasteride. Int J Dermatol 38:92–930

Chein E (1998) Age reversal, from hormones to telomeres. WorldLink Medical Publishing

Olsen EA, DeLong ER, Weiner MS (1987) Long-term follow-up of men with male pattern baldness treated with topical minoxidil. J Am Acad Dermatol 16:688–695

Olsen EA, Weiner MS, Amara IA, DeLong ER (1990) Five-year follow-up of men with androgenetic alopecia treated with topical minoxidil. J Am Acad Dermatol 22:643–646

Olsen EA, Dunlap FE, Funicella T et al (2002) A randomized clinical trial of 5% topical minoxidil versus 2% topical minoxidil and placebo in the treatment of androgenetic alopecia in men. J Am Acad Dermatol 47:377–385

Rundegren J (2004) Pattern alopecia: what clinical features determine the response to topical minoxidil treatment? IHRS2004 abstract B2.4. JDDG 2:500

Stough DB, Potter TS (1997) Philosophy and technique in hair restoration surgery. Curr Probl Dermatol 9:113–136

Whiting DA, Olsen EA, Savin R et al (2003) Efficacy and tolerability of finasteride 1 mg in men aged 41 to 60 years with male pattern hair loss. Eur J Dermatol 13:150–160

Hair Aging: Dorian Gray Syndrome

Brosig B, Kupfer J, Niemeier V et al (2001) The "Dorian Gray Syndrome": psychodynamic need for hair growth restorers and, other "fountains of youth". Int J Clin Pharmacol Ther 39:279–283

Cash TF (1990) Losing hair, losing points? The effects of male pattern baldness on social impression formation. J Appl Soc Psychol 20:154–167

Muscarella F, Cunningham MR (1996) The evolutionary significance and social perception of male pattern baldness and facial hair. Ethol Sociobiol 17:99–117

Phillips KA (1996) The broken mirror: understanding and treating body dysmorphic disorder. Oxford University Press, Oxford/New York

Roll S, Verinis JS (1971) Stereotypes of scalp and facial hair as measured by the semantic differential. Psychol Rep 28:975–980

Sarwer DB, Wadden TA, Pertschuk MJ et al (1998) The psychology of cosmetic surgery: a review and reconceptualization. Clin Psychol Rev 18:1–22
Sarwer DB, Grossbart TA, Didie ER (2003) Beauty and society. Semin Cutan Med Surg 22:79–92
Thompson JK, Heinberg LJ, Altabe M et al (1990) Exacting beauty: theory, assessment and treatment of body image disturbance. American Psychological Association, Washington, DC, pp 19–47

Alopecia with Scarring Phenomena: Inflammatory Phenomena and Fibrosis in Male Androgenetic Alopecia

Jaworsky C, Kligman AM, Murphy GF (1992) Characterisation of inflammatory infiltrates in male pattern alopecia: implication for pathogenesis. Br J Dermatol 127:239–246
Mahé YF, Michelet JF, Billoni N et al (2000) Androgenetic alopecia and microinflammation. Int J Dermatol 39:576–584
Philpott MP, Sander DA, Bowen J, Kealey T (1996) Effects of interleukins, colony stimulating factor and tumour necrosis factor on human hair follicle growth in vitro: a possible role for interleukin-1 and tumour necrosis factor-a in alopecia areata. Br J Dermatol 135:942–948
Whiting DA (1993) Diagnostic and predictive value of horizontal sections of scalp biopsy specimens in male pattern androgenetic alopecia. J Am Acad Dermatol 128:755–763

Alopecia with Scarring Phenomena: Male Frontal Fibrosing Alopecia

Armenores P, Shirato K, Reid C, Sidhu S (2010) Frontal fibrosing alopecia associated with generalized hair loss. Australas J Dermatol 51:183–185
Chew AL, Bashir SJ, Wain EM, Fenton DA, Stefanato CM (2010) Expanding the spectrum of frontal fibrosing alopecia: a unifying concept. J Am Acad Dermatol 63:653–660
Miteva M, Camacho I, Romanelli P, Tosti A (2010) Acute hair loss on the limbs in frontal fibrosing alopecia: a clinicopathological study of two cases. Br J Dermatol 163:426–428
Ramaswamy P, Mendese G, Goldberg LJ (2012) Scarring alopecia of the sideburns: a unique presentation of frontal fibrosing alopecia in men. Arch Dermatol 148:1095–1096
Stockmeier M, Kunte C, Sander CA, Wolff H (2002) Kossard frontal fibrosing alopecia in a man. Hautarzt 53:409–411

Alopecia with Scarring Phenomena: Fibrosing Alopecia in a Pattern Distribution (Cicatricial Pattern Hair Loss)

Eichmuller S, van der Veen C, Moll L et al (1998) Clusters of perifollicular macrophages in normal murine skin: physiological degeneration of selected hair follicles by programmed organ deletion. J Histochem Cytochem 46:361–370
Kossard S (1994) Postmenopausal frontal fibrosing alopecia: scarring alopecia in a pattern distribution. Arch Dermatol 130:770–774
Kossard S, Lee MS, Wilkinson B (1997) Postmenopausal frontal fibrosing alopecia: a frontal variant of lichen planopilaris. J Am Acad Dermatol 36:59–66
Olsen EA (2005) Female pattern hair loss and its relationship to permanent/cicatricial alopecia: a new perspective. J Investig Dermatol Symp Proc 10:217–221
Trüeb RM, Toricelli R (1998) Lichen planopilaris unter dem Bild einer postmenopausalen frontalen fibrosierenden Alopezie (Kossard). Hautarzt 49:388–391
Zinkernagel MS, Trüeb RM (2000) Fibrosing alopecia in a pattern distribution. Patterned lichen planopilaris or androgenetic alopecia with a lichenoid tissue reaction pattern? Arch Dermatol 136:205–211

Alopecia with Scarring Phenomena: Inflammatory Scarring Alopecias

Chicarilli ZN (1987) Follicular occlusion triad: hidradenitis suppurativa, acne conglobata, and dissecting cellulitis of the scalp. Ann Plast Surg 18:230–237
Donovan JC, Samrao A, Ruben BS, Price VH (2010) Eyebrow regrowth in patients with frontal fibrosing alopecia treated with intralesional triamcinolone acetonide. Br J Dermatol 163:1142–1144
Elston DM, McCollough ML, Angeloni VL (1995) Vertical and transverse sections of alopecia biopsy specimens. Combining the two to maximize diagnostic yield. J Am Acad Dermatol 32:454–457
Harries MJ, Trueb RM, Tosti A et al (2009) How not to get scar(r)ed: pointers to the correct diagnosis in patients with suspected primary cicatricial alopecia. Br J Dermatol 160:482–501
Häusermann P, Walter RB, Halter J, Biedermann BC, Tichelli A, Itin P, Gratwohl A (2008) Cutaneous graft-versus-host disease: a guide for the dermatologist. Dermatology 216:287–304
Headington JT (1996) Cicatricial alopecia. Dermatol Clin 14:773–782
Laymon CW (1947) The cicatricial alopecias: historical and clinical review, and histologic investigation. J Invest Dermatol 8:99–122
Ljubojevic S, Pasic A, Lipozencic J, Skerlev M (2005) Perifolliculitis capitis abscedens etsuffodiens. J Eur Acad Dermatol Venereol 19:719–721

Matard B, Meylheuc T, Briandet R, Casin I, Assouly P, Cavelier-balloy B, Reygagne P (2012) First evidence of bacterial biofilms in the anaerobe part of scalp hair follicles: a pilot comparative study in folliculitis decalvans. J Eur Acad Dermatol Venereol 27:853–860

Navarini AA, Kolios AG, Prinz-Vavricka BM et al (2011) Low-dose excimer 308-nm laser for treatment of lichen planopilaris. Arch Dermatol 147:1325–1326

Nayar M, Schomberg K, Dawber RPR, Millard PR (1993) A clinicopathological study of scarring alopecia. Br J Dermatol 128:533–536

Olsen EA, Bergfeld WF, Cotsarelis G et al (2003) Summary of North American Hair Research Society (NAHRS) – sponsored Workshop on Cicatricial Alopecia, Duke University Medical Center, February 10 and 11, 2001. J Am Acad Dermatol 48:103–110

Price V, Mirmirani P (2011) Cicatricial alopecia. An approach to diagnosis and management. Springer, New York/Dordrecht/Heidelberg/London

Ross EK, Tan E, Shapiro J (2005) Update on primary cicatricial alopecias. J Am Acad Dermatol 53:1–37

Solomon AR (1994) The transversely sectioned scalp biopsy specimen: the technique and a algorithm for its use in the diagnosis of alopecia. Adv Dermatol 9:127–157

Sperling LC (2001) Scarring alopecia and the dermatopathologist. J Cutan Pathol 28:333–342

Sperling LC, Solomon AR, Whiting DA (2000) A new look at scarring alopecia. Arch Dermatol 136:235–242

Spitzer L (1903) Dermatitis follicularis et perifollicularis conglobata. Dermatologische Z 110:109–120

Templeton SF, Solomon AR (1994) Scarring alopecia: a classification based on microscopic criteria. J Cutan Pathol 21:97–109

Trachsler S, Trueb RM (2005) Value of direct immunofluorescence for differential diagnosis of cicatricial alopecia. Dermatology 211:98–102

Alopecia with Scarring Phenomena: Alopecia Mucinosa

Bi MY, Curry JL, Christiano AM, Hordinsky MK, Norris DA, Price VH, Duvic M (2011) The spectrum of hair loss in patients with mycosis fungoides and Sézary syndrome. J Am Acad Dermatol 64:53–63

Brown HA, Gibson LE, Pujol RM, Lust JA, Pittelkow MR (2002) Primary follicular mucinosis: long-term follow-up of patients younger than 40 years with and without clonal T-cell receptor gene rearrangement. J Am Acad Dermatol 47:856–862

Fierro MT, Marenco F, Novelli M, Fava P, Quaglino P, Bernengo MG (2010) Long-term evolution of an untreated primary cutaneous follicle center lymphoma of the scalp. Am J Dermatopathol 32:91–94

Gerami P, Rosen S, Kuzel T, Boone SL, Guitart J (2008) Folliculotropic mycosis fungoides: an aggressive variant of cutaneous T-cell lymphoma. Arch Dermatol 144:738–746

Gulia A, Saggini A, Wiesner T, Fink-Puches R, Argenyi Z, Ferrara G, Müller CS, Vale E, Cerroni L (2011) Clinicopathologic features of early lesions of primary cutaneous follicle center lymphoma, diffuse type: implications for early diagnosis and treatment. J Am Acad Dermatol 65:991–1000

Trüeb R, Bruckner-Tuderman L (1990) Generalized follicular mucinosis. Hautarzt 41:625–627

Alopecia with Scarring Phenomena: Alopecia Neoplastica

Carson HJ, Pellettiere EV, Lack E (1994) Alopecia neoplastica simulating alopecia areata and antedating the detection of primary breast carcinoma. J Cutan Pathol 21:67–70

Chen W, Yang CC, Todorova A, Al Khuzaei S, Chiu HC, Worret WI, Ring J (2010) Hair loss in elderly women. Eur J Dermatol 20:145–151

Chiu CS, Lin CY, Kuo TT, Kuan YZ, Chen MJ, Ho HC, Yang LC, Chen CH, Shih IH, Hong HS, Chuang YH (2007) Malignant cutaneous tumors of the scalp: a study of demographic characteristics and histologic distributions of 398 Taiwanese patients. J Am Acad Dermatol 56:448–452

Cohen PR (2009) Primary alopecia neoplastica versus secondary alopecia neoplastica: a new classification for neoplasm-associated scalp hair loss. J Cutan Pathol 36:917–918

Katz TM, Silapunt S, Goldberg LH, Jih MH, Kimyai-Asadi A (2005) Analysis of 197 female scalp tumors treated with Mohs micrographic surgery. J Am Acad Dermatol 52:291–294

Lin WL, Lin WC, Jung SM et al (2007) Breast cancer metastasized to the scalp mimicking alopecia areata: alopecia neoplastica. Breast J 13:94–95

Mallon E, Dawber RP (1994) Alopecia neoplastica without alopecia: a unique presentation of breast carcinoma scalp metastasis. J Am Acad Dermatol 31:319–321

Peison B (1971) Metastasis of carcinoma of the prostate to the scalp. Simulation of a large sebaceous cyst. Arch Dermatol 104:301–303

Richmond HM, Duvic M, Macfarlane DF (2010) Primary and metastatic malignant tumors of the scalp: an update. Am J Clin Dermatol 11:233–246

Schorr WF, Swanson PM, Gomez F, Reyes CN (1970) Alopecia neoplastica. Hair loss resembling alopecia areata caused by metastatic breast cancer. JAMA 213:1335–1337

Dystrophic Anagen Effluvium: Thomas More Syndrome

Elston DM, Clayton AS, Meffert JJ, McCollough ML (2000) Migratory poliosis: a forme fruste of alopecia areata? J Am Acad Dermatol 42:1076–1077

Ephraim A (1959) On sudden or rapid whitening of the hair. AMA Arch Derm 79:228–236

Goldenhersh MA (1992) Rapid whitening of the hair first reported in the Talmud: possible mechanisms of this intriguing phenomenon. Am J Dermatopathol 14:367–368

Guin JD, Kumar V, Petersen BH (1981) Immunofluorescence findings in rapid whitening of scalp hair. Arch Dermatol 117:576–578

Helm F, Milgrom H (1970) Can scalp hair suddenly turn white? A case of canities subita. Arch Dermatol 102:102–103

Hoffmann E (1957) Sudden turning gray of the hair caused by fright, canities subita psychogenica. Z Haut Geschlechtskr 22:74–78

McBride AK, Bergfeld WF (1990) Mosaic hair color changes in alopecia areata. Cleve Clin J Med 157:354–356

Metchnikoff E (1901) On the process of hair turning white. Proc R Soc Lond 69:156

Navarini AA, Trüeb RM (2010) Why Henry III of Navarre's hair probably did not turn white overnight. Int J Trichology 2:2–4

Navarini AA, Nobbe S, Trüeb RM (2009) Marie Antoinette syndrome. Arch Dermatol 145:656

Paus R, Slominski A, Czarnetzki BM (1993) Is alopecia areata, an autoimmune response against melanogenesis-related proteins, exposed by abnormal MHC class I expression in the anagen hair bulb? Yale J Biol Med 66:541–554

Trüeb RM, Navarini AA (2010) Thomas More syndrome. Dermatology 220:55–56

Xavier S (1934) Sudden blanching of the hair as described in literature. Chron Med 41:116–120

Dystrophic Anagen Effluvium: Treatment Algorithm for Alopecia Areata

Abell E, Munro DD (1973) Intralesional treatment of alopecia areata with triamcinolone acetonide by jet injector. Br J Dermatol 88:55–59

Cipriani R, Perini GI, Rampinelli S (2001) Paroxetine in alopecia areata. Int J Dermatol 40:600–601

Delamere FM, Sladden MM, Dobbins HM, Leonardi-Bee J (2008) Interventions for alopecia areata. Cochrane Database Syst Rev (2):CD004413

Hordinsky MK (2011) Treatment of alopecia areata: "What is new on the horizon?". Dermatol Ther 24:364–368

Joly P (2006) The use of methotrexate alone or in combination with low doses of oral corticosteroids in the treatment of alopecia totalis or universalis. J Am Acad Dermatol 55:632–636

Nakajima T, Inui S, Itami S (2007) Pulse corticosteroid therapy for alopecia areata: study of 139 patients. Dermatology 215:320–324

Park H, Kim CW, Kim SS, Park CW (2009) The therapeutic effect and the changed serum zinc level after zinc supplementation in alopecia areata patients who had a low serum zinc level. Ann Dermatol 21:142–146

Pericin M, Trüeb RM (1998) Topical immunotherapy of severe alopecia areata with diphenylcyclopropenone: evaluation of 68 cases. Dermatology 196:418–421

Perini G, Zara M, Cipriani R et al (1994) Imipramine in alopecia areata. A double-blind, placebo-controlled study. Psychother Psychosom 61:195–198

Petukhova L, Duvic M, Hordinsky M, Norris D, Price V, Shimomura Y, Kim H, Singh P, Lee A, Chen WV, Meyer KC, Paus R, Jahoda CA, Amos CI, Gregersen PK, Christiano AM (2010) Genome-wide association study in alopecia areata implicates both innate and adaptive immunity. Nature 466:113–117

Ricciardi A, Ruberto A, García-Hernández MJ et al (2006) Alopecia areata with comorbid depression: early resolution with combined paroxetine-triamcinolone treatment. J Eur Acad Dermatol Venereol 20:1000–1001

Trost LB, Bergfeld WF, Calogeras E (2006) The diagnosis and treatment of iron deficiency and its potential relationship to hair loss. J Am Acad Dermatol 54: 824–844

Tosti A, Piraccini BM, Pazzaglia M, Vincenzi C (2003) Clobetasol propionate 0.05% under occlusion in the treatment of alopecia totalis/universalis. J Am Acad Dermatol 49:96–98

Tosti A, Iorizzo M, Botta GL, Milani M (2006) Efficacy and safety of a new clobetasol propionate 0.05% foam in alopecia areata: a randomized, double-blind placebo-controlled trial. J Eur Acad Dermatol Venereol 20:1243–1247

Willemsen R, Vanderlinden J, Deconinck A, Roseeuw D (2006) Hypnotherapeutic management of alopecia areata. J Am Acad Dermatol 55:233–237

Willemsen R, Haentjens P, Roseeuw D, Vanderlinden J (2010) Hypnosis in refractory alopecia areata significantly improves depression, anxiety, and life quality but not hair regrowth. J Am Acad Dermatol 62:517–518

Willemsen R, Haentjens P, Roseeuw D, Vanderlinden J (2011) Hypnosis and alopecia areata: long-term beneficial effects on psychological well-being. Acta Derm Venereol 91:35–39

Dystrophic Anagen Effluvium: Postoperative Pressure Alopecia

Abel R, Lewis G (1960) Postoperative (pressure) alopecia. Arch Dermatol Syphilol 81:34–42

Dominguez E, Eslinger MR, McCord SV (1999) Postoperative (pressure) alopecia: report of a case after elective cosmetic surgery. Anesth Analg 89:1062–1063

Lawson N, Mills N, Oscher J (1976) Occipital alopecia following cardiopulmonary bypass. J Thorac Cardiovasc Surg 71:342–347

Dystrophic Anagen Effluvium: Radiation-Induced Temporary Epilation After Neuroradiologically Guided Embolization Procedure

Huda W, Peters KR (1994) Radiation-induced temporary epilation after a neuroradiologically guided embolization procedure. Radiology 193:642–644

Krasovec M, Trüeb RM (1998) Temporary roentgen epilation after embolization of a cerebral arteriovenous malformation. Hautarzt 49:307–309

Panizzon RG, Goldtschmitdt H (1991) Radiation reactions and sequelae. In: Goldschmidt H, Panizzon RG (eds) Modern radiation therapy. Springer, Berlin

Dystrophic Anagen Effluvium: Chemotherapy-Induced Hair Loss

Baker B, Wilson C, Davis A et al (1991) Busulphan/cyclophosphamide conditioning for bone marrow transplantation may lead to failure of hair regrowth. Bone Marrow Transplant 7:43–47

Betticher DC, Delmore G, Breitenstein U, Anchisi S, Zimmerli-Schwab B, Müller A, von Moos R, Hügli-Dayer AM, Schefer H, Bodenmann S, Bühler V, Trüeb RM (2013) Efficacy and tolerability of two scalp cooling systems for the prevention of alopecia associated with docetaxel treatment. Support Care Cancer 21:2565–2573

Grevelman EG, Breed WPM (2005) Prevention of chemotherapy-induced hair loss by scalp cooling. Ann Oncol 16:352–358

McGarvey EL, Baum LD, Pinkerton RC et al (2001) Psychological sequelae and alopecia among women with cancer. Cancer Pract 9:283–289

Mundstedt K, Manthey N, Sachsse S et al (1997) Changes in self-concept and body image during alopecia induced cancer chemotherapy. Support Care Cancer 5:139–143

Rosman S (2004) Cancer and stigma: experience of patients with chemotherapy-induced alopecia. Patient Educ Couns 52:333–339

Tran D, Sinclair RD, Schwarer AP et al (2000) Permanent alopecia following chemotherapy and bone marrow transplantation. Australas J Dermatol 41:106–108

Trüeb RM (2007) Chemotherapy-induced anagen effluvium: diffuse or patterned? Dermatology 215:1–2

Trüeb RM (2009) Chemotherapy-induced alopecia. Semin Cutan Med Surg 28:11–14

Vowels M, Chan LL, Giri N et al (1993) Factors affecting hair regrowth after bone marrow transplantation. Bone Marrow Transplant 12:347–350

Wang J, Lu Z, Au JLS (2006) Protection against chemotherapy-induced alopecia. Pharm Res 23: 2505–2514

Dystrophic Anagen Effluvium: Side Effects from Molecularly Targeted Therapies for Cancer

Donovan JC, Ghazarian DM, Shaw JC (2008) Scarring alopecia associated with use of the epidermal growth factor receptor inhibitor gefitinib. Arch Dermatol 144:1524–1525

Graves JE, Jones BF, Lind AC, Heffernan MP (2006) Nonscarring inflammatory alopecia associated with the epidermal growth factor receptor inhibitor gefitinib. J Am Acad Dermatol 55:349–353

Hansen T, Little AJ, Miller JJ, Ioffreda MD (2013) A case of inflammatory nonscarring alopecia associated with the tyrosine kinase inhibitor nilotinib. JAMA Dermatol 149:330–332

Hepper DM, Wu P, Anadkat MJ (2011) Scarring alopecia associated with the epidermal growth factor receptor inhibitor erlotinib. J Am Acad Dermatol 64: 996–998

Lacouture ME, Schadendorf D, Chu CY, Uttenreuther-Fischer M, Stammberger U, O'Brien D, Hauschild A (2013) Dermatologic adverse events associated with afatinib: an oral ErbB family blocker. Expert Rev Anticancer Ther 13:721–728

Nakamura-Wakatsuki T, Yamamoto T (2012) Purpuric drug eruption and alopecia induced by erlotinib. Dermatol Online J 18:16

Pongpudpunth M, Demierre MF, Goldberg LJ (2009) A case report of inflammatory nonscarring alopecia associated with the epidermal growth factor receptor inhibitor erlotinib. J Cutan Pathol 36:1303–1307

Toda N, Fujimoto N, Kato T, Fujii N, Nakanishi G, Nagao T, Tanaka T (2012) Erosive pustular dermatosis of the scalp-like eruption due to gefitinib: case report and review of the literature of alopecia associated with EGFR inhibitors. Dermatology 225:18–21

Wu CY, Chen GS, Lan CC (2008) Erosive pustular dermatosis of the scalp after gefitinib and radiotherapy for brain metastases secondary to lung cancer. Clin Exp Dermatol 33:106–107

Yang BH, Bang CY, Byun JW, Han SH, Song HJ, In SG, Shin JH, Choi GS (2011) A case of cicatricial alopecia associated with erlotinib. Ann Dermatol 23(Suppl 3): S350–S353

Dystrophic Anagen Effluvium: Toxic Alopecia

Aldosary BM, Sutter ME, Schwartz M, Morgan BW (2012) Case series of selenium toxicity from a nutritional supplement. Clin Toxicol (Phila) 50:57–64

Bågedahl-Strindlund M, Ilie M, Furhoff AK, Tomson Y, Larsson KS, Sandborgh-Englund G, Torstenson B, Wretlind K (1997) A multidisciplinary clinical study of patients suffering from illness associated with mercury release from dental restorations: psychiatric aspects. Acta Psychiatr Scand 96:475–482

Bailer J, Rist F, Rudolf A, Staehle HJ, Eickholz P, Triebig G, Bader M, Pfeifer U (2001) Adverse health effects related to mercury exposure from dental amalgam fillings: toxicological or psychological causes? Psychol Med 31:255–263

Bratel J, Haraldson T, Meding B et al (1997) Potential side effects of dental amalgam restorations. An oral and medical investigation. Eur J Oral Sci 105: 234–243

Feldman J, Levisohn DR (1993) Acute alopecia: clue to thallium toxicity. Pediatr Dermatol 10:29–31

Furhoff AK, Tomson Y, Ilie M, Bågedahl-Strindlund M, Larsson KS, Sandborgh-Englund G, Torstenson B, Wretlind K (1998) A multidisciplinary clinical study of patients suffering from illness associated with release of mercury from dental restorations. Medical and odontological aspects. Scand J Prim Health Care 16:247–252

Langworth S, Björkman L, Elinder CG, Järup L, Savlin P (2002) Multidisciplinary examination of patients with illness attributed to dental fillings. J Oral Rehabil 29:705–713

Lindberg NE, Lindberg E, Larsson G (1994) Psychologic factors in the etiology of amalgam illness. Acta Odontol Scand 52:219–228

Lopez RE, Knable AL Jr, Burruss JB (2010) Ingestion of a dietary supplement resulting in selenium toxicity. J Am Acad Dermatol 63:168–169

Piérard GE (1979) Toxic effects of metals from the environment on hair growth and structure. J Cutan Pathol 6:237–242

Rusyniak DE, Furbee RB, Kirk MA (2002) Thallium and arsenic poisoning in a small midwestern town. Ann Emerg Med 39:307–311

Senthilkumaran S, Balamurugan N, Vohra R, Thirumalaikolundusubramanian P (2012) Paradise nut paradox: alopecia due to selenosis from a nutritional therapy. Int J Trichology 4:283–284

Sundström A, Bergdahl J, Nyberg L, Bergdahl M, Nilsson LG (2011) Stressful negative life events and amalgam-related complaints. Community Dent Oral Epidemiol 39:12–18

Vinceti M, Wei ET, Malagoli C, Bergomi M, Vivoli G (2001) Adverse health effects of selenium in humans. Rev Environ Health 16:233–251

Loose Anagen Hair and Short Anagen Hair of Childhood: Loose Anagen Hair

Baden HP, Kvedar JC, Magro CM (1992) Loose anagen hair as a cause of hereditary hair loss in children. Arch Dermatol 128:1349–1353

Hamm H, Traupe H (1989) Loose anagen hair of childhood: the phenomenon of easily pluckable hair. J Am Acad Dermatol 20:242–248

Pham CM, Krejci-Manwaring J (2010) Loose anagen hair syndrome: an underdiagnosed condition in males. Pediatr Dermatol 27:408–409

Price VH, Gummer CL (1989) Loose anagen syndrome. J Am Acad Dermatol 20:249–256

Shelley WB, Shelley ED (1985) Uncombable hair syndrome: observations on response to biotin and occurrence in siblings with ectodermal dysplasia. J Am Acad Dermatol 13:97–102

Tosti A, Peluso AM, Misciali C et al (1997) Loose anagen hair. Arch Dermatol 133:1089–1093

Trüeb RM, Burg G (1992) Loose anagen hair. Hautarzt 43:505–508

Loose Anagen Hair and Short Anagen Hair of Childhood: Short Anagen Hair

Antaya RJ, Sideridou E, Olsen EA (2005) Short anagen syndrome. J Am Acad Dermatol 53(2 Suppl 1):S130–S134

Barraud-Klenovsek MM, Trüeb RM (2000) Congenital hypotrichosis due to short anagen. Br J Dermatol 143:612–617

Giacomini F, Starace M, Tosti A (2011) Short anagen syndrome. Pediatr Dermatol 28:133–134

Herskovitz I, de Sousa IC, Simon J, Tosti A (2013) Short anagen hair syndrome. Int J Trichology 5:45–46

Kersey PJW (1987) Tricho-dental syndrome: a disorder with a short hair cycle. Br J Dermatol 116:259–263

Thai KE, Sinclair RD (2003) Short anagen hair with persistent synchronized pattern of scalp hair growth. J Am Acad Dermatol 49:949–951

van Egmond S, Hoedemaker C, Sinclair R (2007) Short anagen hair naevus: improvement after treatment with 5% topical minoxidil. Int J Dermatol 46:757–759

Psychocutaneous Disorders of the Hair and Scalp

Bloch MH, Panza KE, Grant JE, Pittenger C, Leckman JF (2013) N-acetylcysteine in the treatment of pediatric trichotillomania: a randomized, double-blind, placebo-controlled add-on trial. J Am Acad Child Adolesc Psychiatry 52:231–240

Blum NJ, Barone VJ, Friman PC (1993) A simplified behavioral treatment of trichotillomania: report of two cases. Pediatrics 91:993–995

Braun-Falco O, Vogel PG (1968) Trichotemnomanie. Eine besondere manifestation eines hirnorganischen psychosyndroms. Hautarzt 119:551–553

Cotterill JA (1996a) Dermatologic nondisease. Dermatol Clin 14:439–445

Cotterill JA (1996b) Body dysmorphic disorder. Dermatol Clin 14:457–463

Delsmann BM, Nikolaidis N, Schomacher PH (1993) Trichobezoar als seltene Ursache eines Dünndarmileus. Dtsch Med Wochenschr 118:1361–1364

Fabisch W (1980) Psychiatric aspects of dermatitis artefacta. Br J Dermatol 102:29–34

Fruensgaaard K (1986) Neurotic excoriations: a controlled psychiatric examination. Acta Psychiatr Scand Suppl 69:1–52

Fruensgaaard K (1991a) Psychotherapeutic strategy and neurotic excoriations. Int J Dermatol 30:198–203

Fruensgaaard K (1991b) Psychotherapy and neurotic excoriations. Int J Dermatol 30:262–265

Gandy DT (1953) The concept and clinical aspects of factitious dermatitis. South Med J 46:551–555

Grant JE, Odlaug BL, Kim SW (2009) N-acetylcysteine, a glutamate modulator, in the treatment of trichotillomania: a double-blind, placebo-controlled study. Arch Gen Psychiatry 66(7):756–763

Grant JE, Odlaug BL, Chamberlain SR, Kim SW (2011) Dronabinol, a cannabinoid agonist, reduces hair pulling in trichotillomania: a pilot study. Psychopharmacology (Berlin) 218:493–502

Griesemer RD (1978) Emotionally triggered disease in a dermatology practice. Psychiatr Ann 8:49–56

Harris BA, Sherertz EF, Flowers FP (1987) Improvement of chronic neurotic excoriations with oral Doxepin therapy. Int J Dermatol 26:541–543

Hollender MH, Abram HS (1973) Dermatitis factitia. South Med J 66:1279–1285

Koblenzer CS (1993a) Psychiatric syndromes of interest to dermatologists. Int J Dermatol 32:82–88

Koblenzer CS (1993b) Pharmacology of psychotropic drugs useful in dermatologic practice. Int J Dermatol 32:162–168

Koo J (1995) Psychodermatology: a practical manual for clinicians. Curr Probl Dermatol VII:199–234

Lochner C, Seedat S, Niehaus DJ, Stein DJ (2006) Topiramate in the treatment of trichotillomania: an open-label pilot study. Int Clin Psychopharmacol 21:255–259

Lyell A (1979) Cutaneous artifactual disease. A review amplified by personal experience. J Am Acad Dermatol 1:391–407

McGehee FT, Buchanan GR (1980) Trichophagia and trichobezoar: etiologic role of iron deficiency. J Pediatr 97:946–948

Meiers HG, Rechenberger HG, Rechenberger I (1973) Trichotillomanie. Untersuchungen zur Ätiologie, Diagnostik und Therapie. Hautarzt 24:248–252

Muller SA (1990) Trichotillomania: a histopathologic study in sixty-six patients. J Am Acad Dermatol 23:56–62

Oranje AP, Peereboom-Wynia JDR, de Raeymaecker DMJ (1986) Trichotillomania in childhood. J Am Acad Dermatol 15:614–619

Pericin M, Kündig TM, Trüeb RM (1996) Trichotillomanie in Verbindung mit Alopecia areata. Z Hautkrankh 12:921–924

Reinhardt V, Reinhardt A, Houser D (1986) Hair pulling and eating in captive rhesus monkey troops. Folia Primatol (Basel) 47:158–164

Sheikha SH, Wagner KD, Wagner RF (1993) Fluoxetine treatment of trichotillomania and depression in a prepubertal child. Cutis 51:50–52

Shome S, Bhatia MS, Gautam RK (1993) Culture-bound trichotillomania. Am J Psychiatr 150:674

Sneddon I, Sneddon J (1975) Self-inflicted injury: a follow-up study of 43 patients. Br Med J 2:527–530

Swed SE, Lenane MC, Leonard HL (1993) Long-term treatment of trichotillomania (hair pulling). N Engl J Med 329:141–142

Taylor S, Hyler SE (1993) Update on factitious disorders. Int J Psychiatry Med 23:81–94

Tribó MJ, Ros S, Toll A et al (2005) Trichotillomania: about five cases. 11th International Congress Dermatology and Psychiatry Abstract Book: 84

Trüeb RM (1993) Differential diagnosis in pediatric dermatology: trichotillomania/battered child syndrome. Eur J Pediatr Dermatol 3:134–139

Trüeb RM, Cavegn B (1996) Trichotillomania in connection with alopecia areata. Cutis 58:67–70

Van Moffaert M (1991) Localization of self-inflicted dermatological lesions: what do they tell the dermatologist. Acta Derm Venereol Suppl (Stockh) 156:23–27

Weller EB, Weller RA, Carr S (1989) Imipramine treatment of trichotillomania and co-existing depression in a seven-year-old. J Am Acad Child Adolesc Psychiatry 28:952–953

Psychocutaneous Disorders of the Hair and Scalp: Trichodynia

Arck PC, Handjiski B, Hagen E et al (2001) Indications for a 'brain-hair follicle axis (BHA)': inhibition of keratinocyte proliferation and up-regulation of keratinocyte apoptosis in telogen hair follicles by stress and substance P. FASEB J 15:2536–2538

Burstein R, Cutrer MF, Yarnitsky D (2000) The developmental of cutaneous allodynia during a migraine attack clinical evidence for the sequential recruitment of spinal and supraspinal nociceptive neurons in migraine. Brain 123:1703–1709

Chizh BA, Göhring M, Tröster A, Quartey GK, Schmelz M, Koppert W (2007) Effects of oral pregabalin and aprepitant on pain and central sensitization in the electrical hyperalgesia model in human volunteers. Br J Anaesth 98:246–254

Ericson M, Gabrielson A, Worel S et al (1999) Substance P (SP) in innervated and non-innervated blood vessels in the skin of patients with symptomatic scalp. Exp Dermatol 8:344–345

Gazerani P, Au S, Dong X, Kumar U, Arendt-Nielsen L, Cairns BE (2010) Botulinum neurotoxin type A (BoNTA) decreases the mechanical sensitivity of nociceptors and inhibits neurogenic vasodilation in a craniofacial muscle targeted for migraine prophylaxis. Pain 151:606–616

Grimalt R, Ferrando J, Grimalt F (1998) Trichodynia (letter). Dermatology 196:374

Hafizi S, Chandra P, Cowen J (2007) Neurokinin-1 receptor antagonists as novel antidepressants: trials and tribulations. Br J Psychiatry 191:282–284

Hoss D, Segal S (1998) Scalp dysesthesia. Arch Dermatol 134:327–330

Kramer MS, Cuttler N, Feighner J et al (1998) Distinct mechanism for antidepressant activity by blockade of central substance P receptors. Science 281:1640–1645

Lonne-Rahm SB, Fischer T, Berg M (1999) Stinging rosacea. Acta Derm Venereol 79:460–461

Lucioni A, Bales GT, Lotan TL, McGehee DS, Cook SP, Rapp DE (2008) Botulinum toxin type A inhibits sensory neuropeptide release in rat bladder models of acute injury and chronic inflammation. BJU Int 101:366–370

Mustafa G, Anderson EM, Bokrand-Donatelli Y, Neubert JK, Caudle RM (2013) Anti-nociceptive effect of a conjugate of substance P and light chain of botulinum neurotoxin type A. Pain 154(11):2547–2553, pii: S0304-3959(13)00409-0

Panconesi E, Hartmann G (1996) Psychophysiology of stress in dermatology. The psychologic pattern of psychosomatics. Dermatol Clin 14:399–421

Rebora A (1997) Telogen effluvium. Dermatology 195:209–212

Rebora A, Semino MT, Guarrera M (1996) Trichodynia (letter). Dermatology 192:292–293

Rebora A, Semino MT, Guarrera M (1998) Reply to Trüeb RM. Telogen effluvium and trichodynia (letter). Dermatology 196:374–375

Rollman GB, Lautenbacher S, Jones KS (2000) Sex and gender differences in responses to experimentally induced pain in humans. Sex, gender, and pain. In: Fillingim RB (ed) Progress in pain research and management, vol 17. IASP Press, Seattle

Trüeb RM (1997) Trichodynie. Hautarzt 48:877–880

Trüeb RM (1998) Telogen effluvium and trichodynia (letter). Dermatology 196:374–375

Willimann B, Trüeb RM (2002) Hair pain (trichodynia): frequency and relationship to hair loss and patient gender. Dermatology 205:374–377

Psychocutaneous Disorders of the Hair and Scalp: Trichoteiromania

Freyschmidt-Paul P, Hoffmann R, Happle R (2001) Trichoteiromanie. Eur J Dermatol 11:369–371

Reich S, Trüeb RM (2003) Trichoteiromanie. J Dtsch Dermatol Ges 1:22–28

Concept of Multitargeted Treatment: Value of Nutritional Supplementation Therapy

Ahrens J (1994) Systemische Behandlung des diffusen Haarausfalls. Therapiewoche Schweiz 10:551–554

Budde J, Tronnier H, Rahlfs VW, Frei-Kleiner S (1993) Systemische Therapie von diffusem Effluvium und Haarstrukturschäden. Hautarzt 144:380–384

Buhl AE, Waldon DJ, Kawabe TT, Holland JM (1989) Minoxidil stimulates mouse vibrissae follicles in organ culture. J Invest Dermatol 92:315–320

D'Agostini F, Balansky R, Pesce C et al (2000) Induction of alopecia in mice exposed to cigarette smoking. Toxicol Lett 114:117–123

D'Agostini F, Fiallo P, Pennisi TM, De Flora S (2007) Chemoprevention of smoke-induced alopecia in mice by oral administration of L-cystine and vitamin B6. J Dermatol Sci 46:189–198

Finner AM (2013) Nutrition and hair: deficiencies and supplements. Dermatol Clin 31:167–172

Frenkel MJ, Gillepsie JM, Reis PJ (1974) Factors influencing the biosynthesis of the tyrosine-rich proteins of wool. Aust J Biol Sci 27:31–38

Garneata L (2008) Intravenous iron, inflammation, and oxidative stress: is iron a friend or an enemy of uremic patients? J Ren Nutr 18:40–45

Gillespie JM, Reis PJ (1966) Dietary regulated biosynthesis of high-sulfur wool proteins. Biochem J 98: 669–677

Gummer CL (1985) Diet and hair loss. Semin Dermatol 4:35–39

King SM, Donangelo CM, Knutson MD, Walter PB, Ames BN, Viteri FE, King JC (2008) Daily supplementation with iron increases lipid peroxidation in young women with low iron stores. Exp Biol Med 233:701–707

Petri H, Perchalla P, Tronnier H (1990) Die Wirksamkeit einer medikamentösen Therapie bei Haarstrukturschäden und diffusen Effluvien – vergleichende Doppelblindstudie. Schweiz Rundsch Med Prax 79:1457–1462

Reis PJ, Tunks DA, Sharry LF (1973) Plasma amino acid patterns in sheep receiving abomasal infusions of methionine and cystine. Aust J Biol Sci 26:635–644

Rushton DH (2002) Nutritional factors and hair loss. Clin Exp Dermatol 27:396–404

Schümann K, Ettle T, Szegner B, Elsenhans B, Solomons NW (2007) On risks and benefits of iron supplementation recommendations for iron intake revisited. J Trace Elem Med Biol 21:147–168

Senol E, Ersoy A, Erdinc S, Sarandol E, Yurtkuran M (2008) Oxidative stress and ferritin levels in haemodialysis patients. Nephrol Dial Transplant 23:665–672

Yoshimura K, Nakano H, Yokoyama K, Nakayama M (2005) High iron storage levels are associated with increased DNA oxidative injury in patients on regular hemodialysis. Clin Exp Nephrol 9:158–163

Concept of Multitargeted Treatment: Targeting the Inflammatory Component in Androgenetic Alopecia

Berger RS, Fu JL, Smiles KA, Turner CB, Schnell BM, Werchowski KM, Lammers KM (2003) The effects of minoxidil, 1% pyrithione zinc and a combination of both on hair density: a randomized controlled trial. Br J Dermatol 149:354–362

Piérard-Franchimont C, De Doncker P, Cauwenbergh G, Piérard GE (1998) Ketoconazole shampoo: effect of long-term use in androgenic alopecia. Dermatology 196:474–477

Trüeb RM (2002) Molecular mechanisms of androgenetic alopecia. Exp Gerontol 37:981–990

Concept of Multitargeted Treatment: Combination Treatments

Rajput RJ (2010) Controversy: is there a role for adjuvants in the management of male pattern hair loss? J Cutan Aesthet Surg 3:82–86

Follow-up

4

There is no medicine like hope, no incentive so great, and no tonic so powerful as expectation of something better tomorrow

Orison Swett Marden (1850–1924)

4.1 Global Photographic Assessment

Global photographic assessment has successfully been established as a standard method for objectively monitoring hair growth in the course of the finasteride trials in men since 1992. Since its introduction the technique has proven to be essential for follow-up of hair loss patients undergoing long-term treatment in daily clinical practice as well.

For clinical study purposes, the method is used in tandem with the phototrichogram technique. While the latter yields a quantitative measure of the hair number (n), hair density (n/cm^2), ratio of anagen to telogen phase hairs (%), hair thickness (μm), and linear hair growth rate (mm/day) within a defined area of the scalp, the former reflects the overall clinical changes in the patient over time in a standardized manner.

Global photographs represent head shots taken at short distance from the patient and are therefore different from the closeup photographs used in the phototrichogram technique. For this purpose, the patient's head is positioned in a stereotactic device in which the patient's chin and forehead are fixed and on which a given camera and flash device are mounted (Fig. 4.1), ensuring that the view, magnification, and lighting are the same at consecutive visits, thus enabling precise follow-up of the same scalp area of interest. The stereotactic camera device can be converted to the scalp area of interest with frontal and vertex (center of the scalp whorl) views.

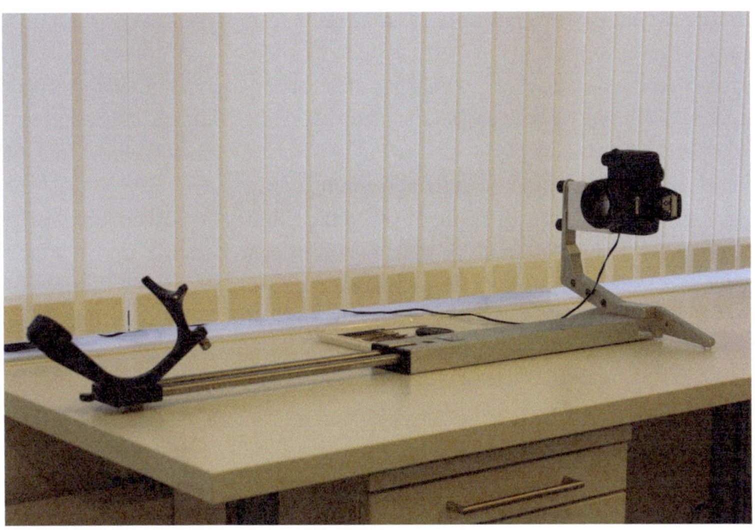

Fig. 4.1 Stereotactic device with mounted camera

R.M. Trüeb, W.-S. Lee, *Male Alopecia*,
DOI 10.1007/978-3-319-03233-7_4, © Springer International Publishing Switzerland 2014

The length, color, shape, and combing of the hair must remain as constant as possible throughout follow-up. Patients must be informed not to change their hairstyle much, as different hairstyles can change how the hair looks. They should also not use cosmetic treatments like having a perm or coloring or use hair thickening products. Patient's hair should be washed on the morning of photography and no hair styling products, such as mousse, gel, or spray should be used. No water should be applied to the hair during hair preparation for the photograph, since this affects the appearance of hair density, especially when the hair is thin. Usually, the hair is neatly parted in the middle. Ultimately, the result of global photographs is easily falsified, if photographs are taken with different degrees of flash lighting for each photograph. More light reflectance on the skin and hair can give the impression of less hair, while correspondingly less lighting can give the impression of more hair. As a result, photographs taken without fixing the photographic system and maintaining consistency in the way the photographs are taken can look very different and bias the results.

Trüeb et al. conducted a 6-month, prospective, open, multicenter cohort study in 265 men with male pattern hair loss treated with oral finasteride 1 mg/day in the office of 52 Swiss dermatologists. The patient's head was placed in a stereotactic device, and photographs were taken of the vertex and frontal areas. Study endpoints were to determine treatment efficacy in an office-based environment, and reliability and acceptance of the photographic method. The photographic method was well accepted by the physicians. The office-based photographic system allowed reliable assessment of change during treatment of male pattern hair loss with oral finasteride. The data generated in this manner corresponded to the antecedent results of the multicenter, placebo-controlled studies with oral finasteride.

The original supplier of this kind of equipment is Canfield Scientific. Clinical studies with minoxidil and finasteride both used photographic apparatus from Canfield Scientific.

Global photographs can be combined with any other quantitative hair growth method complementing clinical data.

> In daily clinical practice, a combination of global photography with trichoscopic examination and photography is recommended.

4.2 Hair Loss-Related Life Quality Index

Finlay et al. were the first to quantify the effect of hair loss on quality of life (QoL) using the Dermatology Life Quality Index (DLQI). It represents a 10-item questionnaire with the aim to measure how much a skin problem has affected the patient's life over the preceding week. For the study patients were recruited from an alopecia support group. With a 90 % response rate, 70 questionnaires were returned.

> DLQI scores in responders with hair loss were comparable to those formerly recorded in patients with severe psoriasis. Forty percent of patients also felt dissatisfied with the way in which their doctor dealt with them.

The authors concluded that the study specifically identified the feelings of loss of self-confidence, low self-esteem, and heightened self-consciousness in people affected by hair loss. The hair loss continued to have a significant impact on life quality well after the initial event. For daily clinical practice, the Dermatology Life Quality Index (DLQI) questionnaire and instructions for use and scoring can be downloaded from www.dermatology.org.uk/quality/dlqi/quality-dlqi-questionnaire.html.

Fischer et al. alternatively developed the Hairdex as a tool for evaluation of disease-specific life quality in hair patients following the Skindex questionnaire for patients with skin diseases. It consists of a 48-item questionnaire with hair-specific questions. For use, readers must to refer to the original publication (in German).

4.3 Patient Compliance Issues

Treatment success relies on patient compliance that, on its part, relies on confidence and motivation. Noncompliance is a major obstacle to the delivery of effective hair loss treatment.

> More often than being a failure of the patient, patient noncompliance results from failure of the physician to ensure that essential confidence and motivation for successful treatment.

Patient compliance describes the degree to which a patient correctly follows medical advice and instruction. It most commonly refers to drug prescriptions, but it can also apply to the use of medical devices, self-care, or therapeutic sessions. Patient perception of the balance between the necessity for treatment and concerns over its use is a powerful predictor of adherence with treatment. This perception of the risk–benefit ratio of treatment explains why compliance with therapy for long-term conditions can be particularly poor. Since both the patient and the healthcare provider affect compliance, a positive physician–patient relationship and regular follow-up visits are the most important factor in determining the degree of patient compliance. The major barriers to compliance are listed in Table 4.1.

In general, efforts to improve compliance have been aimed at simplifying medication packaging, providing effective medication reminders, improving patient education, incl. handouts, and limiting the number of medications prescribed simultaneously. Major recommendations for improvement of patient compliance are listed in Table 4.2.

Table 4.1 Major barriers to patient compliance

Denial of the problem
Lack of comprehension of treatment benefits
Occurrence or fear of side effects
Cost of the treatment
Complexity of treatment regimen
Poor previous experience
Poor communication and lack of trust
Neglect and forgetfulness

Table 4.2 Recommendations for improvement of patient compliance

Only recommending treatments that are effective in circumstances when they are required
Prescribing the minimum number of different medications, e.g., combining active ingredients into a single compound
Simplifying dosage regimen by selecting different treatment or using a preparation that needs fewer doses during the day
Selecting treatments with lower levels of side effects or fewer concerns for long-term risks
Discussing possible side effects, and whether it is important to continue medication regardless of those effects
Advice on minimizing or coping with side effects
Regular follow-up for reassurance on drug safety and treatment benefits
Developing trust so patients don't fear embarrassment or anger if unable to take a particular drug, allowing the doctor to propose a more acceptable alternative

In the treatment of male alopecia, there are short-term compliance issues and long-term compliance issues to be taken into account. Accordingly, regular follow-up visits at 3, 6, and 12 months are recommended, later twice a year, typically in February and August, when due to seasonal variations of hair growth and shedding, telogen rates are the lowest and highest, respectively.

An additional visit at 1 month is optional in regard to drug tolerance issues, especially in the elderly put on topical minoxidil.

Short-term compliance issues that are addressed by the physician within the first 3 months of therapy are: winning the patient's confidence in the diagnosis and treatment plan and detecting problems relating to the prescribed treatment regimen or drug tolerance.

Table 4.3 Four steps to patient adherence

1. *Begin from the patient's perspective:* use the patient's story as the starting place. Listen for the patient's meanings, language, and values as he tells his story. Use the patient's language as much as possible. Translate biomedical terms into terms the patient understands
2. *Include feelings in the discussion:* ask the patient how he feels about his situation. Actively listen, using the patient's terms to reflect on what he is saying. Show the patient you care by expressing your feelings about his progress, problems, etc.
3. *Base treatment goals on the patient's values:* ask the patient how much he prefers to participate in medical decision making. Allow the patient to participate to the extent that he is willing. Guide the patient to set goals, establish steps he is willing to take, and identify barriers to self-care based on his own needs and values
4. *Support patient learning:* ask the patient what other sources he has consulted for information about his condition, and help him make accurate sense of it. Provide or direct the patient to the information he is seeking

From: Stone MS, Bronkesh SJ, Gerbarg ZB, Wood SD (1998) Improving patient compliance. Strategic medicine

The overall goal is to gain short-term compliance as a prerequisite to long-term adherence to treatment.

Based on health communication research, the four steps in Table 4.3 have been suggested to help establish the right conditions for patient adherence to treatment.

The difference between the terms compliance and adherence is not just semantic, it is at the heart of the physician's relationship with patients. While compliance implies an involuntary act of submission to authority, the physician needs to influence patients to become and remain adherents of good self-care. To do this, three key conditions need to be established in the communication with patients: shared values, shared language, and mutual respect.

The following open-ended questions, developed by the Bayer Institute for Health Care Communications, can help gain the patient's adherence under various circumstances:

To clarify the patient's expectations and meanings:
"What were you hoping I would be able to do for you today?"
"You have quite a bit of experience with doctors, what works best for you?"
"Why did you come to see me at this time?"

To clarify what you need from the patient:
"I'd like to be your doctor and to help you with this problem/condition. For me to be effective, though, I'm going to need your help. Would you be willing to []?"

To acknowledge differences in values or points of view:
"I find it difficult to proceed knowing that you have a different view of the situation than I do."
"I'm wondering if we are working together as well as we might be able to."

To encourage problem-solving:
"I want to solve this problem we seem to be having. My thoughts about the situation are []. What are your thoughts?"
"Is there something that I can do at this point to help us work together more effectively?"

To express empathy:
"That must be very difficult for you. I'm sorry."

To acknowledge the patient's difficulty:
"This appears to be difficult for you to talk about. Is there some way I can make it easier?"
"I understand that you are scared at the thought of surgery. Let's talk more about it."

To agree on a diagnosis:
"I've arrived at one explanation of what the difficulty is. [Provide the explanation.] How does that fit in with what you have been thinking?"

Long-term compliance issues that are addressed at 6 and 12 months of follow-up and thereafter are treatment efficacy and sustainability, long-term toxicities, and treatment costs.

Ultimately, in the long-term treatment of an oligosymptomatic condition, neglect may become a problem, since the patient may take the pharmacologically induced condition for granted. On the other hand, forgetfulness is a frequent cause of noncompliance in the elderly.

Further Reading

Global Photographic Assessment

Canfield D (1996) Photographic documentation of hair growth in androgenetic alopecia. Dermatol Clin 14:713–721

DiBernardo BE, Giampapa VC, Vogel J (1996) Standardized hair photography. Dermatol Surg 22:945–952

Olsen EA (2003) Current and novel methods for assessing efficacy of hair growth promoters in pattern hair loss. J Am Acad Dermatol 48:253–262

Trüeb RM, Itin P, Itin and Swiss Trichology Working Group (2001) Photographic documentation of the effectiveness of 1 mg. oral finasteride in treatment of androgenic alopecia in the man in routine general practice in Switzerland. Praxis (Bern 1994) 90:2087–2093

Hair-Loss-Related Life Quality Index

Chren MM (2012) The Skindex instruments to measure the effects of skin disease on quality of life. Dermatol Clin 30:231–236

Fischer TW, Schmidt S, Strauss B, Elsner P (2001) Hairdex: a tool for evaluation of disease-specific quality of life in patients with hair diseases. Hautarzt 52:219–227

Williamson D, Gonzalez M, Finlay AY (2001) The effect of hair loss on quality of life. J Eur Acad Dermatol Venereol 15:137–139

Patient Compliance Issues

Keller V, White MK, Carroll JG, Segal E (1995) "Difficult" physician-patient relationships workbook. Bayer Institute for Health Care Communication, West Haven

Marinker M, Shaw J (2003) Not to be taken as directed. BMJ 326:348–349

Ngoh LN (2003) Health literacy: a barrier to pharmacist-patient communication and medication adherence. J Am Pharm Assoc 49:e132–e146

Stone MS, Bronkesh SJ, Gerbarg ZB, Wood SD (1998) Improving patient compliance. Strategic medicine. www.patientcompliancemedia.com/Improving_Patient_Compliance_article.pdf

White MK, Keller V, Carroll JG (1995) Physician-patient communication workbook. Bayer Institute for Health Care Communication, West Haven

World Health Organization (2003) Adherence to long-term therapies: evidence for action. WHO, Geneva. http://www.who.int/chp/knowledge/publications/adherence_full_report.pdf

5 Patient Expectation Management

It is far more important to know what person the disease has than what disease the person has.

Hippocrates (460–370 BC)

Few dermatologic problems carry as much emotional overtones as the complaint of hair loss. Adding to some patient's worry may be prior frustrating experiences with physicians, who tend to trivialize complaints of hair loss or dismiss them completely. This attitude on the part of physicians is related either to lack of comprehension of the impact of hair loss on quality of life or to lack of confidence in the treatment of alopecia.

> Treatment options are available, though limited, both in terms of indications and of efficacy. Success depends not only on comprehension of the underlying pathology but also on unpatronizing sympathy from the part of the physician.

A detailed patient history focusing on chronology of events, examination of the scalp and pattern of hair loss, a simple pull test, dermoscopy of the scalp and hair, a few pertinent screening blood tests, and a scalp biopsy in selected cases – as outlined in the respective chapters – will usually establish a specific diagnosis.

> Once the diagnosis is certain, treatment appropriate for that diagnosis is likely to control the problem.

In addition, patients need to be educated about the basics of the hair cycle and why considerable patience is required for effective cosmetic recovery.

5.1 Beyond Evidence-Based Medicine

The Latin maxim TUTO CELERITER IUCUNDE stands for "safely, swiftly, and gladly" and was originally coined by Asclepiades of Bithynia (124–56 BC), personal physician and near friend of notable personalities of Ancient Rome, such as Cicero and Marc Anthony.

While the foreign Greek physicians were originally encountered with much distrust by ancient Romans and especially its aristocracy, Asclepiades managed to convince through his high learning, brilliant medical achievements, and worldly wisdom. Above all, he was always attentive and sympathetic to the individual needs of his patients. Asclepiades was born in Prusa. He travelled much when young and at first settled at Rome as a rhetorician. Though he did not succeed in that profession, he eventually acquired great reputation as a physician. Asclepiades began by vilifying the principles and practices of his predecessors and by asserting that he had discovered a more effective method of treating diseases than had been before known to the world. His remedies were directed to the restoration of harmony.

R.M. Trüeb, W.-S. Lee, *Male Alopecia*,
DOI 10.1007/978-3-319-03233-7_5, © Springer International Publishing Switzerland 2014

A part of the great popularity which Asclepiades enjoyed depended upon his attending to every need of his patients and indulging their inclinations.

Finally, Asclepiades advocated humane treatment of mental disorders. His teachings are surprisingly modern; therefore Asclepiades is considered to be a pioneer physician in both the medical sciences and psychotherapy.

The same way Asclepiades won the Roman populace and aristocracy for his cause, the physician must advance to build up his reputation and to secure the confidence of his patients.

A liaison with patients, respect for their individuality, and professional expertise are preliminary to creating an atmosphere of mutual trust, which on the one side enables the physician's professional contribution to the healing process, and on the other side assists patients to draw also from their own mental self-healing capacities. This is where, at times, success in treating hair loss disorders may supersede evidence-based medicine (EBM).

Although EBM is becoming regarded as the gold standard for clinical practice, there are a number of limitations of its use. EBM guidelines do not remove the problem of extrapolation to different populations or longer timeframes. Even if several top-quality studies are available, questions always remain about how far, and to which populations, their results may be generalized. Certain groups have been historically under-researched, such as racial minorities and people with many comorbid diseases, and thus the literature is sparse in areas that do not allow for generalizing.

EBM applies to groups of people, but this does not preclude clinicians from using their personal experience in deciding how to treat an individual subject.

Ex cathedra statements by the medical expert are considered to be the least valid form of evidence. Nevertheless, knowledge gained from clinical research does not directly answer the primary clinical question of what is best for the patient at hand and suggests that EBM should not discount the value of clinical experience. Good medical practice means integrating individual clinical expertise with the best available external clinical evidence from EBM.

Finally, one must remain open-minded for the possibility of a multitude of cause relationships underlying hair loss, and accordingly for the potential of combination treatments.

5.2 Listening to the Patient

Communication is an important component of patient care. Traditionally, communication in medical school curricula is incorporated informally as part of rounds and faculty feedback, but without a specific focus on skills of communicating. Communication skills are not a question of talent. One's effectiveness in communication can be improved through training and through experience.

For a successful encounter at an office visit, one needs to be sure that the patient's key concerns have been directly and specifically solicited and addressed.

To be effective, the physician must gain an understanding of the patient's perspective on his ailment. Patient concerns can be wide ranging, including fear of hair loss and disfigurement; apprehension of scalp symptoms; distrust of the medical profession or of pharmacologic agents; concern about loss of wholeness, role, status, or independence; denial of reality of medical conditions; grief; and other uniquely personal issues. Patient values, cultures, and preferences need to be explored. Gender is another element that needs to be taken into consideration. Ensuring key issues are verbalized openly is fundamental to effective patient–doctor communication. Appropriate reassurance or pragmatic suggestions to help with problem solving and setting up a structured plan of action may be an important part of the patient care that is required.

The physician should be careful not to be judgmental or scolding because this may rapidly close down communication. Sometimes the patient gains therapeutic benefit just from venting concerns in a safe environment with a caring physician.

Hair loss is a common dermatologic problem. Psychological research confirms a negative effect of visible hair loss on social perceptions and body image satisfaction. Therefore, a thorough evaluation, a specific diagnosis, effective treatment, and appropriate counselling all have some psychological efficacy.

In 1992, Cash examined psychological effects of androgenetic alopecia in men and found that although most men regard hair loss to be an unwanted, distressing experience that diminishes their body image, bald men actively cope and generally retain the integrity of their personality functioning (Table 5.1).

In contrast, Maffei et al. found the prevalence of personality disorders in subjects with androgenetic alopecia to be significantly higher than in the general population and found the existence of three distinct personality profiles:

- Suspicious, with grandiose sense of self-importance, obsessive, and socially withdrawn
- Impulsive, identity disordered, and socially maladjusted
- Dramatic, emotional, and dependent.

Physicians should recognize that androgenetic alopecia in men goes well beyond the simple physical aspects of hair loss and growth.

It must be kept in mind that patients' psychological reactions to hair loss are less related to physicians' ratings than to patients' own perceptions of the extent of their hair loss. Irrespective of the extent, hair loss may be imbued with considerable emotional bearing that the physician should not ignore.

Table 5.1 Percentage of men attributing specific effects to the occurrence of androgenetic alopecia

	Extent of hair loss	
Reported experience	Low	High
Cognitive preoccupation		
Wish for more hair	52	84
Notice bald/balding men	54	82
Spend time looking in mirror at hair/head	54	69
Wonder what others think	47	67
Negative socio-emotional events		
Get teased by peers	45	79
Feel self-conscious	42	78
Look older than actual age	40	55
Worry that others will notice	39	56
Feel helpless about baldness	37	56
Worry about aging	37	46
Feel less attractive	31	51
Envy good-looking men	33	34
Behavioral coping		
Try to improve hairstyle	63	66
Try to improve physique	41	36
Dress more nicely	26	45
Wear hats or caps	23	41
Seek reassurance about looks	23	39
Grow beard or moustache	18	36

From: Cash TF (1992) The psychological effects of androgenetic alopecia in men. J Am Acad Dermatol 26:926–931

Androgenetic alopecia is clearly not uniform in its psychological impact.

Cash identified several variables predictive of greater androgenetic alopecia-related distress among men:

- Younger men (under 26 years old) with earlier-onset hair loss
- Romantically unattached men
- Those who view their alopecia as socially noticeable and expect it to progress

- Men with a heightened social (public) self-consciousness, a vulnerable sense of self-acceptability, and a higher psychological investment in their appearance.

Finally, patients with personality disorders tend to experience more distress from hair loss than non-disordered patients, since these individuals lack a secure sense of self and effective coping skills, and therefore may be especially vulnerable to the adverse effects of androgenetic alopecia.

> The psychological effects of hair loss may be hard to differentiate clinically form pre-existing psychopathology.

Often, hair loss may first become apparent at particularly demanding periods of life, such as during the period of mate selection or at the onset of a challenging career. At such times, men may find hair loss especially upsetting and even use it as a scapegoat for a lack of satisfaction in other areas of life.

Left to their own resources, individuals with androgenetic alopecia engage in a number of strategies to cope with the unwanted conditions, such as:

- Styling the remaining scalp hair to conceal thinning areas
- Using cosmetic products to camouflage hair loss
- Wearing caps or hats to conceal the condition
- Avoiding situations that aggravate distress by making the hair loss more socially recognizable, e.g., wet hair, windy or brightly lit environments
- Compensating for the diminished body image by growing a beard or improving grooming and physique
- Paradoxically shaving the entire head do hide hair loss

Patients who have concluded that the above strategies, or over-the-counter treatments, are insufficient to abate their distress, finally consult professionals for medical or surgical solutions. With the advent of pharmacologic agents, such as topical minoxidil solution and oral finasteride, and improved surgical hair transplantation procedures for effective treatment of male androgenetic alopecia, the options for managing androgenetic alopecia and androgenetic alopecia-related distress have expanded.

> In 1991, van der Donk et al. conducted a prospective study of the psychological changes in men who received either 2 % topical minoxidil solution or placebo and found favorable changes in psychological adjustment and self-image among responders to topical minoxidil solution compared to placebo recipients, but only in the group aged above 35 years.

Ultimately, psychosocial assessment was an aspect of the double-blind, placebo-controlled trials submitted to the US Food and Drug Administration (FDA) for approval of over-the-counter 5 % topical minoxidil solution for treating androgenetic alopecia in men.

In 2011, a study was performed in Japan by Tsuboi et al. in order to ascertain whether treatment with 1 mg oral finasteride can improve the quality of life of male patients with androgenetic alopecia. Patients aged 19–76 years (average, 33.8) answered Visual Analogue Scale (VAS), Dermatology Life Quality Index (DLQI), WHO/QOL-26, and State-Trait Anxiety Inventory (STAI) questionnaires before and after administration of oral finasteride for 6 months. The changes in these indices before and after treatment were statistically analyzed, and the improved values of the indices in the high treatment responders (excellent or good) and the low treatment responders (moderate or no change) from baseline were compared. There was a statistical difference in the VAS and DLQI indices before and after administration of oral finasteride, while no significant change was found for the WHO/QOL-26 and STAI indices. Interestingly, comparison of high and low responders failed to reveal any statistical difference in the improvement of VAS and DLQI scores.

The authors concluded that oral finasteride improves the quality of life of men treating androgenetic alopecia, and VAS and DLQI are useful for the evaluation of patients' quality of life. However, oral finasteride failed to improve the patients' anxiety nor did its efficacy correlate with the level of reported anxiety.

5.3 Tackling Side Effects

A side effect is an effect that is secondary to the one intended. The term is primarily used to describe unwanted or adverse effects. In the broader sense, the term can also apply to unintended, but beneficial effects from the use of the drug. An example is the hair growth-promoting effect of minoxidil that was originally a drug intended to lower the blood pressure but proved to be a powerful trichotrophic agent.

Occurrence or fear of side effects is a major barrier to patient compliance. Therefore it is of upmost importance to inform patients on potential side effects, their frequencies, and appropriate management.

Some side effects are directly related to the pharmacologic effect of the drug, others to a patient's individual allergic or idiosyncratic disposition, to drug–drug interactions, or to simply not following instructions for proper use of the medication. Patients should be aware of possible allergies to active ingredients or additives and report other medical conditions and medications. Therefore, it is highly recommended, even when treatment can be purchased without a doctor's prescription, that the patient visits a physician for proper indication, exclusion of contraindications, instructions for proper use, and follow-up. Adverse reactions to topical minoxidil solution and oral finasteride are listed in Tables 5.2 and 5.3, respectively.

Table 5.2 Adverse reactions to 2 or 5 % topical minoxidil solution

Common
Hair shedding (during initial 4–6 weeks of treatment)
Unwanted hair growth elsewhere on the body (usually facial in women, within 3–6 weeks of treatment)
Itching, redness, or irritation at the treated area (usually due to propylene glycol)
Changes in hair color or texture
Burning or irritation of the eyes
Rare (treatment should be withheld immediately)
Severe allergic reactions: rash, hives, itching, difficulty breathing, tightness in the chest, swelling of the mouth, face, lips, or tongue
Cardiovascular effects: chest pain, dizziness, fainting, increased heart rate, pounding heartbeat, sudden, unexplained weight gain, swollen hands or feet
Unexplained: breast tenderness, changes in vision or hearing
Thrombocytopenia and leukopenia (WBC $<3{,}000/mm^3$) have very rarely been reported with oral minoxidil

Table 5.3 Adverse reactions to 1 mg oral finasteride

Common (frequency between ≥1/100 and 1/10)
Sexual dysfunction (finasteride 3.8 % vs. 2.1 % within first 12 months of treatment, 1 % of men withdrew finasteride because of sexual dysfunction within first 12 months of treatment, thereafter frequency decreased to 0.6 % during following 4 years of treatment)
Diminished libido (finasteride 1.8 % vs. placebo 1.3 %)
Erectile dysfunction (finasteride 1.3 % vs. placebo 0.7 %)
Occasional (frequency between ≥1/1,000 and <1/100)
Abnormal ejaculation
Decreased ejaculatory volume
Rare (frequency between ≥1/10,000 and <1/1,000)
Testicular pain
Breast tenderness
Gynecomastia (may persist for months to years after cessation of finasteride treatment)
Allergic reactions: rash, itching, hives, swelling of the mouth, face, lips, or tongue (angioedema)
Very rare (frequency between <1/10,000)
Depression
Male breast cancer
Unknown (frequency cannot be estimated from existing data)
Persistent diminished libido or erectile dysfunction (after cessation of finasteride treatment)
Male infertility (usually in association with preexistent subfertility)

(continued)

Table 5.3 (continued)

Decrease in quality of semen (there are reports on normalization or improvement of semen quality following withdrawal of drug)
Post-finasteride syndrome
Cause relationship unresolved
High Gleason grade tumor (7–10) in the event of prostate carcinoma in men > 55 years treated with 5 mg oral finasteride daily for benign prostatic hyperplasia (finasteride 6.4 % vs. placebo 5.1 %)

Topical minoxidil solution and foam are used to promote hair growth in the treatment of androgenetic alopecia. Minoxidil is not indicated for treatment of telogen effluvium or alopecia areata, lest androgenetic alopecia represents a comorbidity. Efficacy and safety data are not available before the age of 18 years and after the age of 65 years. Nevertheless, minoxidil can be safely used before 18 or after 65 years at the discretion of the prescriber (off-label use).

> Children are at higher risk of adverse cardiovascular effects of topical minoxidil solution.

Therefore, before the age of 12 years, the dosage should be halved. Any of the following health problems should caution to the use of topical minoxidil: active diseases of the scalp, e.g., eczema, infection, and cuts, as well as heart problems, e.g., chest pain, heart attack, and heart failure.

Before applying minoxidil to the scalp, the area should be clean and dry. The product may be applied to damp hair. To use the solution, the applicator is filled with 1 ml of medication. The hair in the area of thinning is parted, and the solution is applied evenly to the affected area of the scalp and gently rubbed in. The solution or foam is applied twice a day. The solution is allowed to dry completely before using other styling products, e.g., gels or mousse, or before going to bed. If a dose is missed, the missed dose is to be skipped and the usual dosing schedule resumed. The dose should not be doubled to catch up.

The best thing to do is to treat through until the shedding stops (usually within 6 weeks), and

> Upon initiation of treatment with topical minoxidil, patients may experience temporary increased shedding of hair (shedding phase). Patients should be prepared and informed that this represents a physiological response to treatment, since minoxidil not only increases the duration of anagen in the hair cycle but triggers an immediate telogen release.

new hair growth is seen (usually at 3 months). Patients should also be aware that it takes time for hair to regrow. Most people need to use this medication regularly for at least 8 weeks to see a benefit. If the condition does not improve or worsens after using this medication for 3–6 months, the condition and treatment need to be reevaluated by the physician. The effect of minoxidil builds up until 12 months of treatment. Once it is established that minoxidil is effective, treatment should thereafter continue indefinitely since positive results will be reversed within 6 weeks to 3 months once treatment is stopped.

> Itching, redness, or irritation at the treated area is far more frequent due to an irritant dermatitis to propylene glycol or the alcohol-based solution of minoxidil.

If irritant scalp dermatitis is a problem, either minoxidil foam or a minoxidil compound should be used that are free of propylene glycol:

Rp.	
Minoxidil	2.0, 3.0, or 5.0 g
Glycerine	10.0 g
Water	20.0 g
Ethanol	96 % ad 100.0 g
M.D.S. Apply twice daily 1 ml to the affected area	

After applying minoxidil onto the scalp, exposure to the sun should be avoided, since it may cause sunburns. Minoxidil should not be used on skin that is red, painful, irritated, scraped, cut, or infected, since doing so may cause the drug to be absorbed into the body and result in systemic side effects. Hands should be thoroughly washed after application. Caution is to be given to avoiding getting the medication in eyes. If this occurs, eyes should be rinsed with large amounts of cool water.

Very few minoxidil users are truly allergic to the active ingredient. While irritant dermatitis usually develops early in the course of treatment, allergic reactions are usually acquired later.

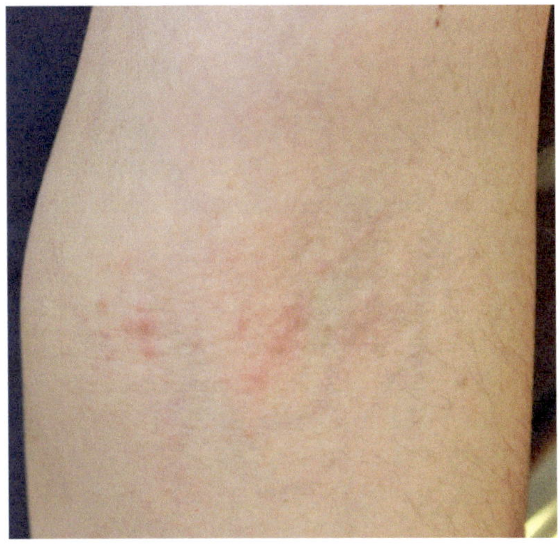

Fig. 5.1 Positive ROAT to minoxidil

If an allergic reaction to minoxidil is suspected, this can be clarified by performing a repeated open application test (ROAT) to the forearm: minoxidil is applied twice daily to an area of 5 × 5 cm on the inner aspect of the forearm for a duration of 7 days. In the event of a contact allergic reaction, an erythematous rash with papules will become apparent usually within 48–72 h (Fig. 5.1). Severe allergic reactions and unexplained other adverse reactions to topical minoxidil are exceedingly rare.

One milligram oral finasteride received FDA approval for treatment of male pattern baldness in 1997. In several clinical studies, oral finasteride, like topical minoxidil solution, was shown to work on both the crown area and the hairline but is most successful in the crown area. Again, finasteride is effective only for as long as it is taken. The hair gained or maintained is lost within 6–12 months of stopping treatment.

In a more recent 10-year study of 118 men between 20 and 61 years of age treated with 1 mg oral finasteride daily for androgenetic alopecia, Rossi et al. found that 86 % of men continued to benefit from treatment over the entire course of 10 years. In the opinion of the authors, the result after the first year could help in predicting the effectiveness of the treatment; however, many of those unchanged after 1 year of treatment were found to improve later on. Interestingly, better improvements were observed in patients older than 30 years with Hamilton–Norwood grades IV and V. Treatment efficacy was not reduced over time (including those over 40 years of age). Adverse effects were reported in 5.9 % of patients; however some of them went on with treatment because of the good results.

In the most recent study published in 2012, Sato and Takeda reported on efficacy and safety of 1 mg oral finasteride for treatment of male androgenetic alopecia in the so far largest population study. The study enrolled 3,177 Japanese men treated with oral finasteride from January 2006 to June 2009 at the Tokyo Memorial Clinic Hirayama Department of Plastic and Aesthetic Surgery, School of Medicine, Kitasato University, Tokyo, Japan. Efficacy was evaluated by global photographic assessment, and safety data were assessed by interviews and laboratory tests. The overall effect on hair growth was seen in 87.1 %, in whom hair increased greatly in 11.1 %, moderately in 36.5 %, and slightly in 39.5 %. The response rate improved with increasing duration of treatment. Adverse reactions occurred in 0.7 % of men. Seven men discontinued treatment based on risk–benefit considerations. No specific safety problems associated with long-term use were observed. The authors concluded that in Japanese men with androgenetic alopecia, 1 mg oral finasteride used for long-term treatment maintains progressive hair regrowth without recognized side effect.

Nevertheless, since the original report of persistent diminished libido, erectile dysfunction, and depression among former users of oral finasteride by Traish et al. in 2011, there have been several reports on sexual side effects that may persist despite discontinuation of finasteride medication. These subjects also reported a wide range of symptoms including changes in cognition, ejaculate quality, and genital sensations. Ultimately, Irwig reported depressive symptoms and suicidal thoughts among former users of finasteride with persistent sexual side effects. The author concluded that prescribers of finasteride and men contemplating its use should be made aware of these potential adverse medication effects.

With respect to finasteride and male fertility, early studies did not show any significant influence of finasteride on parameters of semen quality, whereas some later case reports suggested that in subfertile patients, the effects of the drug might be amplified. Therefore, respective counselling may be particularly challenging for male partners of couples who are attempting to become pregnant.

Some users, in an effort to save money, buy 5 mg finasteride tablets instead of the original 1 mg pill and split them into several parts to approximate the 1 mg dosage. Also, finasteride 1 mg capsules formulated with an active ingredient of unknown origin are marketed unofficially to treat androgenetic alopecia in men. Navarro Guerrero et al. performed a galenic-pharmaceutical study of pieces of Proscar® (5 mg finasteride) tablets and finasteride 1 mg capsules versus Propecia® in the treatment of androgenetic alopecia, with the effort to ascertain the pharmaceutical quality of these alternative preparations. The results obtained demonstrated a high variability in the dosage of pieces of tablets ranging from 0.49 to 1.81 mg of finasteride, only 10 % being within the dosage range, which is ± 5 %, as compared with the authorized 1 mg dose. Applying the criteria of the mass uniformity test, set down in the European Pharmacopoeia, to the set of Proscar® pieces and to the value of the standard deviation percentage (18 %) obtained the batch would have to be rejected. The finasteride 1 mg capsules showed variable in vitro availability values between 51 and 86 % as compared to Propecia®, which has 92 % availability. Some of these formulations again do not meet the availability specifications established by standard pharmacopoeias. Furthermore, the dissolution efficiency of the capsules (from 27 to 76 %) was significantly lower than that of the reference proprietary drug with 82 % (unpublished data).

Finally, the 1 mg finasteride pills are coated to prevent contact with the active ingredient during handling, and the dust or crumbs from broken 5 mg finasteride tablets should be kept away from pregnant women or women who may become pregnant due to teratogenicity.

> Splitting 5 mg finasteride tablets to treat androgenetic alopecia is an inappropriate practice from the point of view of safety and dosage variability. With regard to the finasteride 1 mg capsules marketed unofficially, any finasteride formulation purportedly similar to the reference proprietary drug must prove its bioequivalence or interchangeability with respect to the availability of the active ingredient.

Due to interference with doping assays, many sports organizations had banned oral finasteride because it could be misused to mask steroid abuse. Not until 2009, finasteride was removed from the World Anti-Doping Agency's list of banned substances. Prominent athletes who used finasteride for treatment of their hair loss and were banned from international competition include: skeleton racer Zach Lund, bobsledder Sebastien Gattuso, footballer Romário, and ice hockey goaltender José Théodore.

The Prostate Cancer and Prevention Trial (PCPT) was a landmark study that sought to reduce the morbidity and mortality of prostate cancer with the use of oral finasteride to prevent disease. The investigators randomly assigned 18,882 men 55 years of age or older with a normal digital rectal examination and a prostate-specific antigen (PSA) level of 3.0 ng per milliliter or lower to treatment with finasteride (5 mg per day) or placebo for 7 years. Prostate biopsy was performed if the annual PSA level, adjusted for the effect of finasteride, exceeded 4.0 ng per milliliter, or if the digital rectal examination was abnormal. Prostate cancer was detected in 803 of the 4,368 men in the finasteride group who had data for the final analysis (18.4 %) and in 1,147 of the 4,692 men in the placebo group who had such data (24.4 %), for a 24.8 % reduction in prevalence over the 7-year period (95 % confidence interval, 18.6–30.6 %; $p<0.001$). Tumors of Gleason grade 7 or more were more common in the finasteride group (280 of 757 tumors [37.0 %], or 6.4 % of the 4,368 men included in the final analysis) than in the placebo group (237 of 1,068 tumors [22.2 %], $p<0.001$ for the comparison between groups; or 5.1 % of the 4,692 men included in the final analysis, $p=0.005$ for the comparison between groups). Sexual side effects were more common in finasteride-treated men, whereas urinary symptoms were more common in men receiving placebo.

To seek to alleviate the concern of the increase of number of high-grade cancers detected in the original PCPT, Thompson et al. examined long-term all-cause mortality among PCPT participants. The results were reassuring with an overall 15-year rate of death of 22 % in both the finasteride group and the control group. The investigators were unable to report prostate-cancer-specific mortality.

In men 55 years or older, 5 mg oral finasteride prevents or delays the appearance of prostate cancer, but this possible benefit and a reduced risk of urinary problems must be weighed against sexual side effects. The increased risk of high-grade prostate cancer detected with finasteride in the original Prostate Cancer Prevention Trial did not prove to affect the overall 15-year rate of death in both the finasteride and the control group in a subsequent study, and the investigators were unable to report prostate-cancer-specific mortality.

For a comprehensive list of reported adverse reactions to other drugs used for treatment of alopecia, readers are encouraged to refer to the respective information for consumers and healthcare professionals accompanying the drug.

When a drug is used for unapproved indications, it is termed *off-label use*. Off-label use of drugs is legal, but the promotion of drugs toward unapproved indications is illegal.

An example for off-label use is oral finasteride for hormone replacement therapy in male-to-female transsexuals in combination with a form of estrogen treatment due to its antiandrogenic properties. However, little clinical research on finasteride use for this indication has been conducted and evidence for efficacy is limited. Moreover, finasteride is a substantially weaker antiandrogen in comparison to conventional antiandrogens like cyproterone acetate. Furthermore, finasteride has been associated with inducing depression and anxiety in both male and female patients, symptoms that are very common in transsexuals, who are already at a high risk.

As a result, prescription of oral finasteride either for hormone replacement therapy or for treatment of male androgenetic alopecia in male-to-female transsexuals may not be particularly useful or could put them at risk for emotional side effects.

Finasteride has also been shown to reduce alcohol intake and suppress alcohol preference in male mice; studies on effects on alcohol consumption and withdrawal in humans are ongoing.

The prescribing physician should always be aware that the off-label prescription of drugs occurs at the discretion of the prescriber.

This applies as well to the use of oral dutasteride for treatment of male androgenetic alopecia, as to the use of oral tetracyclines, oral hydroxychloroquine, oral mycophenolate mofetil, or cyclosporine A, or oral pioglitazone in the treatment of lichen planopilaris and related conditions (frontal fibrosing alopecia, fibrosing alopecia in a pattern distribution). The case of the oral antidiabetic pioglitazone that has recently been proposed for treatment of lichen planopilaris sheds light on the risks of liability issues: June 9, 2011, the French Agency for the Safety of Health Products decided to withdraw pioglitazone in regard to high risk of bladder cancer; June 10, 2011, Germany's Federal Institute for Drugs and Medical Devices advised doctors not to prescribe the medication until further investigation of the cancer risk had been conducted; ultimately, June 15, 2011, the US FDA announced that pioglitazone use for more than 1 year may be associated with an increased risk of bladder cancer and that the information about this risk will be added to the Warnings and Precautions section of the label for pioglitazone-containing medicines.

For adverse effects of cosmetic hair treatments refer to Sect. 6.7.

5.3.1 Nocebo Effect

In a strict sense, a nocebo reaction refers to undesirable effects a subject experiences after receiving an inert dummy drug or placebo. Nocebo reactions are not chemically generated and are due only to the subject's pessimistic belief and expectation that treatment will produce negative consequences. In a wider sense, the term is being increasingly used for unexpected negative reactions to an active drug.

The term nocebo (from Latin for "I will harm") was originally coined in 1961 by W. Kennedy for the counterpart of placebo (from Latin for "I will please"), which refers to desirable effects a subject experiences after receiving an inert dummy drug. In both cases, there is no real pharmacologically active substance involved, but the actual negative or positive consequences, resp., of the administration of the drug, which may be physiological, behavioral, emotional, or cognitive, are nonetheless real. Kennedy emphasized that his specific usage of the term nocebo does not refer to the iatrogenic action of the drug, but insisted that a nocebo reaction is subject-centered and that the term nocebo reaction specifically refers to a quality inherent in the patient rather than in the drug. Kennedy was precisely speaking of an outcome that is totally generated by a subject's negative expectation of a drug administration and is the exact counterpart of a placebo response that would be generated by a subject's positive expectation.

In 2007, Mondaini et al. addressed the question how many of sexual side effects associated with oral finasteride treatment are related to a nocebo phenomenon: 120 sexually active male patients with an International Index of Erectile Function-erectile function (IIEF-EF) domain ≥ 25 and a clinical diagnosis of benign prostatic hyperplasia were randomized to receive 5 mg oral finasteride concealed as an "X compound of proven efficacy for the treatment of benign prostatic hyperplasia" for 1 year with (group 2) or without (group 1) counselling on the drug sexual side effects. The phrase used to inform group 2 patients was "may cause erectile dysfunction, decreased libido, problems of ejaculation but these are uncommon." The estimation of side effects was conducted at 6 and 12 months using the male sexual function-4 (MSF-4 item) questionnaire and a self-administered questionnaire. One hundred and seven patients completed the study. Group 2 patients ($n=55$) reported a significant higher proportion of one or more sexual side effects as compared to group 1 ($n=52$) (43.6 % vs. 15.3 %, $p=0.03$). The incidence of erectile dysfunction, decreased libido, and ejaculation disorders was 9.6, 7.7, and 5.7 %, resp., for group 1 and 30.9, 23.6, and 16.3 %, resp., for group 2 ($p=0.02$, $p=0.04$, and $p=0.06$). The authors concluded that blinded administration of finasteride was associated with a significantly higher proportion of sexual dysfunction in patients informed on sexual side effects as compared to those in which the same information was omitted. A scenario is likely to occur in clinical practice, where the patient is counselled by the physician and has access to the drug information sheet. The burden of this nocebo effect has to be taken into account when managing finasteride sexual side effects.

> The influence of the prescribing physician should be kept in mind, since inspiring confidence versus skepticism and fear clearly impacts the outcome of treatment.

Ultimately, some patients with somatoform disorder and specific personality disorders, e.g., anxious, negativistic, histrionic, or paranoid, are more prone to nocebo reactions and should be recognized as such.

5.3.2 Post-Finasteride Syndrome

The post-finasteride syndrome has been claimed to occur in men who have taken oral finasteride to treat either hair loss or benign prostatic hyperplasia. Reported symptoms include loss of libido, erectile dysfunction, reduction in penis size, penile curvature or reduced sensation, gynecomastia, muscle atrophy, cognitive impairment, severely dry skin, and depression. The condition allegedly may have a life-altering impact on sufferers and their families, such as job loss and the breakup of romantic relationships or marriages, while also being linked to suicides.

As yet, the condition is not recognized by the scientific community, although individuals who suffer from the syndrome do present with very distinctive and relatively homogenous symptoms.

While the incidence of persistent sexual, mental, and physical side effects which continue despite quitting finasteride is unknown, it is likely that over 1,000 men worldwide are experiencing the effects. This estimate is based on the number of registered users of the Internet forum www.propeciahelp.com.

Persistent neurologic effects from other drugs are well recognized, such as the tardive dyskinesias related to the use of phenothiazines for treatment of chronic schizophrenia. There is a growing body of scientific evidence from studies in rodents, that finasteride may reduce the concentration of several neuroactive steroids important for neurogenesis and neuronal survival. An important neurosteroid is allo-pregnanolone (ALLO), a metabolite of dihydroprogesterone. ALLO is a potent ligand of the inhibitory GABA-barbiturate receptor. $GABA_A$ receptors have variable sensitivities to ALLO in the settings of neurosteroid withdrawal, stress, social isolation, and aging. Less ALLO, as a consequence of finasteride treatment, could alter GABAergic transmission with implications for neuronal progenitors and young neurons. Interestingly, the mechanisms of irreversible tardive dyskinesias from phenothiazines may be similar to the mechanisms underlying the persistent side effects of finasteride: in rats treated with the phenothiazine haloperidol to induce orofacial dyskinesias, coadministration of progesterone prevented this side effect, while pretreatment of the rats with finasteride reversed this protective effect, demonstrating an important role of the progesterone pathway and its metabolites.

The Post-Finasteride Syndrome Foundation (www.pfsfoundation.org) is a nonprofit organization dedicated to helping fund research on the characterization, underlying biological mechanisms and treatments of the post-finasteride syndrome, while improving public awareness of the condition.

Up to date there are no predictive factors for the risk of development of post-finasteride syndrome and no known treatment for the disorder. For the time being, as a general rule:

- Refrain from prescribing oral finasteride to a patient with a personal history of depression, sexual dysfunction, or fertility problems.
- When fertility is an issue, may consider performing a sperm count before and during treatment with oral finasteride.
- In any case of adverse effects, stop oral finasteride treatment.
- In all men 45 and over, perform PSA before, after starting therapy with oral finasteride, and thereafter on twice yearly basis. The level should drop by ca. 50 % upon initiation of therapy. In case of increase >0.4 ng/ml per year, refer to urologist to check prostate condition.

- For men who choose regular prostate cancer screening, the use of oral finasteride meaningfully reduces the risk of prostate cancer.

In men aged 35 years or more, a successful switch from oral finasteride to topical minoxidil may be considered in anticipation of age-related more frequent sexual function-related problems (Fig. 5.2a–c).

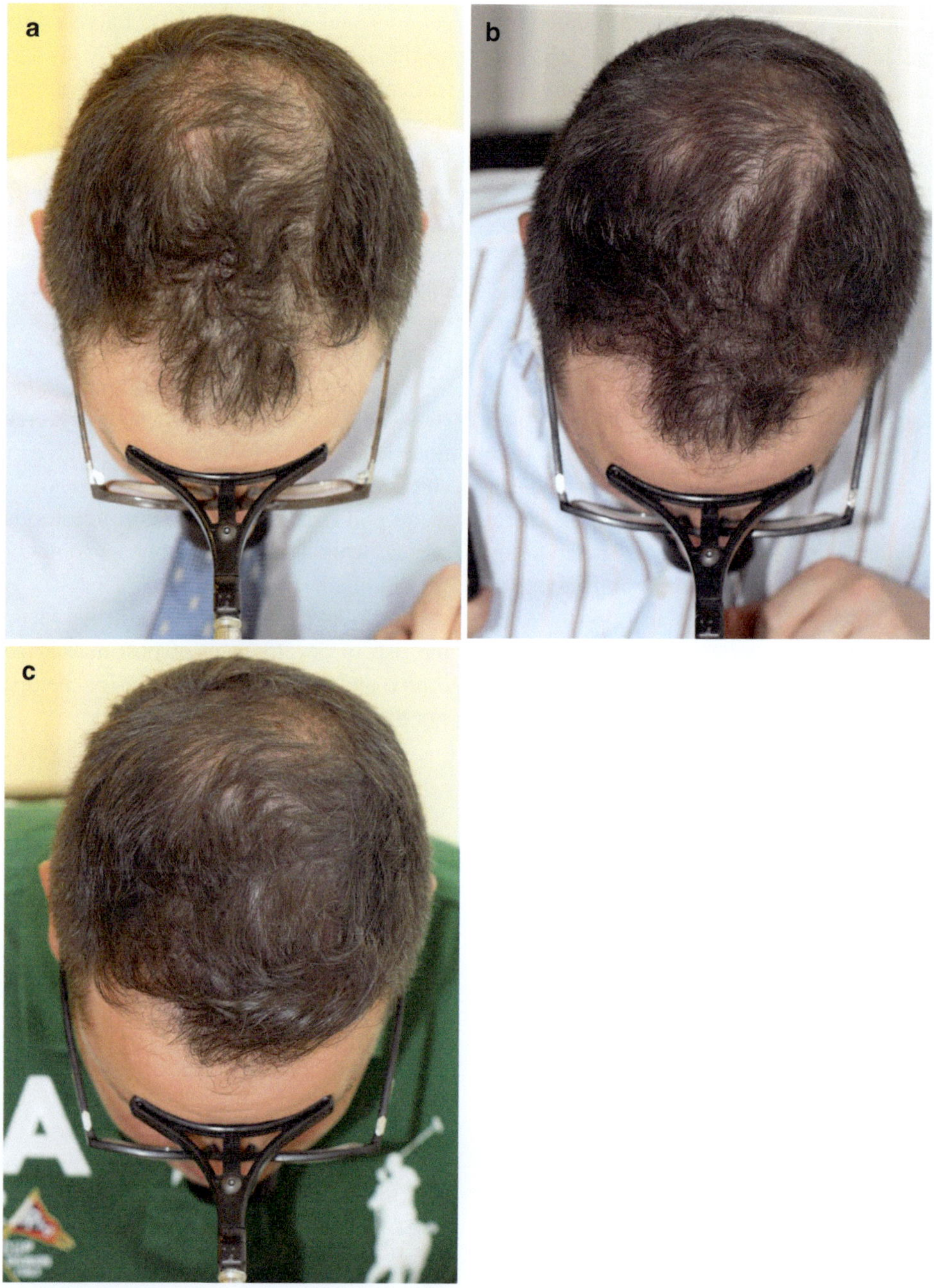

Fig. 5.2 (**a–c**) Successful switch in a 38-year-old male from (**a**, **b**) 1 mg oral finasteride, to (**c**) topical 5 % minoxidil solution bid

5.4 Cosmetic Camouflage and Hair Prosthesis

Cosmetic camouflage is the application of makeup creams and/or powders to conceal irregularities or abnormalities of the body surface. It offers an option to solve problems of congenital, traumatic, or dermatologic origin. Furthermore, cosmetic camouflage may help alleviate the psychological problems potentially related to a skin imperfection. A number of products are available on the market for hair loss camouflage (Fig. 5.3a, b), ranging from fibers (Toppik®, Hair Magic®, Nanogen Nanofibers®), sprays (Mane®, ProThik®, Fullmore®, X-tra Hair®), and creams (Couvre®), to powder cakes (Derm Match®).

Van der Velden et al. performed a 10-year study to assess the usefulness of the treatment of eyebrows loss due to alopecia areata with dermatography as a relatively quick and simple method to obtain a cosmetically satisfactory result (Fig. 5.4). For this purpose the eyebrow areas were covered with a halftone pattern of tiny dots of color pigments, using a Van der Velden Derma-injector, without anesthesia. On average, two to three dermatography sessions of 1 h were required. The follow-up was 4 years. Thirty three patients, most of whom had been previously treated with topical immunotherapy, were treated in this way. Four patients had also been treated by a beautician with a crude form of tattooing. The results in 30 patients were excellent. In three patients the results were good. The authors concluded that the technique offered a good alternative for time-consuming, troublesome treatment modalities that have potential adverse effects, while with dermatography no side effects were found. A reservation to be made is that the makeup look seems less suitable for male than for female patients.

A hair or cranial prosthesis is a custom-made wig specifically designed for patients who have lost their hair as a result of medical conditions or treatments, such as alopecia totalis, trichotillomania, chemotherapy, or any other

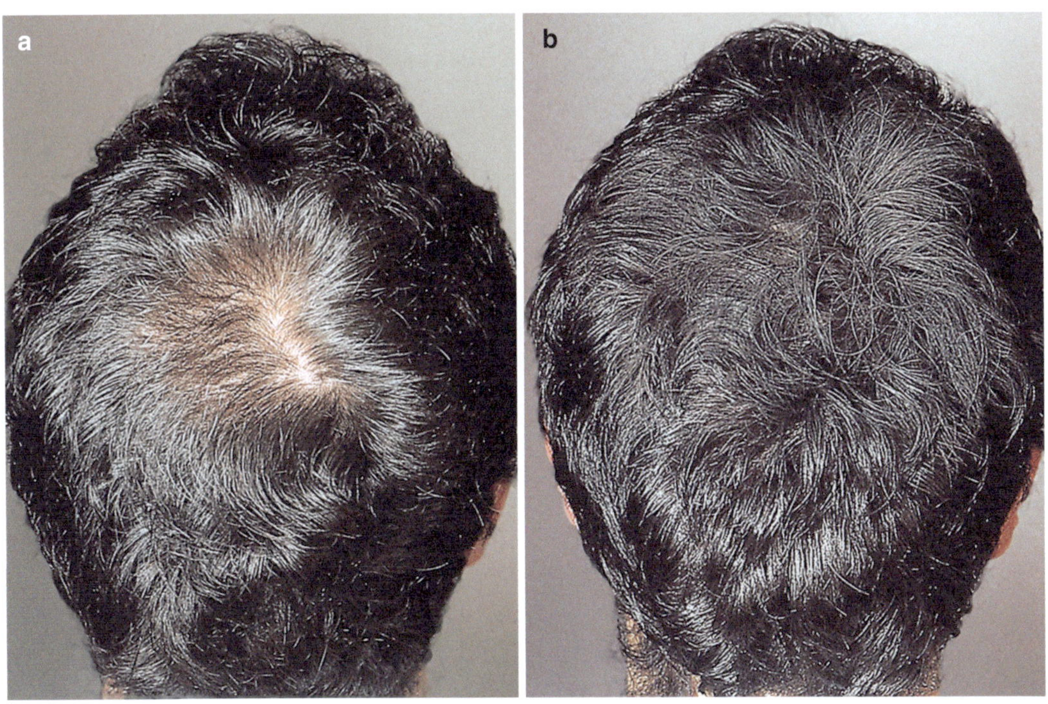

Fig. 5.3 (**a**, **b**) Cosmetic camouflage (spray) of vertex alopecia

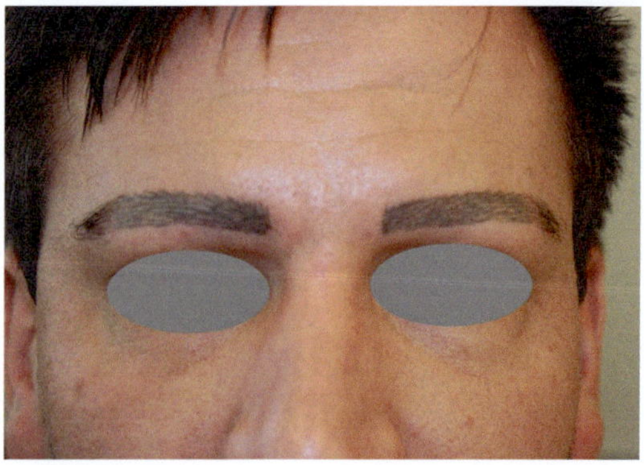

Fig. 5.4 Dermatography (permanent makeup) of eyebrows in alopecia areata

clinical disease or treatment resulting in hair loss. The terminology is used when applying for medical insurance or tax deduction status. Physicians have been prescribing these prostheses since the 1950s. Cranial prostheses do not only have the purpose to disguise hair loss but also help to protect the unprotected scalp from the sun and to regulate body temperature. Many of the manufacturers today are designing excellent high quality wigs that provide comfortable caps, high quality synthetic fibers, durable human hair, and special materials to achieve a secure fit. Many of these products will be extremely light weight and have a very natural appearance. While wigs covers the whole head, hair pieces and hair integrations intend to complement the proper hair.

Little research has be done and published on the psychosocial effect of the various methods of hair-loss management: all existing studies pertain to the pharmacologic treatments, and none has evaluated hair transplantation or nonsurgical methods, such as hair loss camouflage or hair additions.

Further Reading

Evidence-Based Medicine

Rawson E (1982) The life and death of asclepiades of bithynia. Class Q 32:358–370

www.wikipedia.org/wiki/Evidence-based_medicine

Listening to the Patient

Cash TF (1992) The psychological effects of androgenetic alopecia in men. J Am Acad Dermatol 26:926–931

Cash TF (1999) The psychosocial consequences of androgenetic alopecia: a review of the research literature. Br J Dermatol 141:398–405

Maffei C, Fossati A, Rinaldi F, Riva E (1994) Personality disorders and psychopathologic symptoms in patients with androgenetic alopecia. Arch Dermatol 130:868–872

Neumann M, Scheffer C, Tauschel D, Lutz G, Wirtz M, Edelhäuser F (2012) Physician empathy: definition, outcome-relevance and its measurement in patient care and medical education. GMS Z Med Ausbild 29:Doc11

Teutsch C (2003) Patient-doctor communication. Med Clin North Am 87:1115–1145

Yamazaki M, Miyakura T, Uchiyama M, Hobo A, Irisawa R, Tsuboi R (2011) Oral finasteride improved the quality of life of androgenetic alopecia patients. J Dermatol 38:773–777

Tackling Side Effects

Altomare G, Capella GL (2002) Depression circumstantially related to the administration of finasteride for androgenetic alopecia. J Dermatol 29:665–669

Baibergenova A, Walsh S (2012) Use of pioglitazone in patients with lichen planopilaris. J Cutan Med Surg 16:97–100

Finn DA, Long SL, Tanchuck MA, Crabbe J (2004) Interaction of chronic ethanol exposure and finasteride: sex and strain differences. Pharmacol Biochem Behav 78:435–443

Georgala S, Befon A, Maniatopoulou E, Georgala C (2007) Topical use of minoxidil in children and systemic side effects. Dermatology 214:101–102

Glina S, Neves PA, Saade R, Netto NR Jr, Soares JB, Galuppo AG (2004) Finasteride-associated male infertility. Rev Hosp Clin Fac Med Sao Paulo 59: 203–205

Gorin RE, Crabbe JC, Tanchuck MA, Long SL, Finn DA (2005) Effects of finasteride on chronic and acute ethanol withdrawal severity in the WSP and WSR selected lines. Alcohol Clin Exp Res 29:939–948

Hepp U, Kraemer B, Schnyder U, Miller N, Delsignore A (2005) Psychiatric comorbidity in gender identity disorder. J Psychosom Res 58:259–261

Irwig MS (2012) Depressive symptoms and suicidal thoughts among former users of finasteride with persistent sexual side effects. J Clin Psychiatry 73:1220–1223

Irwig MS (2013) Decreased alcohol consumption among former male users of finasteride with persistent sexual side effects: a preliminary report. Alcohol Clin Exp Res doi:10.1111/acer.12177. [Epub ahead of print]

Irwig MS, Kolukula S (2011) Persistent sexual side effects of finasteride for male pattern hair loss. J Sex Med 8:1747–1753
Mirmirani P, Karnik P (2009) Lichen planopilaris treated with a peroxisome proliferator-activated receptor gamma agonist. Arch Dermatol 145:1363–1366
Morrow J (1999) New profits in old bottles; companies find bonus in drugs that cure several ills. The New York Times, 19 March
Overstreet JW, Fuh VL, Gould J, Howards SS, Lieber MM, Hellstrom W, Shapiro S, Carroll P, Corfman RS, Petrou S, Lewis R, Toth P, Shown T, Roy J, Jarow JP, Bonilla J, Jacobsen CA, Wang DZ, Kaufman KD (1999) Chronic treatment with finasteride daily does not affect spermatogenesis or semen production in young men. J Urol 162:1295–1300
Ramot Y, Czarnowicki T, Zlotogorski A (2009) Finasteride induced gynecomastia: case report and review of the Literature. Int J Trichol 1:27–29
Ricci G, Martinelli M, Luppi S, Lo Bello L, De Santis M, Skerk K, Zito G (2012) Finasteride and fertility: case report and review of the literature. J Drugs Dermatol 11:1511–1513
Rossi A, Cantisani C, Scarnò M, Trucchia A, Fortuna MC, Calvieri S (2011) Finasteride, 1 mg daily administration on male androgenetic alopecia in different age groups: 10-year follow-up. Dermatol Ther 24:455–461
Sandomir R (2006) Skin deep; fighting baldness, and now an olympic ban. The New York Times, 19 January
Sato A, Takeda A (2012) Evaluation of efficacy and safety of finasteride 1 mg in 3177 Japanese men with androgenetic alopecia. J Dermatol 39:27–32
Thompson IM, Goodman PJ, Tangen CM, Lucia MS, Miller GJ, Ford LG, Lieber MM, Cespedes RD, Atkins JN, Lippman SM, Carlin SM, Ryan A, Szczepanek CM, Crowley JJ, Coltman CA Jr (2003) The influence of finasteride on the development of prostate cancer. N Engl J Med 349:215–224
Thompson IM Jr, Goodman PJ, Tangen CM, Parnes HL, Minasian LM, Godley PA, Lucia MS, Ford LG (2013) Long-term survival of participants in the prostate cancer prevention trial. N Engl J Med 369:603–610
Traish AM, Hassani J, Guay AT, Zitzmann M, Hansen ML (2011) Adverse side effects of 5α-reductase inhibitors therapy: persistent diminished libido and erectile dysfunction and depression in a subset of patients. J Sex Med 8:872–884

Tackling Side Effects: Nocebo Effect

Kennedy WP (1961) The nocebo reaction. Med World 95:203–205
Mondaini N, Gontero P, Giubilei G, Lombardi G, Cai T, Gavazzi A, Bartoletti R (2007) Finasteride 5 mg and sexual side effects: how many of these are related to a nocebo phenomenon? J Sex Med 4:1708–1712

Tackling Side Effects: Post-finasteride Syndrome

Irwig MS (2012) Persistent sexual side effects of finasteride: could they be permanent? J Sex Med 9: 2927–2932
LeFevre M (2013) A role for finasteride in the prevention of prostate cancer? N Engl J Med 369:670–671
www.pfsfoundation.org
www.propeciahelp.com

Cosmetic Camouflage and Hair Prosthesis

Delamere FM, Sladden MM, Dobbins HM, Leonardi-Bee J (2008) Interventions for alopecia areata. Cochrane Database Syst Rev (2):CD004413
Draelos ZD (2013) Shampoos, conditioners, and camouflage techniques. Dermatol Clin 31:173–178
Vandegrift KV (1994) The development of an oncology alopecia wig program. J Intraven Nurs 17:78–82
van der Velden EM et al (1998) Dermatography as a new treatment for alopecia areata of the eyebrows. Int J Dermatol 37:617–621

Hair Care and Cosmetics 6

My hair was slicked down with a part.
But that was before I discovered the blow-dryer.
Now I'm fabulous.

Barry Manilow (1943–)

Hair care, color, and style play an important role in people's physical appearance and self-perception. Hair defines an individual's gender, age, sexual attitude, and social status. There are no significant differences in the number of hair follicles between men and women or between different races. Differences in the appearance of hair are due to the type of hair produced by the follicle and to the type of hair care and cosmetics practiced by the individual.

Healthy hair is usually perceived to be shiny with a smooth texture and clean-cut end or tapered tips. Hair texture and shine relate to hair surface properties, while the integrity of hair ends relates to the hair cortex.

Hair consists of an outer hydrophobic lipid epicuticle, a layer of flattened overlapping cuticle cells surrounding the elongated polyhedral cortical cells. The cortical cells surround an optional and often discontinuous central medulla. The surface of the hair is covered in a covalently bound, monomolecular layer of a unique, branched, fatty acid, 18-methyl eicosanoic acid (18-MEA) or the f-layer. The intact cuticle has a smooth appearance, allowing light reflection and limiting friction between the hair shafts. It is responsible for the luster and smoothness of hair. Finally, the cortex consists of closely packed spindle-shaped cortical cells filled with keratin filaments that are oriented parallel to the longitudinal axis of the hair shaft and an amorphous matrix of high sulfur proteins. The keratin chains have a large number of sulfur-containing cysteine residues, which form covalent disulfide bonds in adjacent keratin filaments. The disulfide bonds contribute to the shape, stability, and texture of the hair.

The condition of the hair fiber is dependent on hereditary and ethnic factors, age and sex, nutritional and overall health status, condition of the scalp, hair length, hair care and styling habits, and external factors and hair damage including those from cosmetic hair treatments.

Manipulation of the normal hair structure is dictated by culture, and although cosmetic procedures are inherently aimed to be safe, there remains a potential for damage to the hair shaft.

For permanent changes to the color or style of hair, the chemical reaction of coloring, perming, or straightening must occur in the cortex. The f-layer is removed from the surface with any chemical procedure, and the internal disulfide bonds of the cortex are broken in hair styling and permanent waves.

Loss of luster, frizz, split ends, and other hair problems are particularly prevalent among subjects who repeatedly alter the natural state of their hair.

While medicinal treatments of hair aim at specific problems relating to the superficial condition of the scalp, such as dandruff, itchiness, and hair loss, cosmetic hair treatments aim at cleansing the hair, conditioning hair, styling hair, changing hair color, and perming hair. Table 6.1 lists the main types of hair cosmetics.

In the study on the significance of scalp hair and treatment of hair loss in Swiss men performed by Trüeb et al. in 2001, the results of the questionnaire on hair care products used are reproduced in Fig. 6.1.

R.M. Trüeb, W.-S. Lee, *Male Alopecia*,
DOI 10.1007/978-3-319-03233-7_6,

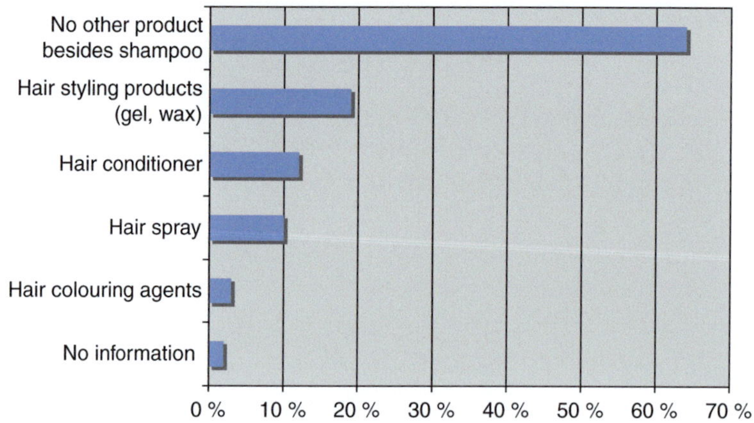

Fig. 6.1 Hair care products used by men in Switzerland on a regular basis (From: Trüeb RM, de Viragh PA, and Swiss Trichology Study Group (2001) Significance of scalp hair and therapy of alopecia in men in Switzerland. Praxis (Bern 1994) 90:241–248)

Table 6.1 Hair cosmetics

Hair shampoos: to remove sebum and environmental dirt without decreasing cosmetic appearance of hair
Hair conditioners: to improve hair manageability, decrease hair static electricity, add luster, and enhance styling ease
Hair styling aids: to maintain hair in a fashionable arrangement while improving the quality of hair fibers
Hair dyes: to lighten or darken hair color while covering gray hair
Permanent hair waving/straightening: to reposition hair keratin disulfide bonds in a new curly or straight position

6.1 Hair Weathering

Hair weathering is the progressive hair damage resulting from external factors, basically the "wear and tear" from environment and cosmetic procedures that mainly affect the free end of the growing hair fiber: friction damage from combing and brushing, damage from excessive heat "blown" or from curling irons; structural and chemical damage from chemical treatment of hair, i.e., bleaching, coloring, perming, and straightening; and finally effects of ultraviolet radiation or photoaging.

Hair is porous, and damaged hair is increasingly so. Water absorption causes hair shaft swelling. Wet hair has higher combing friction than dry hair; therefore, combing wet hair is more likely to stretch brittle hair to the point of breaking. When wet, hair can be stretched by 30 % of its original length without damage. Irreversible changes occur when hair is stretched between 30 and 70 %, ultimately, stretching to 80 % causes fracturing.

Although all hair exhibits some degree of weathering, longer hair, subjected to repeated insults, inevitably shows more severe changes of weathering.

Negroid hair has a larger diameter, lower water content, and flattened elliptical cross section. It is usually black or dark brown, tightly curled, low in shine, and high in sebum. It has increased grooming friction, which combined with low tensile strength makes it more difficult to manage.

Features of hair weathering include damaged cuticles (Fig. 6.2a), longitudinal fissures or split ends (trichoptilosis, Fig. 6.2b), and transverse fissures (trichorrhexis nodosa, Fig. 6.2c). These result from alterations in the ultrastructure and physical and chemical properties of the hair fiber, i.e., mechanical abrasion of the cuticle, damage of the hair cortex with alterations of viscoelastic properties and tensile strength of the hair fiber, and a depletion of specific amino acids: methionine (by minus 50 %), tryptophan (−50 %), cystine (−20 %), histidine (−20 %), tyrosine (−15 %), and lysine (−10 %). Scrutinizing very long hair (length > 2.4 m) that has undergone little or no aggression from chemical agents such as bleaching or dyeing from the root to the tip, Thibaut et al. from L'OREAL Recherche, Clichy, France demonstrated the deterioration process, which gradually takes place from the outside to the inside of the hair shaft: first, a progressive abrasion of the cuticle, while the cortex structure remains unaltered, is evidenced along a length of roughly 1 m onwards together with constant shine, hydrophobicity, and friction characteristics. Further, along the fiber, a significant damage to

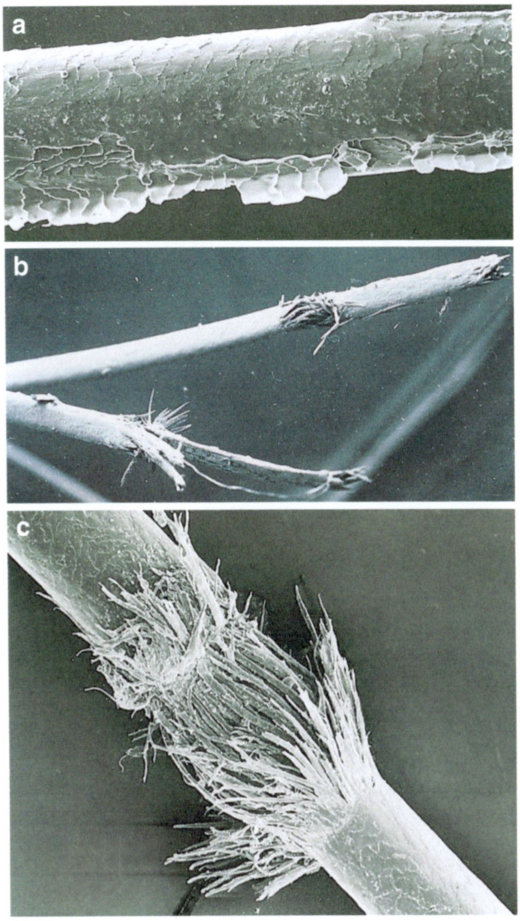

Fig. 6.2 (**a**–**c**) Hair weathering. (**a**) Damaged cuticles. (**b**) Split ends (trichoptilosis). (**c**) Transverse breakage (trichorrhexis nodosa)

cuticle scales occurs, which correlated well with ceramides and 18-MEA decline and progressive decrease in keratin-associated protein content.

Finally, hair may be intrinsically weak in the less common inherited abnormalities in hair fiber formation. Hofbauer et al. originally described acquired hair fragility in pili annulati with a causal relationship with androgenetic alopecia. Pili annulati are defined by characteristic alternating light and dark banding in the hair shaft, due to air-filled spaces between the macrofibrillar units of the hair cortex, and are regarded as a congenital hair shaft disorder without increased hair fragility. In the presented cases of pili annulati, fragility of hair developed with the onset of androgenetic alopecia. Accordingly, trichorrhexis-nodosa-like hair fracturing was limited to the androgenetic region. With the onset of hair thinning due to androgenetic alopecia, progressive reduction of hair shaft diameter may cause increased fragility in pili annulati. In this case, hair shaft fracturing occurs within the area of androgenetic alopecia and colocalizes with the air-filled cavities of pili annulati.

As a general rule, trichorrhexis nodosa is an unspecific finding related to excess stress of hair in relation to its fragility.

For treatment, hair care products that improve the structural integrity of damaged hair fibers and increase tensile strength are available, as are products that increase hair volume, reduce frizz, and improve overall hair manageability.

6.2 Shampoos

Shampoo treatments are the most commonly used means of managing hair and scalp conditions. Until the introduction of the first non-alkaline shampoos in 1933, soap was the only available cleanser for the hair.

Today shampoos are expected to be more than mere cleansing agents.

They are expected to not dry out the hair, to produce lather in hard and soft water and when applied to oily hair, to be nonirritating to skin and mucous membranes, to be chemically and physically stable, to possess conditioning benefits, and to be biodegradable and affordable. A shampoo is expected to improve the hair cosmetically while being tailored to the needs of various hair types as well as age and individual habits. Scalp condition is another important factor in individual health and well-being; the scalp should neither be oily nor should dandruff develop.

Accordingly, shampoos have evolved into high-tech products consisting of 10–30 ingredients that are combined in precise formulations to meet consumer demands (Fig. 6.3, Table 6.2).

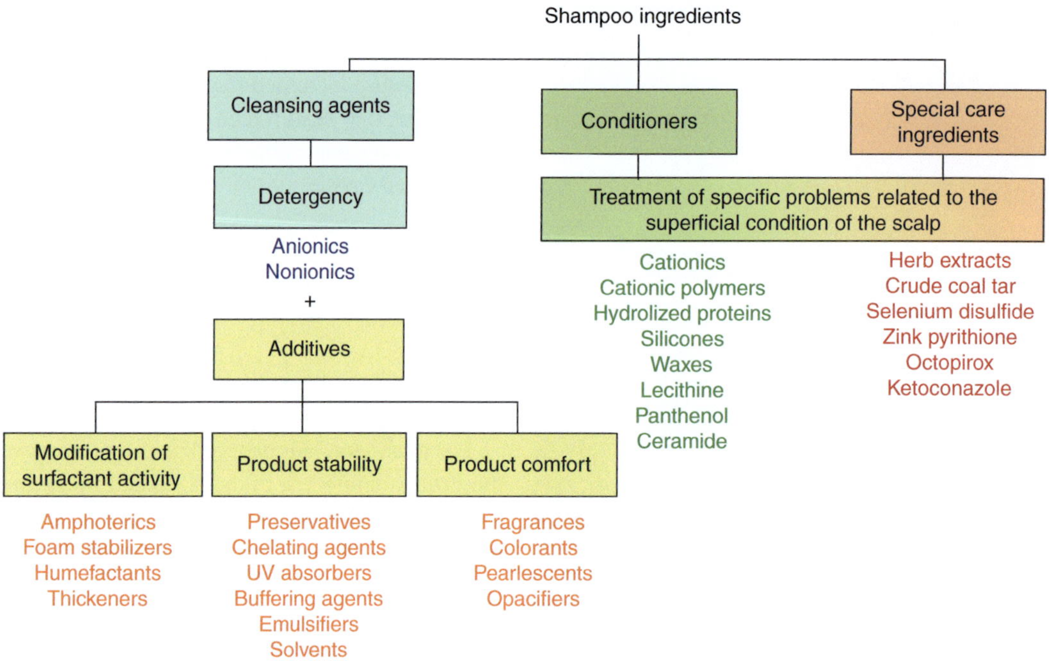

Fig. 6.3 Shampoo ingredients

Table 6.2 Shampoo ingredients and effects on hair and scalp condition

Shampoo ingredients include:
Detergents, i.e., surfactants
Conditioning and active ingredients for hair manageability
Additives that
Modify the surfactant effect (viscosity control agents, foam stabilizers)
Stabilize the product (preservatives)
Increase its appeal (fragrances, dyes, ingredients for consistency and pearlescent appearance)
The most important effects of shampoo on the hair are:
Moisturizing
Adsorption and/or penetration of the hair
Cleansing, removal of oils, lipid regeneration
The following effects of shampoo influence scalp condition:
Restoration of alkali neutralization ability (pH)
Dryness
Seborrhea
Scalp microbial flora (*Malassezia* spp., *Propionibacterium* spp.)
Enzyme activity of the scalp
Scalp circulation

6.2.1 Shampoo Surfactants

The cleansing ability of a shampoo depends on the surface activity of its detergents. Surface-active ingredients, or surfactants, facilitate the removal of environmental dirt by reducing surface tension between water and dirt; dirt is suspended in the water phase and adsorption prevented. This is achieved by a special molecular structure consisting of a hydrophilic and a lipophilic group. Sebum and dirt are bound and surrounded at the center of a micelle structure with the hydrophilic molecule ends pointing outward. Dirt particles become water soluble and can be removed from the hair shaft.

> The cleansing ability of a shampoo depends on how well it removes grease as well as the type and amount of surfactants used.

Surfactants are classified according to hydrophilic polar group as anionic, cationic, amphoteric (zwitterionic), and nonionic. Various surfactants are used in shampoos in order to accommodate different hair types. In most products, the shampoo base consists of anionic and amphoteric surfactants. Depending on individual product requirements, non-ionic and cationic surfactants are added to modify the effects of the surfactants or as conditioning agents for hair with surface damage.

Anionic surfactants are characterized by a negatively charged hydrophilic polar group. Well into the twentieth century, natural soaps were the most commonly used anionic hair cleansing substances. Soap consists of salts that are extracted from naturally occurring animal or vegetable fatty acids. Synthetic surfactants have now replaced soap as a hair cleanser. Because soap is sensitive to hard water, it leaves insoluble salts on the hair, forming a film which causes a dull look. Soap's alkaline pH can make it irritating to the skin and mucous membranes. The first shampoos introduced on the market in 1933 were alkyl sulfate surfactants. These were still sensitive to hard water and were not adequately tolerated by the skin. They have since been replaced by sodium alkyl ether sulfates which are now the leading surfactants. These are superior with regard to sensitivity to water hardness as well as skin and mucous membrane tolerability and are virtually the only surfactants that can also be used alone in a shampoo as raw ingredients. The best known anionic surfactants are sulfated fatty alcohols, alkyl sulfates, and their polyethoxylated analogues, alkyl ether sulfates. They possess an outstanding cleansing ability and produce rich lather. A number of anionic surfactants, such as alkyl ether carboxylate, acyl peptides, alkyl sulfosuccinate, and olefin sulfonate, which are well tolerated by the skin, are used together with other anionic and amphoteric surfactants to optimize shampoo properties.

Amphoteric (zwitterionic) surfactants contain both negatively and positively charged hydrophilic polar groups. At low pH values they behave as cationic agents and at higher pH values as anionic agents and are thus classified between cationic and anionic surfactants. Amphoteric surfactants form complexes with anionic surfactants and reduce their tendency to attach to proteins. In combination with anionic surfactants, amphoteric surfactants are mainly used to optimize anionic-based shampoos: amphoteric acetates/diacetates in particular demonstrate excellent skin and mucous membrane tolerability, have a conditioning benefit on the hair, and are suitable for use in mild shampoos. Examples include betaine, sulfonate betaine, and amphoteric acetate/diacetate.

Nonionic surfactants differ from other surfactants in that they do not possess a charged polar group and are hence compatible with all other surfactants. They are also among the mildest form of surfactant; they make good cleansers with dispersion and emulsification properties, but lather poorly. In combination with alkyl ether sulfates or amphoteric surfactants, they serve to enhance tolerability in very mild cleansers such as baby shampoos. Examples of nonionic surfactants are fatty alcohol ethoxylates, sorbitan ether esters, and alkyl polyglucosides.

Cationic surfactants are quaternary ammonium compounds which are characterized by a positively charged hydrophilic polar group. Given its amino acid structure, the keratin found in human hair has an excess of negatively charged acid groups. The positively charged quaternary ammonium compounds of cationic surfactants thus attach by salt bonds to the negatively charged hair and remain after rinsing. Due to its high level of cysteine, damaged hair contains a higher number of negatively charged acid groups and thus absorbs more quaternary ammonium compounds than intact hair.

> Because of this quality, quaternary ammonium compounds (quats) are used as conditioning agents in shampoos for damaged hair.

Although they make hair easier to comb and manage, and they have antistatic properties, they are poor cleansers and do not lather well. They are also potentially strong irritants and are thus

Table 6.3 Shampoo surfactants

Surfactant type (polar group charge)	Chemical class/examples	Characteristics	Purpose
Anionics (negative)	Lauryl sulfates, laureth sulfates, sarcosines, sulfosuccinates	Deep cleansing, may leave hair harsh	Cleansing
Cationics (positive)	Long-chain amino esters, ammonioesters	Poor cleansing, poor lather, impart softness and manageability	Conditioning
Amphoterics (both)	Betaines, sultaines, imidazolinium derivatives	Nonirritating to eyes, mild cleansing, impart manageability	Additive for modification of surfactant activity
Nonionics (none)	Polyoxyethylene fatty alcohols, polyoxyethylene sorbitol esters, alkanolamides	Mildest cleansing, impart manageability	Cleansing

only used with less irritating nonionic surfactants in shampoos designed for chemically treated or very dry hair. Their incompatibility with anionic surfactants limits their use in other shampoo formulations.

Table 6.3 lists the surfactant types according to their polar group charge, chemical classes and examples, their characteristics, and purposes in a shampoo formulation.

6.2.2 Shampoo Additives

Shampoo products are also expected to possess stability and to have an appealing quality, making the use of a number of additives necessary.

In addition to selection and combination of surfactants, additives also help reduce skin irritation. Moisturizers and humectants are added to make the hair silkier:

- Moisturizers include natural oils, fatty acid esters, and alkanolamides.
- Humectants include propylene glycol, polyethylene glycol, glycerin, sorbitol, and lactate.

Ensuring shampoo stability requires:

- Use of preservatives to protect against bacterial contamination: organic acids and their derivatives, e.g., para-hydroxybenzoic acid ester, salicylic and sorbic acid, and methylparaben, formaldehyde releasers, e.g., DMDM hydantoin
- UV absorbers to stabilize dyes against light: benzophenone derivatives
- Antioxidants to protect oxidation-sensitive substances: ascorbic acid, α-tocopherol, and butyl hydroxyanisole
- Buffers to ensure pH stability: citrate, lactate, and phosphate buffers
- Co-solvents to keep conditioning oils and fragrances clear in solution
- Dispersing agents to keep otherwise insoluble agents, such as silicone oils and anti-dandruff agents, in suspension: polyvinylpyrrolidone.

Last, but not least, attractiveness of a shampoo is enhanced by fragrances, dyes, and special ingredients that give it a pearlescent appearance:

- Fragrance oils cover up the typically fatty odor of the shampoo base and lend the product an individual and pleasant-smelling scent. An appealing fragrance also helps promote regular use of the product.
- Dyes and liquid crystal concentrates give the shampoo a pearlescent and more "concentrated" appearance. Liquid crystal concentrates also contribute to its moisturizing effect. They usually consist of insoluble crystal particles made up of fatty acid esters of polyols and alkanolamide derivatives of fatty acids that reflect light.

6.2.3 Shampoo Conditioning Agents

Depending on hair length and exogenous factors, the distal end of the continually growing hair shaft exhibits increasing signs of damage (hair weathering).

> The aim of conditioning agents in a shampoo is to maintain the natural condition of newly grown hairs for as long as possible.

Virtually, all standard shampoos used today contain conditioning agents. Damaged hair can, of course, not be restored to the condition of healthy, newly growing hair and more than a reparative effect cannot be expected. Nonetheless, it is possible to increase shine and make hair more manageable and easier to comb by using a shampoo with a high proportion of conditioning agents, i.e., the *conditioner effect*.

Conditioning agents include fatty substances such as vegetable oils, wax, lecithin and lanolin derivatives, protein hydrolysates (collagen, silk, animal proteins), quaternary ammonium compound, and silicones.

There is an increasing use of cationic polymers (polyquaternium) in place of monomer quaternary ammonium compounds, in which the cationic groups are integrated in a polymer structure, e.g., polyquaternium-10 and polyquaternium-16 as well as guar hydroxypropyltrimonium chloride. These adhere more firmly to the hair than monomer bonds and leave a film that coats the surface of the hair fiber, making it appear to be soft and smooth while improving shine and color by altering the refractive index. In addition to their use in conditioners, these cationic polymer finishing agents have become a main component of *2-in-1 shampoos* which combine cleansing and conditioning actions. The amount used must correspond to the condition of the hair since these agents have a high affinity for the hair and with repeated use can build up on the hair shaft.

> Excessive conditioning can make hair less manageable and appear oily.

In addition to cationic polymer finishing agents, silicones are also used, especially dimethicone, which is added along with special dispersing agents to a shampoo base containing a relatively high proportion of surfactants. The strong conditioning effect occurs as a result of extremely fine dimethicone droplets being deposited on the hair as the shampoo is diluted during washing.

> Silicones have a similar effect to that of fats and oils, but without weighing the hair down. Silicones add lubricity and reduce friction that arises from combing, making the hair easier to comb and style and thus also preventing damage. They also give the hair antistatic properties that prevent it from becoming frizzy.

Table 6.4 lists the hair conditioner categories with their primary ingredients, main advantages, and hair grooming benefits.

6.2.4 Shampoo Active Ingredients

Active ingredients are added to shampoos for the management of specific problems affecting the scalp such as seborrhea, itchy or burning scalp, dandruff, seborrheic dermatitis, and psoriasis. The spectrum of active shampoo ingredients is broad and varied, from clinically proven, primarily anti-dandruff agents, to traditionally used substances derived from natural sources, e.g., herbal extracts (Table 6.5).

Ingredients for Managing Scalp Seborrhea. A greasy scalp is a frequent condition, both causing cosmetic embarrassment and a disposition to pathologic conditions such as seborrheic dermatitis and scalp folliculitis. The condition sets in with adolescence, and its frequency declines after the age of 30 years. Oral isotretinoin treatment represents the most effective treatment of seborrhea.

> A significant improvement in seborrhea generally cannot be achieved with over-the-counter shampoos.

Coal tar (*Liquor carbonis detergens*), which reduces sebum production, is virtually the only effective active ingredient in medicated shampoos. Ammonium bituminosulfonate (ichthammol) is comparatively ineffective. To maintain volume, the surface of the hair must be prevented from becoming too smooth, and to avoid lipolytic or peroxidative transformation of scalp or hair lipids, antimicrobial substances are used. This is

Table 6.4 Hair conditioning agents

Hair conditioner category	Primary ingredient	Main advantage	Hair grooming benefit
Fatty ingredients	Fatty alcohols, lanolin derivatives, oils, waxes, lecithins	Increase hair shine, increase hair manageability	Improve appearance of dry hair
Cationic detergents and film formers	Quaternary ammonium compounds (quats)	Smooth cuticle, decrease static electricity	Excellent to restore damaged, chemically processed hair
	Polymers (polyquaternium)	Fill hair shaft defects, decrease static electricity, improve shine	Improve appearance of dry hair, improve grooming of coarse, kinky hair
Protein-containing	Hydrolyzed proteins (keratin, collagen, silk, wheat, soya)	Penetrate hair shaft to minimally increase strength	Temporarily mend splits
Silicones	Dimethicone, cyclomethicone, amodimethicone	Thin coating placed on hair shaft	Decrease static electricity, decrease combing friction, add shine

Table 6.5 Herbal extracts for hair and scalp care

Plant	Botanical	Indication
Soap bark	*Quillaja saponaria*	Cleansing Antimicrobial
Willow bark	*Salix alba*	Dandruff Repellent against head lice
Coltsfoot	*Tussilago farfara*	Dandruff
Seaweed	*Fucus vesiculosus*	Seborrhea
Thyme	*Thymus vulgaris*	Seborrhea
Mallow	*Malva sylvestris*	Conditioning (thin hair)
Linden	*Tilia cordata*	Conditioning (thin hair)
Millet	*Panicum miliaceum*	Conditioning (thin hair)
Horsetail	*Equisetum arvense*	Conditioning (dry, brittle hair)
Avocado	*Persea gratissima*	Conditioning (colored hair)
Sage	*Salvia officinalis*	Conditioning (gray hair)
Chamomile	*Matricaria chamomilla*	Scalp irritation
Heartseed	*Cardiospermum halicacabum*	Scalp irritation
Witch hazel	*Hamamelis virginiana*	Scalp irritation
He Shou Wu	*Polygonum multiflorum*	Antiaging

usually achieved with a mild, generally anionic surfactant base consisting of effective cleansing substances with low substantivity. Inhibition of microbial lipolysis can also be achieved by the surfactants forming the shampoo base. Antimicrobial agents that are effective against *Malassezia* spp. are suited for use in seborrhea and dandruff.

While Piérard-Franchimont et al. have found that ketoconazole shampoo appears to decrease the sebum casual level, selenium disulfide is contraindicated in scalp seborrhea since it increases sebaceous gland excretion.

Additional conditioners, especially moisturizers and cationic polymers, should be avoided in hair that has a tendency to become oily, since they weigh it down. The use of herbal extracts containing tannin, e.g., oak bark (*Quercus* spp.) extract, can have a positive influence holding a style by roughening the surface of the hair.

Special Care Ingredients for Managing the Itchy or Burning Scalp. Special care ingredients with some degree of efficacy in treating itchiness or burning sensations of the scalp are piroctone olamine (anti-dandruff agent with antipruritic properties), menthol (antipruritic agent), polidocanol (local anesthetic agent), and plant extracts with anti-inflammatory properties, such as chamomile (*Matricaria chamomilla*), heartseed (*Cardiospermum halicacabum*), or witch hazel (*Hamamelis virginiana*).

Witch hazel is an astringent produced from the leaves and bark of the North American Witch-hazel shrub, originally used for medicinal purposes by Native Americans, who produced witch hazel extract by boiling the stems of the shrub and producing a decoction, which was used to treat inflammatory conditions. Early Puritan settlers in New England adopted this remedy from the natives. A missionary, Dr. Charles Hawes, eventually learned of the preparation's therapeutic properties and further determined that the product of the plant's twigs was even more efficacious. Hawes' process was further refined by Tomas Newton Dickinson, Sr., who is credited with starting the commercial production of witch-hazel extract in 1866 and establishing its wide use. The main constituents of the extract include tannin, gallic acid, catechins, proanthocyanidins, flavonoids (kaempferol, quercetin), essential oils (carvacrol, eugenol, hexenol), choline, and saponins. It is a strong antioxidant and astringent, which makes it useful as a natural remedy for acne, psoriasis, eczema, aftershave applications, ingrown nails, cracked or blistered skin, and for treating insect bites.

In shampoo form, witch hazel is particularly useful in the treatment of the red scalp syndrome and in preventing or soothing scalp irritation resulting from sustained use of ethanolic topical minoxidil solutions.

6.2.5 Dandruff

A study with 1,000 men reported that 18 % of respondents had mild dandruff and 4.5 % severe dandruff. In a smaller study with 500 students, 70 % reported having dandruff.

The specific anatomic features of the scalp skin, such as the large number of terminal hair follicles and the enlarged epidermal surface due to numerous hair canals, contribute to a higher rate of exfoliation. Even a healthy scalp will develop dandruff within 1 or 2 weeks, if the hair is not washed.

Pathologic dandruff results from accelerated proliferation of epidermal cells and thus increased exfoliation of variously large collections of abnormally keratinizing epidermal cells. This leads to breakdown of the normal columnar structure of the stratum corneum and increased formation of cell aggregates which determine the size of the flakes. The process results from focal inflammation of the scalp with parakeratosis which causes abnormal exfoliation and an altered light refractive index of the keratinized cell aggregates (Fig. 6.4). The clinical appearance of dandruff is determined by the size, adherence, and light refractive characteristics of the flakes. Among the factors that lead to inflamed patches on the scalp are physical/chemical stimuli, microbial colonization, and sebum production and composition.

The lipophilic yeast *Malassezia* spp. normally inhabits the scalp, making up about 45 % of its resident microflora. In patients with dandruff, it is the predominant yeast type with about 75 % and in patients with seborrheic eczema 83 %. Modern classification and nomenclature of *Malassezia* spp. is based on DNA typing. The most common types found on the scalp are *M. restricta* and *M. globosa*, the latter of which in particular has a major role in the development of dandruff given its high level of lipase activity.

Dandruff is clinically divided into the following types:

- *Simple dandruff* (Fig. 6.5a) typically occurs with dry skin as a result of atopic dermatitis or age-related dry skin. It can be caused by excessive hair cleansing or the use of a shampoo designed for oily hair. Typical findings include dry, bran-like scales, and patients often complain of itching. Most authors also cite the coexistence of overgrowth of *Malassezia* spp. in simple dandruff as evidence of its role in pathogenesis.
- *Oily dandruff* (Fig. 6.5b) is associated with seborrhea of the scalp. It often occurs with inadequate personal hygiene, and *Malassezia* spp. is widely believed to be involved in pathogenesis. Firmly adherent, oily, bran-like scales are found, often on the anterior hairline, external ear, preauricular area, and around the eyes.
- *Asbestos-like scaling* or *pityriasis amiantacea* (Fig. 6.5c) frequently occurs as an idiopathic

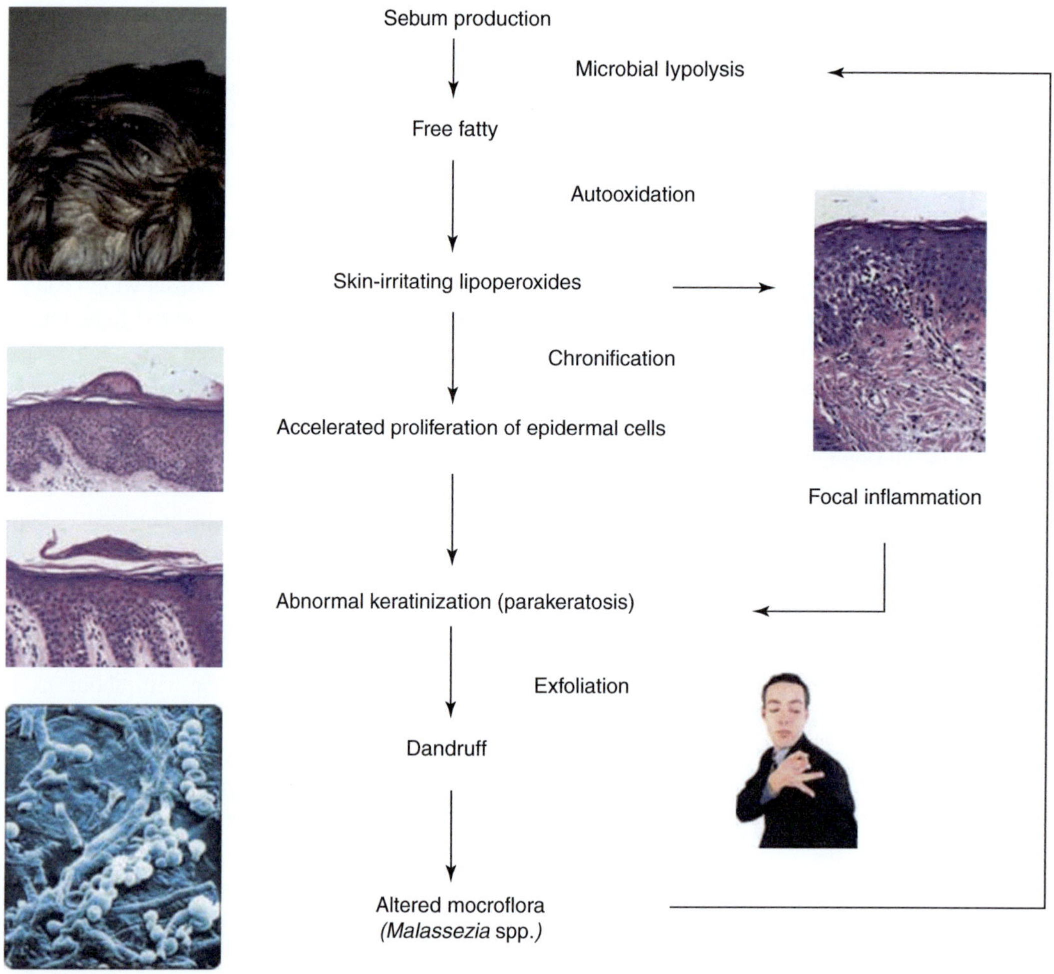

Fig. 6.4 Pathogenesis of dandruff (From: Trüeb RM (2007) Shampoos: ingredients, efficacy and adverse effects. J Dtsch Dermatol Ges 5:356–365)

disorder in girls but can also be related to lacking personal hygiene. It presents with well-circumscribed areas of thick, asbestos-like, firmly attached scales with focal hair loss and no itching. Concomitant postauricular skin cracks are typical. Underlying specific dermatologic disease such as eczema, psoriasis, tinea capitis, and – rarely – pemphigus foliaceus should be excluded.

Medicated shampoos containing anti-dandruff ingredients are essential in treating dandruff and exfoliative scalp disorders such as seborrheic eczema and psoriasis. The choice and frequency of shampooing are determined by the underlying cause, i.e., dry skin (sebostasis) or seborrhea. Patients with dry skin should be advised to wash their hair less frequently and avoid using oily hair shampoos. For oily dandruff, on the contrary, daily hair cleansing alone can lead to improvement.

Table 6.6 lists active ingredients used in the treatment of dandruff according to their mode of action.

Zinc pyrithione demonstrates a strong anti-dandruff effect with a low potential for irritation or sensitization. Clinical studies have shown it to

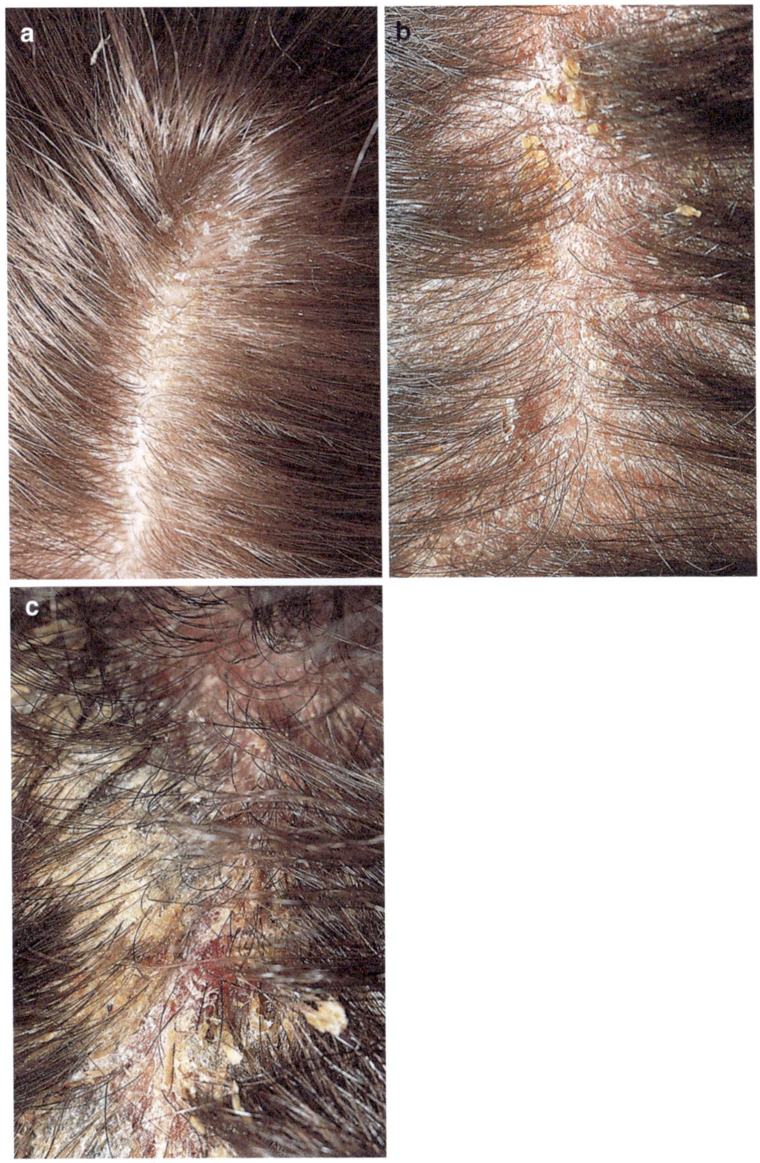

Fig. 6.5 (**a–c**) Dandruff. (**a**) Simple dandruff (pityriasis simplex). (**b**) Oily dandruff (pityriasis oleosa). (**c**) Asbestos-like scaling (pityriasis amiantacea)

be superior to coal tar, selenium disulfide, and piroctone olamine.

In one study, the effect of 2 % ketoconazole was better and longer-lasting than 1 % zinc pyrithione, but improving shampoo formulation can increase the effectiveness of anti-dandruff agents. In particular, the effectiveness of zinc pyrithione could be significantly improved with the use of micronized ingredients, especially given the legal maximum of 1 %. The zinc pyrithione molecule is present as a crystalline suspension in glycol distearate and is not water soluble. The formulation allows even distribution of zinc pyrithione crystals in shampoo and the use of nonspherical crystals measuring only 2.5 μm allows better adsorption and more even distribution on the scalp. This is particularly effective in inhibiting *Malassezia* yeasts, even with a short contact time and rinsing. The combination of zinc pyrithione with zinc carbonate leads to reduced dissociation of the active ingredients into zinc and pyrithione, which alone have a lower anti-dandruff effect.

In terms of minimal inhibitory concentrations (MIC) on *Malassezia* spp., there are considerable differences in the potency of the various anti-dandruff agents (in brackets): crude coal tar

Table 6.6 Anti-dandruff shampoo ingredients

Keratostatic agents that inhibit overproduction of keratinizing cells: coal tar and ammonium bituminosulfonate (pale sulfonated shale oil as a coal tar substitute)
Keratolytic agents that break down cell aggregations: colloidal sulfur and salicylic acid
Antimicrobial agents that inhibit *Malassezia* yeasts: selenium disulfide, zinc pyrithione, piroctone olamine, ketoconazole, and ciclopirox olamine
Combinations of these

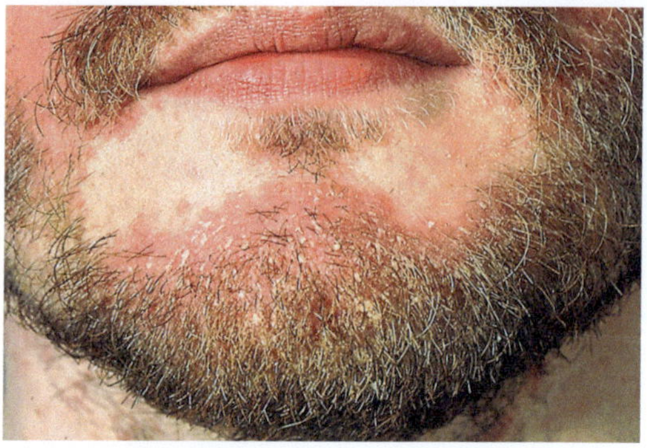

Fig. 6.6 Seborrheic dermatitis of the beard area

(MIC: 250–5,000), salicylic acid (MC: >100), selenium disulfide (MIC: 1.56–3.3), zinc pyrithione (MIC: 0.78–1.66), and ketoconazole (MIC: 0.1). Potency in terms of MIC's is important, but it is not the sole factor that determines efficacy. Other influential aspects of treatment pharmacology include delivery, retention, bioavailability, mildness, and aesthetics. Finally, dandruff must be controlled through regular treatment.

> Patients are compliant for only 30 s. Shampoos that achieve antimycosis on contact lead to a more successful management of dandruff.

6.2.6 Seborrheic Dermatitis of the Scalp

Seborrheic dermatitis represents a chronic recurrent condition characterized by scaling and poorly defined erythematous patches with a predilection for areas rich in sebaceous glands. The scalp is almost invariably affected; other areas of skin involved (in order of frequency) are the face, chest, and intertriginous areas. On the scalp, lesions may vary from fine white scales (dandruff) to yellow, greasy scales with erythema of the underlying scalp. On the face, the condition mainly affects the medial aspects of the eyebrows, the glabella, the nasolabial fold, and in men, the hair-bearing areas, such as the beard (Fig. 6.6), moustache, or sideburns. Seborrheic blepharoconjunctivitis may occur, as well as seborrheic dermatitis of the external auditory meatus, either in isolation or in association with skin or scalp lesions. Occasionally, marginated lesions may occur on the male external genital and present as a puzzling persistent penile plaque. Itching is usually limited to the scalp and the external auditory meatus, where it can be particularly annoying.

Seborrheic dermatitis is a common disorder that may also occur in association with other health conditions, particularly HIV infection with CD4 counts below 400 cells per cubic millimeter, parkinsonism, and trisomy 21. It has been reported to be triggered by stress, with a stress responder rate of 41 %.

The differential diagnosis may have to consider scalp psoriasis, atopic dermatitis *of the head and neck type* (with specific IgE antibodies to *Malassezia* spp.), tinea capitis in children, and actinic field cancerization of the scalp in the elderly, or rare conditions, such as dermatomyositis, and Langerhans cell histiocytosis (Fig. 6.7a, b).

> A lesional biopsy is rarely needed for diagnosis of seborrheic dermatitis, but it may be useful in the occasional refractory case to rule out other diagnoses.

The cause of seborrheic dermatitis is understood to be analogous to the pathogenesis of dandruff: again, fungi of the genus *Malassezia* have been implicated as being pathogenic, since they are present on affected skin, and antifungal agents are useful in treatment. The inflammatory

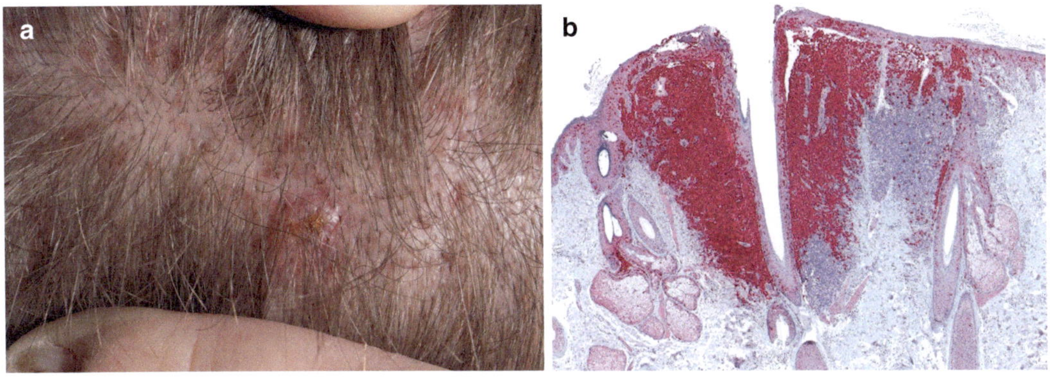

Fig. 6.7 (**a**) Langerhans cell histiocytosis of scalp mimicking seborrheic dermatitis (**b**) CD1a positive stain

process is believed to be mediated by fungal metabolites, specifically free fatty acids released from sebaceous triglycerides.

Accordingly, antifungal agents are the mainstay of treatment of seborrheic dermatitis, with a number of well-performed studies proving superiority of ketoconazole and ciclopirox olamine shampoo over placebo for treatment of seborrheic dermatitis of the scalp. In contrast, data on the efficacy of systemic antifungal agents for seborrheic dermatitis are limited. While no major side effects have been reported with the topical antifungal agents, with the exception of the rare event of contact sensitivity with long-term use, the safety profile of systemic antifungal agents must be weighed-out for treatment of a chronic condition such as seborrheic dermatitis.

With respect to the use of topical corticosteroids for treatment of seborrheic dermatitis, either as lotion, cream, or foam, there is a consensus that they are useful in the short term, mainly to control erythema und itching. No data are available regarding the question whether the combination of topical antifungal agents with topical corticosteroid results in a greater benefit than single-agent therapy.

A typically successful therapy for seborrheic dermatitis of the scalp would be using a 2 % ketoconazole or a 1.5 % ciclopirox olamine shampoo every other day during the first 2 weeks and thereafter twice weekly, depending on severity, either as monotherapy or in the more severe cases in combination with systemic itraconazole 200 mg daily during the first 7 days of treatment, and topical clobetasol propionate 0.05 % foam as needed.

Hair shedding has been reported to be affected by dandruff and seborrheic dermatitis, and sometimes patients blame their anti-dandruff shampoos to cause hair shedding. To study the effect of anti-dandruff shampoos on hair shedding, Piérard-Franchimont et al. examined 150 men presenting with telogen effluvium related to androgenetic alopecia and associated with the complaint of dandruff. They were randomly allocated to three groups receiving each one of three shampoos containing either 1 % ketoconazole (KTZ), 1 % piroctone olamine (PTO), or 1 % zinc pyrithione (ZPT). Shampoos were used 2–3 times a week for a duration of 6 months. Hair shedding during shampoo was evaluated semiquantitatively, hair density on the vertex was evaluated on photographs, and trichograms were used to determine the anagen hair percentage. The three treatments cleared pruritus and dandruff rapidly. At end point, hair density was unchanged, although hair shedding was decreased (KTZ: −17.3 %, PTO: −16.5 %, ZPT: −10.1 %), and the anagen hair percentage was increased (KTZ: 4.9 %, PTO: 7.9 %, ZPT: 6.8 %).

The authors concluded that (inflammatory) telogen effluvium related to androgenetic alopecia and associated with the complaint of dandruff was controlled by either ketoconazole, piroctone olamine, or zinc pyrithione shampoos.

6.2.7 Methods for Measuring Efficacy of Hair Care Products

Modern hair care products must be safe and nonirritating, but they must also demonstrate efficacy. Cosmetics laboratories have developed objective methods for measuring efficacy. Measurements are made using individual hair fibers as well as strands of hair. Compared to measurements of individual hair fibers, those conducted on groups of hairs are more valuable, yet the degree of abstraction remains high given that consumers are not concerned with strands of hair, but with overall appearance. Nevertheless, they supply important information. Measurement methods encompass a large number of computerized and sometimes robot methods which are used to quantify cosmetic phenomena and effects such as buildup, bounce, body, manageability, entanglement, causes of damage, and conditioning benefits. By using a carefully selected variety of methods, refining the method park and conducting dialogues with experts on subjective tests with end consumers, hair care effects can be precisely described and optimized to suit practical considerations and economic targets. Testing of various hair types in climate chambers with different levels of humidity is aimed at developing global hair care product lines.

6.2.8 Product Safety

The public is keenly interested in knowing of any health risks potentially associated with everyday products such as shampoo.

> The effects of shampoo ingredients such as crude coal tar, halogenated organic compounds, formaldehyde, formaldehyde releasers, and musk on personal health and/or the environment are only a few of the issues that have received recent media attention.

The product safety rating of a shampoo is based on an evaluation of the data for all ingredients with regard to skin and mucous membrane tolerability, sensitization potential, acute and chronic toxicity, mutagenicity, skin penetration and accumulation potential, biodegradability, and aquatic toxicity.

Carcinogenicity. Opponents of tar-based products, concerned with the risk of carcinogenicity, grew even more vocal with the first publications on percutaneous absorption of polycyclic aromatic hydrocarbons (PAH) from tar-based shampoo. In fact, in the roughly 100 years since tar-based products have been used for dermatologic indications, the incidence of related skin cancer is very rare and no relationship has been reported with the use of coal tar-based shampoos. Containing up to 79 μg/g benzoapyrene, the main PAH in tar-based shampoos, only a fraction of 79 μg PAH per hair washing is absorbed. By way of comparison, the benzo(a)pyrene in a pound of grilled ground beef is about 10 μg.

Skin and Mucous Membrane Irritation. Critical assessment of validated data on the frequency of contact allergies to shampoo demonstrates their low risk.

> Given that shampoos are diluted by water, have a short contact time, and are rinsed off, the risk of sensitization is low.

Nevertheless, in patients who are already sensitized, exposure could conceivably trigger eczema. Patients should therefore be advised of all the ingredients contained in the shampoo; a complete allergy history can also help avoid contact with relevant allergens. Although in most cases testing individual ingredients is sufficient, testing the final formulation for skin and mucous membrane irritation is preferable. Such testing is not mandated by current directives on cosmetic products and is often not performed. Therefore, safety ratings of cosmetic shampoos used for therapeutic indications should be critically assessed on an individual patient basis.

Environmental Safety. Environmental safety requirements for cosmetic products are derived from applicable environmental laws. Water protection regulations mainly address the effects of substances that end up in the water; for a given ingredient to be approved for use, it should not be expected to cause irreversible damage. Rapid and complete biodegradation of surfactants, which are used in large quantities, is required and has been the subject of careful scrutiny and confirmation.

Most knowledge of ecological characteristics of surfactants has come from their use in laundry detergents and cleaners, which are used in far larger quantities, rather than from the comparatively smaller amounts used in shampoos which pose less of a threat to the environment.

6.3 Conditioners

Sebum is the ideal hair conditioner. Excessive removal of sebum in the course of washing the hair and scalp created the need for synthetic sebum-like substances that attempt to supply hair with the positive attributes of sebum while avoiding the greasy appearance of excessive sebum and dirty hair.

Hair conditioners aim at:

- Imparting softness
- Increasing luster and gloss
- Reducing fly-away
- Enhancing disentangling facility
- Alleviating defects related to certain types of hair and hair treatments

They are available as shampoos for dry or damaged hair, conditioning (2-in-1) shampoos, and hair conditioners (liquids, creams, pastes, gels). The hair conditioning agents are basically the same used in conditioning shampoos and listed in Table 6.4.

6.4 Hair Styling Aids

Hair styling aids are intended to maintain hair in a fashionable arrangement while improving the quality of hair fibers. Hair styles are in part dictated by the available technology in hair styling products.

Hair styling aids aim at:

- Maintaining hair in desired position
- Adding increased hold to hair
- Creating illusion of fullness
- Creating a wet, "spiky" look
- Straightening, conditioning, moisturizing, and adding shine to kinky hair

They are available as hair spray, hair styling gel, hair sculpturing gel, hair wax, hair mousse, and ethnic styling aids, such as pomade, brilliantine, oil sheen spray, and curl activator.

Table 6.7 lists available styling products, their formulation, aim, and application.

6.5 Hair Dyes

In the absence of another way to reliably reverse hair graying, hair colorants have remained the mainstay of recovering lost hair color, reaching back as far as to the Ancient Egyptians who colored their hair with henna and indigo, and the Ancient Romans who used lead combs dipped into vinegar. Henna, obtained from the plant *Lawsonia alba*, is a naturally occurring hair colorant still frequently used today. Although the color can add red highlights to hair, occasionally on gray hair it may come out looking orange.

There are several choices open to cover gray hair:

- To apply blond streaks to some of the hair, a procedure called highlighting
- To color only the gray, especially in the beginning when the gray in men affects only the temples or the perimeter in women
- To color about half the hair by wrapping it with a lighter shade producing a natural look
- To color the entire head of hair, usually going two shades lighter than a person's natural color to prevent a harsh look

Table 6.7 Hair styling aids

Styling product	Formulation	Aim	Application
Hair spray	Aerosolized spray polymer (PVP, VA, MEA)	Maintain hair in desired position	Sprayed on finished hair style
Hair styling gel, hair sculpturing gel	Clear gel polymer	Hold hair away from scalp for fullness or "spiky look"	Rubbed with hands on towel-dried hair
Hair wax	Soft opaque formable wax	Add increased hold to hair	Massaged into dry hair after softening in palm
Hair mousse	Aerosolized polymer foam	Hold hair away from scalp for fullness or "spiky look"	Squirted onto hand and dabbed through towel-dried hair
Ethnic styling aids			
Pomade	Ointment of petrolatum	Straighten, condition, moisturize, add shine to kinky hair	Combed with hands through hair
Brilliantine	Liquid oil	Allow ease of styling and proved shine	Massaged with hands through hair
Oil sheen spray	Aerosolized oil	For shine and moisturization	Sprayed onto hair
Curl activator	Clear glycerin gel	For ringlet hairstyles	Massaged with hands through hair

From: Draelos ZD (2005) Hair grooming cosmetics. In: Draelos ZD (ed) Hair care. An illustrated dermatologic handbook. Taylor & Francis, London/New York, p 75

The following major types of synthetic hair colorants are currently used:

- Temporary (textile dyes)
- Natural coloring (henna)
- Semipermanent (low-molecular-weight direct dyes)
- Permanent (aromatic amines)

Temporary hair colorants consist of large complex organic structures that do not penetrate the cuticle. The colors are not intense but are capable of covering gray hair in a subtle way. This may be a good way for an individual to experiment with the coloring idea. The colorant washes out with the next shampoo.

Semipermanent colorants consist of small molecules that penetrate the cuticle. These compounds color gray hair very nicely, are easily applied in a lotion or foam at home, and last for six to ten shampoos.

Permanent hair dye is the most frequently used hair colorant. In permanent hair coloring, the formation of colored molecules from their precursors occurs inside the hair fibers as a result of oxidation by hydrogen peroxide. The most prominent among permanent hair coloring agents are *p*-phenylenediamine (PPD) and *p*-toluenediamine (PTD). The advantage of permanent color is that the color withstands normal hair washing. Because new growth comes out, the roots need to be touched up. Such products are used in a very gratifying manner and safely by millions of individuals worldwide. Besides a cosmetic benefit, hair dyes have been shown to also have a photoprotective effect on the hair fiber.

> There have been studies that raised the possibility that long-term usage of permanent hair dyes (particularly black dyes) may be associated with an increased risk of developing certain cancers. However, taken together the evidence is insufficient to state with certainty whether there is a link between using hair dye and cancer.

6.6 Cosmetic Treatment for Aging Hair

As hair ages changes affecting pigmentation and growth become evident. Aging hair is characterized by loss of follicle rigor, consistent with slowing of other body activities with age. Senescence of the hair is particularly visible and

Table 6.8 Grooming rules for maintaining good looking hair

Manipulate hair as little as possible
Comb hair gently
Avoid combing wet hair
Avoid high-temperature appliances
Select a vented ball tip styling brush
Avoid scratching of hair and scalp
Cut away split ends
Preferably wear short hair style (length of hair should be inverse proportional to age)

From: Draelos ZD (2010) Care of aging hair and photoprotection. In: Trüeb RM, Tobin DJ (eds) Aging hair. Springer, Berlin/Heidelberg, pp 183 ff

consists in failure to pigment the hair shaft (graying), decrease in rapidity of hair growth, and reduction in the diameter of the hair shaft. Senescent alopecia is different from androgenetic alopecia.

Preventive measures begin with early avoidance of factors that cause damage to the hair and scalp such as UV rays, tobacco smoking, poor diet, and stress. UV rays contribute significantly to the aging of the skin and presumably the hair as well.

Cosmetic treatment for aging hair consists in:

- Grooming rules for maintaining good looking hair (Table 6.8)
- Special shampoo selection for aging hair (Table 6.9)
- Conditioner use
- Use of hair styling aids
- Hair photoprotection

The effect of UV radiation on the hair follicles is attributed, among other things to the light activation of porphyrins produced by *Propionibacterium* spp. in the hair canal which triggers a follicular microinflammation. For this reason, the use of an antimicrobial solution has been recommended as one possible preventive measure. Another would be photoprotection of the hair and scalp. Cinnamidopropyltrimonium chloride is a quaternized UV absorber that also has a conditioning effect in shampoo. Solid nanoparticles as carriers of UV blockers are in development for use in hair.

The efficacy of hair growth agents or antiaging substances in shampoo is questionable given

Table 6.9 Special shampoo selection for aging hair

Primary cleanser:
Anionic, usually a lauryl sulfate, in combination with a laureth sulfate
A sarcosine for dry hair, resp.
A sulfosuccinate for greasy hair
Secondary cleanser (for mild shampoos):
Nonionic or amphoteric (in baby shampoos)
Shampoo conditioners:
Mature individuals should select conditioners developed for fine hair, preferably
Silicone (dimethicone)
Panthenol (humectant)
Hydrolyzed proteins (no buildup)
Special antiaging ingredients:
Photoprotective agents
Antioxidants (primarily aims at protecting shampoos from oxidation)
Niacinamide
Melatonin
Energizers (caffeine, guarana, gingko)
Others from TCM (He Shou Wu) or Ayurweda (at least of great commercial interest)

that their dilution with water and short contact time, unless they can be absorbed in effective quantities. Antioxidants and UV absorbers primarily serve to protect oxidation-sensitive oils or dyes against the effects of light. Yet, they are often present in concentrations that are too low to protect the hair. Pantothenic acid is a strong humectant and is therefore considered a conditioner. Finally, topical melatonin has been found to suppress UV-induced erythema and UV-induced reactive oxygen species in a dose-dependent manner.

A majority of current treatments associated with thinning hair, such as androgenetic alopecia and senescent alopecia, are focused on improving scalp hair density and on preventing further damage of the hair fiber. For the former, prescription drugs such as topical minoxidil solution and oral finasteride are available and for the latter over-the-counter cosmetic products as outlined in Sects. 6.2, 6.3, and 6.4.

Since hair fiber diameter has been recognized to represent another key contributor to hair thinning, a novel leave-on technology has been developed at Procter & Gamble that combines caffeine, niacinamide, panthenol, dimethicone, and an acrylate polymer (CNPDA) to affect the diameter and behavior of individual scalp hair fibers as an approach to improve decreasing fiber diameter. Utilizing laser scan micrometer for assessment of fiber diameter measures, tensile break stress, and torsion pendulum testing for assessment of behavioral properties, it was found that CNPDA significantly increased the diameter of individual terminal scalp hair fibers by 2–5 μm, which yields an increase in the cross-sectional area of approximately 10 %. Beyond the increase in hair fiber diameter, the CNPDA-thickened fibers demonstrated enhanced mechanical properties characteristic of thicker fibers, such as increased suppleness/pliability and better ability to withstand force without breaking.

> Although cosmetic treatments will not reverse the process of hair aging, new technologies help to mitigate the effects of age-related thinning of hair.

Therefore, cosmetic products represent a key integral part of management of aging hair, since they may significantly improve the condition of the hair fiber with more immediate effects, while pharmacologic agents take their time.

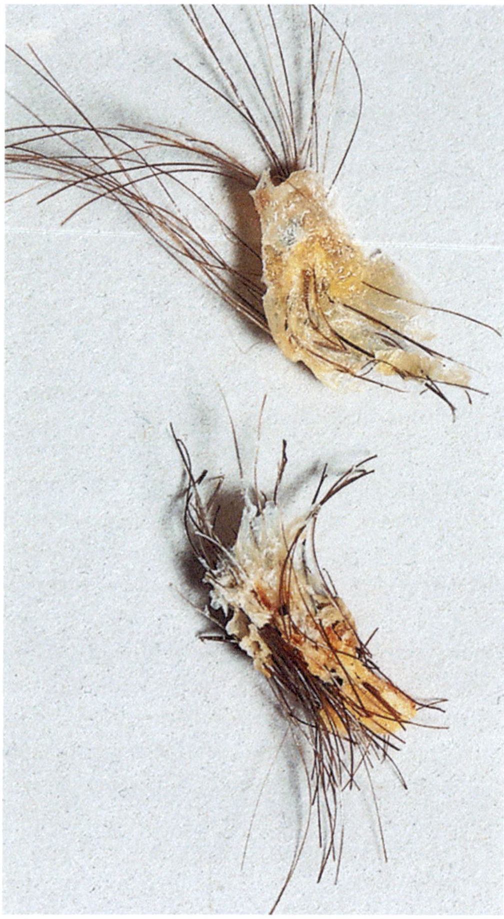

Fig. 6.8 Detached scales containing groups of trapped telogen hairs

6.7 Adverse Effects of Cosmetic Hair Treatments

Besides hair weathering, there exist a number of peculiar adverse effects resulting from inappropriate cosmetic hair treatments. These are:

- Hair matting (from inappropriate hair washing)
- Bubble hair (from inappropriate hair drying)
- Cosmetic hair beads (from inappropriate hair styling)
- Allergic contact dermatitis (from contact sensitivity)

Patients sometimes blame shampoos for their hair loss. Diffuse hair loss due to an inhibition of mitosis associated with long-term use of shampoos containing keratostatic anti-dandruff agents, such as selenium sulfide, has been discussed in the older literature and remains controversial. More frequently, the impression of increased hair shedding is created through the detachment of scales containing groups of trapped telogen hairs (Fig. 6.8).

> Absence of effects of dimethicone- and non-dimethicone-containing shampoos on hair loss rates has systematically been demonstrated.

6.7.1 From Inappropriate Washing: Hair Matting

Hair matting or acute felting of the hair represents a rare condition of irreversible tangling of scalp hair with dramatic onset. It is not a primary hair disorder: physical conditions, chemical agents, and behavioral factors play the main roles. There is invariably a history of previous chemical hair treatment.

Damaged hair, e.g., permanently waved hair, is particularly prone to sudden entanglement, which can occur with the use of viscous fluids such as undiluted shampoo. The piling of long hair on the top of the head while shampooing and the repeated friction of wet hair facilitate the process of matting. The raised cuticle cells of the damaged hair interlock as a result of excessive friction and static electricity, and the hair become tangled. Accordingly, microscopy reveals twisting and bending of the hairs through 180°. An irreversible knot, sometimes referred to as a "bird's nest," forms over a limited area (Fig. 6.9a–d).

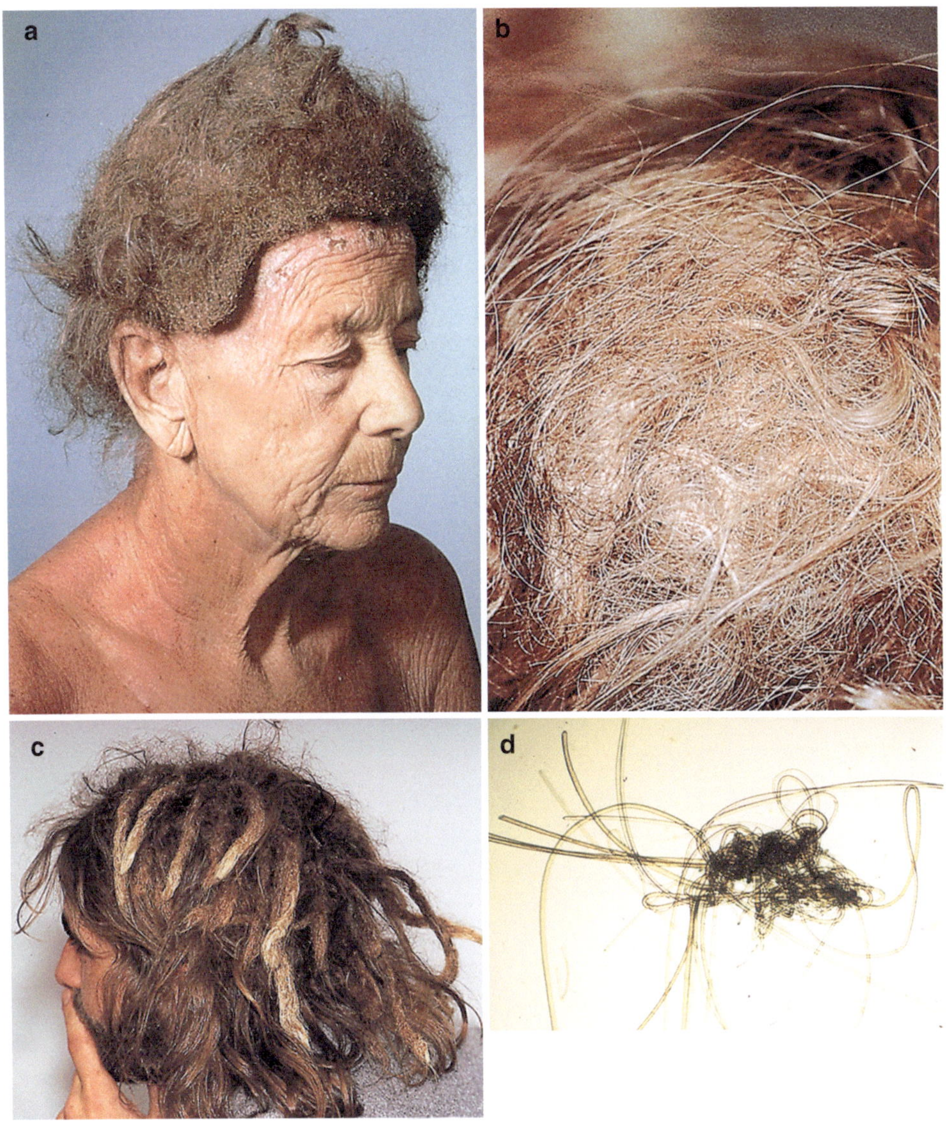

Fig. 6.9 (**a–k**) Adverse reactions to cosmetic hair treatments. (**a–d**) Hair matting: (**a**) Plica polonica (Polish plait). (**b**) Bird's nest hair. (**c**) Deliberate matting of hair: dreadlocks. (**d**) Light microscopy: tangling and knotting of twisted and bent hair through 180°. (**e, f**) Bubble hair, (**f**) light microscopy. (**g, h**) Cosmetic hair beads, (**h**) light microscopy (Courtesy of Prof. P. Itin). (**i–k**) Contact allergy to PPD: (**i**) Allergic contact dermatitis. (**j**) Patch testing. (**k**) Positive patch test

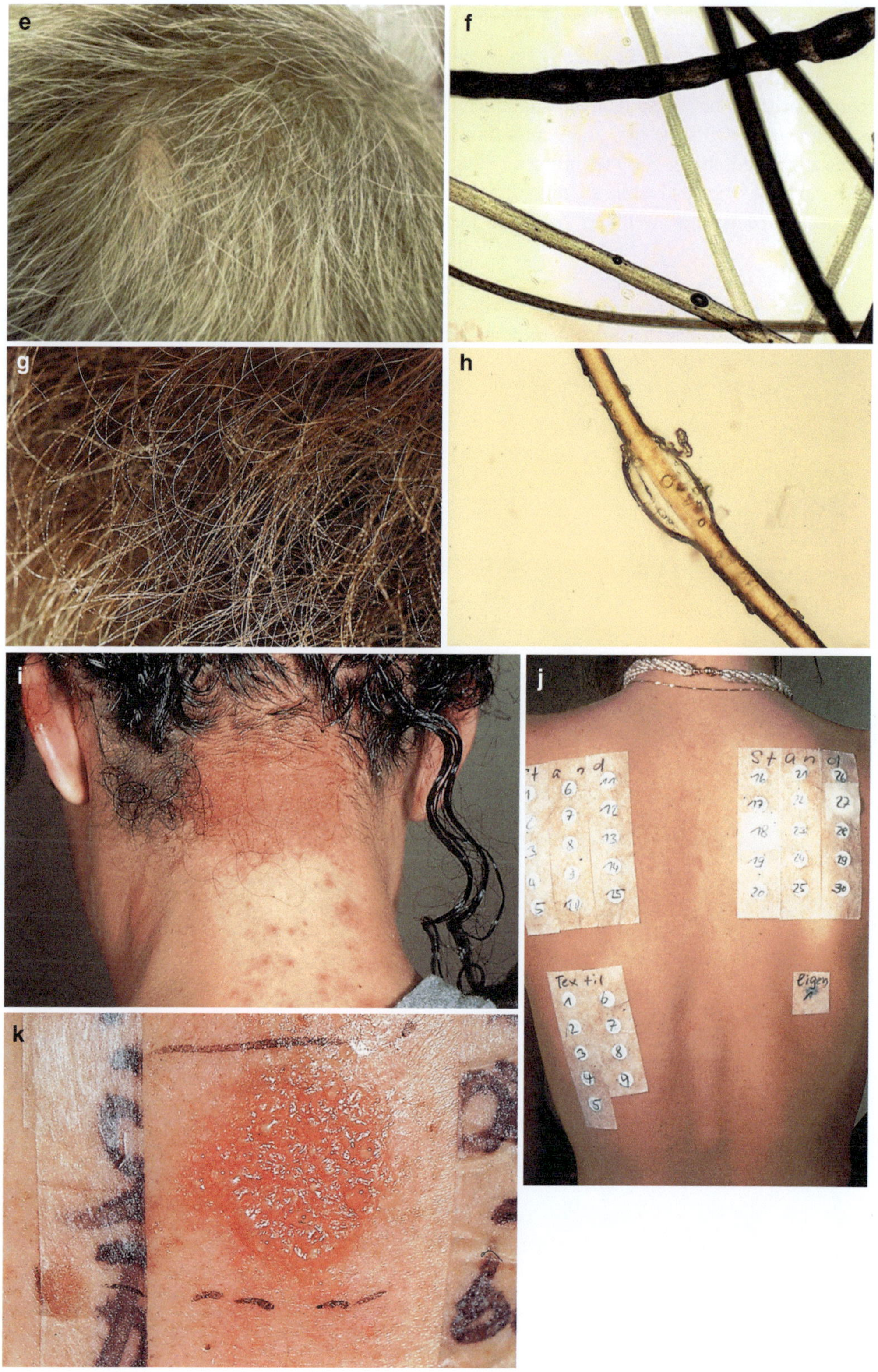

Fig. 6.9 (continued)

Since the structure of the hair is significantly damaged, the only alternative is to cut off the tangled portion.

The best means of preventing hair matting in damaged hair is to follow the instructions for using shampoo products and to regularly use a conditioner, especially for permed hair.

6.7.2 From Inappropriate Drying: Bubble Hair

Bubble hair is an acquired hair shaft abnormality characterized by a localized area of weak, dry, and brittle hair which breaks easily, and bubble-like areas in the hair shaft seen with light microscopy. The overall texture of the hair may change from soft and naturally curly to straight and stiff. Bubble hair is a reproducible hair shaft defect caused by heat. Brief, focal heating of damp hair is sufficient to cause bubbles to form inside the hair fibers (Fig. 6.9e, f).

The use of overheating hair dryers, or any other hair care equipment that overheats, should be avoided.

6.7.3 From Inappropriate Styling: Cosmetically Induced Hair Beads

Cosmetically induced hair beads present as monilethrix-like appearance of hair shafts through buildup of polymers (PVP, vinyl acetate, methacrylates) on hair as a result of excessive use of hair lacquer and hair styling gel. Light microscopy reveals that the hair is encircled by a material with a glassy appearance (Fig. 6.9g, h).

6.7.4 From Contact Sensitivity: Allergic Contact Dermatitis

Allergic contact dermatitis represents the manifestation of an allergic response of the skin caused by contact with a substance the individual is sensitized to.

Allergic reactions to cosmetics are usually overestimated by consumers. Less than 10 % of the population report an intolerance reaction to a cosmetic product; of those 1 % is caused by a contact allergen that is identified with patch testing.

In contrast to irritant contact dermatitis, allergic contact dermatitis represents a hypersensitivity reaction that is atypical within the general population. Common allergens in cosmetics implicated include the following (in order of frequency): fragrances, hair dyes (*p*-phenylenediamine or PPD, and *p*-toluenediamine or PTD), and preservatives (formaldehyde, parabens, quaternium-15, imidazolinylurea, DMDM hydantoin, and bronopol). Allergic contact reactions to *leave-on* products are more frequent than to *wash-off* products. Finally, contact allergy to hairdressing cosmetics poses a bigger problem to hairdressers (hair dressers' hand dermatitis) than to consumers.

In those cases, where an allergic contact dermatitis is suspected, patch testing with the hairdressing series (Table 6.10) is indicated.

Contact sensitivity to parabens is generally overestimated, and the rating "paraben-free" is rather in the interest of marketing purposes than consumer protection. Paraben-sensitive persons, who react to parabens on patch testing and develop dermatitis when paraben-containing products are used on compromised skin, may continue to use paraben-containing product on areas of intact skin, without adverse reaction. This phenomenon has been termed the "paraben paradox" by Fisher in1973. Originally, Fisher included in the definition of "paraben paradox" also the fact that paraben-containing personal products, which are the cause of an allergic contact dermatitis, often produce false-negative patch test reactions when applied to the skin of the back. The explanation for this phenomenon is again that the patch testing is being performed on intact skin.

More important is allergic contact allergy to PPD and PTD (Fig. 6.9i–k) that may result both in allergic contact dermatitis and an acute and diffuse

Table 6.10 Hairdressing series

1. *p*-Phenylenediamine (PPD)
2. Toluene-2,5-diamine sulfate
3. 2-Nitro-*p*-phenylenediamine
4. Ammonium thioglycolate
5. Ammonium persulfate
6. Formaldehyde
7. Nickel sulfate hexahydrate
8. Cobalt(II)chloride hexahydrate
9. Resorcinol
10. *m*-Aminophenol
11. *p*-Aminophenol
12. Hydrogen peroxide
13. Hydroquinone
14. Myroxylon pereirae resin
15. Chloroacetamide
16. Glyceryl monothioglycolate (glyceryl thioglycolate)
17. Cocamidopropyl betaine
18. Methylisothiazolinone + Methylchloroisothiazolinone
19. 2-Bromp-2-nitropropane-1,3-diol (bronopol)
20. Captan
21. *p*-Chloro-*m*-cresol (PCMC)
22. Chloroxylenol (PCMX)
23. Imidazolidinyl urea
24. Quaternium-15 (Dowicil 200)
25. Zinc pyrithione (Zinc Omadine)
26. Diazolidinyl urea
27. Lauryl glucoside
28. Oleamidopropyl dimethylamine

(inflammatory) telogen effluvium following allergic contact reaction approximately by 3 months. Severe cases of allergic contact dermatitis, usually to PPD, are best treated with oral corticosteroids which are tapered gradually, with various dosing schedules ranging from a total of 10–14 days to prevent recurrence of the rash. Sedating antihistamines such as oral hydroxyzine may be added to relieve the intense itching. Persons who develop contact sensitivity to a certain allergen are most likely to have it for the rest of their lives, and detecting the allergen by means of patch testing and avoiding it is mandatory in treating the condition and resolving its symptoms.

Further Reading

Trüeb RM, de Viragh PA, Swiss Trichology Study Group (2001) Significance of scalp hair and therapy of alopecia in men in Switzerland. Praxis (Bern 1994) 90:-241–248, Article in German

Hair Weathering

Hofbauer GF, Tsambaos D, Spycher MA, Trüeb RM (2001) Acquired hair fragility in pili annulati: causal relationship with androgenetic alopecia. Dermatology 203:60–62

Sinclair R (2007) Healthy hair: what is it? J Investig Dermatol Symp Proc 12:2–5

Thibaut S, de Becker E, Bernard BA, Huart M, Fiat F, Baghdadli N, Luengo GS, Leroy F, Angevin P, Kermoal AM, Muller S, Peron M, Provot G, Kravtchenko S, Saint-Léger D, Desbois G, Gauchet L, Nowbuth K, Galliano A, Kempf JY, Silberzan I (2010) Chronological ageing of human hair keratin fibres. Int J Cosmet Sci 1–13

Trüeb RM (2005) Dermocosmetic aspects of hair and scalp. J Investig Dermatol Symp Proc 10:289–292

Shampoos

Ackerman AB, Kligman AM (1969) Some observations on dandruff. J Soc Cosmet Chem 20:81–101

Adams RM, Maibach HI (1985) A five-year study of cosmetic reactions. J Am Acad Dermatol 13: 1062–1069

Baroni A, de Rosa R, de Rosa A et al (2000) New strategies in dandruff treatment: growth control of Malassezia ovalis. Dermatology 201:332–336

Bouillon C (1996) Shampoos. Clin Dermatol 14:113–121

Dawber R (1996) Hair: its structure and response to cosmetic preparations. Clin Dermatol 14:105–112

Faergemann J (2002) Atopic dermatitis and fungi. Clin Microbiol Rev 15:545–563

Georgalas A (2004) Enhanced delivery of antidandruff active in shampoo vehicle. J Cosmet Sci 55 Suppl: S207–S214

Goldschmidt JA, Kligman AM (1968) Increased sebum secretion following selenium sulfide shampoos. Acta Derm Venereol 48:489–491

Griesemer RD (1978) Emotionally triggered disease in a dermatology practice. Psychiatr Ann 8:49–56

Hay RJ, Graham-Brown RAC (1997) Dandruff and seborrhoeic dermatitis: causes and management. Clin Exp Dermatol 22:3–6

Hughes-Formella BJ, Filbry A, Gassmueller J, Rippke F (2002) Anti-inflammatory efficacy of topical preparations with 10 % hamamelis distillate in a UV erythema test. Skin Pharmacol Appl Skin Physiol 15:125–132

Korting HC, Schäfer-Korting M, Klövekorn W et al (1995) Comparative efficacy of hamamelis distillate and hydrocortisone cream in atopic eczema. Eur J Clin Pharmacol 48:461–465

Merk HF, Mukhtar H, Kaufmann I et al (1987) Human hair follicle benzo[a]pyrene and benzo[a]pyrene 7,8-diol metabolism: effect of exposure to a coal tar containing shampoo. J Invest Dermatol 88:71–76

Naldi L, Rebora A (2009) Clinical practice. Seborrheic dermatitis. N Engl J Med 360:387–396, 22

Piérard-Franchimont C, De Doncker P, Cauwenbergh G, Piérard GE (1998) Ketoconazole shampoo: effect of long-term use in androgenic alopecia. Dermatology 196:474–477

Piérard-Franchimont C, Goffin V, Henry F, Uhoda I, Braham C, Piérard GE (2002) Nudging hair shedding by antidandruff shampoos. A comparison of 1 % ketoconazole, 1 % piroctone olamine and 1 % zinc pyrithione formulations. Int J Cosmet Sci 24:249–256

Rushton H, Gummer CL, Flasch H (1994) 2-in-1 shampoo technology: state of the art shampoo and conditioner in one. Skin Pharmacol 7:78–83

Schuster S (1984) The aetiology of dandruff and the mode of action of therapeutic agents. Br J Dermatol 111:235–242

Shapiro J, Maddin S (1996) Medicated shampoos. Clin Dermatol 14:123–128

Sulzberger MB, Witten VH, Hunt JA (1956) Puzzling persistent penile plaques. AMA Arch Dermatol 73: 101–109

Trüeb RM (2007) Shampoos: ingredients, efficacy and adverse effects. J Dtsch Dermatol Ges 5:356–365

Urbano CC (1995) 50 years of hair care development. Cosmet Toiletries 110:85–104

Van Schooten FJ, Moonen EJ, Rhynsburger E et al (1994) Dermal uptake of polycyclic aromatic hydrocarbons after hair wash with coal tar shampoo. Lancet 344:1505–1506

Conditioners

Rushton H, Gummer CL, Flasch H (1994) 2-in-1 shampoo technology: state of the art shampoo and conditioner in one. Skin Pharmacol 17:78–83

Trüeb RM (2005) Dermocosmetic aspects of hair and scalp. J Investig Dermatol Symp Proc 10:289–292

Hairstyling Aids

Draelos ZD (2005) Hair grooming cosmetics. In: Draelos ZD (ed) Hair care. An illustrated dermatologic handbook. Taylor & Francis, London/New York, p 75

Hair Dyes

Bolt HM, Golka K (2007) The debate on carcinogenicity of permanent hair dyes: new insights. Crit Rev Toxicol 37:521–536

Kelsh MA, Alexander DD, Kalmes RM, Buffler PA (2008) Personal use of hair dyes and risk of bladder cancer: a meta-analysis of epidemiologic data. Cancer Causes Control 19:549–558

Mendelsohn JB, Li QZ, Ji BT et al (2009) Personal use of hair dye and cancer risk in a prospective cohort of Chinese women. Cancer Sci 100:1088–1091

Pande CM, Albrecht L, Yang B (2001) Hair photoprotection by dyes. J Cosmet Sci 52:377–389

Rollison DE, Helzlsouer KJ, Pinney SM (2006) Personal hair dye use and cancer: a systematic literature review and evaluation of exposure assessment in studies published since 1992. J Toxicol Environ Health B Crit Rev 9:413–439

Cosmetic Treatment for Aging Hair

Bangha E, Elsner P, Kistler GS (1996) Suppression of UV-induced erythema by topical treatment with melatonin (N-acetyl-5-methoxytryptamine). Arch Dermatol Res 288:522–526

Davis MG, Thomas JH, van de Velde S, Boissy Y, Dawson TL Jr, Iveson R, Sutton K (2011) A novel cosmetic approach to treat thinning hair. Br J Dermatol 165 Suppl 3:24–30

Draelos ZD (2010) Care of aging hair and photoprotection. In: Trüeb RM, Tobin DJ (eds) Aging hair. Springer, Berlin/Heidelberg, pp 183–191

Fischer TW, Scholz G, Knoll B et al (2001) Melatonin reduces UV-induced reactive oxygen species in a dose-dependent manner in IL-3-stimulated leukocytes. J Pineal Res 31:39–45

Gao T, Bedell A (2001) Ultraviolet damage on natural gray hair and its photoprotection. J Cosmet Sci 52:103–118

Wissing SA, Muller RH (2001) Solid lipid nanoparticles (SLN) – a novel carrier for UV blockers. Pharmazie 56:783–786

Adverse Effects of Cosmetic Hair Treatments

Al Ghani MA, Geilen CC, Blume-Peytavi U, Orfanos CE (2000) Matting of hair: a multifactorial enigma. Dermatology 20:101–104

Cashman AL, Warshaw EM (2005) Parabens: a review of epidemiology structure, allergenicity, and hormonal properties. Dermatitis 16:57–66

Gummer CL (1994) Bubble hair: a cosmetic abnormality caused by brief, focal heating of damp hair fibers. Br J Dermatol 131:9801–9903

Itin P, Schiller P, Mathys D, Guggenheim R (1997) Cosmetically induced hair beads. J Am Acad Dermatol 36:260–261

Tosti A, Piraccini BM, van Neste DJ (2001) Telogen effluvium after allergic contact dermatitis of the scalp. Arch Dermatol 137:187–190

7 Epilogue: Male Hair in the Bible

And they had hair as the hair of women,
and their teeth were as [the teeth] of lions.

Revelation 9:8

Any text with the least claim of authority is a mere shadow compared to the authority of the Bible in the history of mankind and civilization. Therefore, it would be negligent not to quote the Bible references to the condition of hair in man.

The Bible, from Koine Greek tà biblía, which means the "the books," is a canonical collection of texts considered sacred in Judaism as well as in Christianity. It has been a major influence on literature and history, especially in the West where it was the first mass printed book.

In modern times, the view that the Bible should be accepted as historically accurate and as a reliable guide to morality has been questioned by many mainstream academics in the field of biblical criticism. Nevertheless, the Bible has retained estimated annual sales of 25 million copies and its authority for all of those who are in the disposition of reading and understanding its profound and timeless wisdom.

7.1 Old Testament

The Old Testament is the Christian term for the collection of religious writings by ancient Israelites. For the Israelites, the writings of the Old Testament told of their own unique relationship with God, but the overarching Messianic nature of Christianity has led Christians from the very beginning of faith to acknowledge the Old Testament as a preparation for the New Covenant and New Testament. The books of the Old Testament can be broadly divided into the Pentateuch, which tells how God selected Israel to be his chosen people; the history books telling the history of the Israelites from their conquest of Canaan to their defeat and exile in Babylon; the poetic and Wisdom books dealing with questions of good and evil in the world; and the books of the Biblical Prophets warning of the consequences of turning away from God.

The following excerpts from the Old Testament relating to the condition of hair in men address such important questions as: the differentiation of common baldness from inflammatory scarring alopecia; the psychological significance of cutting the hair or of the display of long and flowing hair, respectively; and finally the bearing of peer teasing in male pattern baldness.

7.1.1 Tzaraath Breaking Out on the Head

40If a man's hair is gone
this does not make him a leper even though he is bald!
41If the hair is gone from the front part of his head,
he simply has a bald forehead, but this is not leprosy.
42However, if in the baldness there is a reddish white spot, it may be leprosy breaking out.
43In that case the priest shall examine him.

Leviticus 13:40–43

Probably one of thc oldest and most authoritative text on the importance of making a distinction between male pattern baldness and inflammatory scarring alopecia is found in the Old Testament.

R.M. Trüeb, W.-S. Lee, *Male Alopecia*,
DOI 10.1007/978-3-319-03233-7_7, © Springer International Publishing Switzerland 2014

The Hebrew noun *tzaraath*, צרעת, for leprosy originally describes any disfigurative conditions of the skin and body hair mainly referred to in chapters 13–14 of Leviticus. It is only in the Septuagint, a translation of the Hebrew Bible originally used by Greek-speaking Jews and Gentile proselytes, that the term *tzaraath* was translated with Greek lepra, λεπρα, from which the cognate *leprosy* was traditionally used in English Bibles. The New Jewish Publication Society of America Tanakh translates it as a "scaly affection" in Leviticus 13:2.

> It is clear today that Biblical leprosy does not refer to Hansen's disease, but may represent any skin disease fulfilling the criteria for diagnosis of *tzaraath*.

According to Hebrew tradition, patches of the skin are confirmed as *tzaraath* by the occurrence of one of three signs: (1) white hair, if at least two hairs within the confines of the affliction turn white; (2) healthy flesh, if skin of a normal appearance appears within the confines of the patch; (3) spreading, if the patch became enlarged since the time of the initial examination by the priest. From today's medical point of view, we may be dealing with vitiligo.

Whereas common baldness is not a form of *tzaraath*, patches that occur on a bald scalp may be *tzaraath* if they appear in a distinct fashion again regulated in the same fashion as for the glabrous skin; however, it can only occur on men and in one of two places: within what are referred to as a man's posterior baldness and anterior baldness. For a scalp eruption to be *tzaraath*, the lesion must be a white patch tinged with red. The initial symptom of this type of affliction is patches of hair loss. According to Maimonides (1135–1204), scalp and beard afflictions are characterized by hair loss without any change to the skin of the bald spot. The *Tosefta* (compilation of Jewish oral law), however, maintains that the skin of the bald spot does indeed become altered with two confirming signs: (1) thin yellow hair, if at least two and a half hairs from within the bald patch turn yellow, (2) spreading, if the balding spreads, according to Maimonides. According to Abraham ben David (1125–1198) who quotes the *Tosefta*, this spreading would refer to spreading of a skin change as well. From today's medical point of view in the case of Maimonides, we would be dealing with alopecia areata or pseudopelade, and in the case of Abraham ben David, with anything from tinea capitis to cutaneous lupus erythematosus.

The affected individual had to consult the Priest or *Kohen*, who was trained in examining the lesions and determine whether or not they meet the specifications of *tzaraath*. Specifically, he would evaluate the lesion for the criteria mentioned above including the final criterion of spreading diagnosed at a follow-up examination. If characteristics of the lesions met the criteria for *tzaraath*, either at the initial or at the follow-up examination, the *Kohen* declared the individual ritually impure. The individual who is declared impure with *tzaraath* was shunned and had to live alone outside the confines of the community (Leviticus 13:46), had to tear his garments in mourning like those who are in mourning for a close family member, not cut his hair, cover his face until the upper lip in the fashion of mourners, and call out "impure, impure" to warn others to keep their distance.

> Irrespective of the contagiosity of the underlying skin disease or not, the concept of *tzaraath* underscores the social stigmatization that results from affections of the skin and hair and sets it into a moral context.

In as much as the linguistic root of *tzaraath* may mean "smiting," in reference to a Talmudical explanation it serves as a punishment for sin. Accordingly, for the purification process

> The kohen shall command to take for the person undergoing purification two live kosher birds, cedarwood, red string and hyssop.

The items used in the purification ritual were specifically included to deliver a message to the afflicted. Although many sins may lead to this punishment, the most predominant sin to cause *tzaraath* was an "evil tongue." To speak derogatorily about others consistently to one's friends is likened to birds, who chatter endlessly. In a similar vein, the one who speaks ill of others is haughty, holding himself high above others and is likened to the tall cedar. To be healed, the subject concerned must erase arrogance, making themselves lowly like a worm. This is a play on words and means both "red" and "worm" – as well as hyssop.

7.1.2 Samson and Delilah

> 15"How can you say you love me when you don't confide in me?" she (Delilah) whined. "You've made fun of me three times now, and you still haven't told me what makes you so strong!"
>
> 16,17She nagged hat him (Samson) every day until he couldn't stand it any longer and finally told her his secret.
>
> "My hair has never been cut", he confessed, "for I've been a Nazirite to God since before my birth. If my hair were cut, my strength would leave me, and I would become as weak as anyone else."
>
> 18Delilah realized that he had finally told her the truth, so she sent for the five Philistine leaders.
>
> "Come just this once more," she said, "for this time he has told me everything." So they brought the money with them.
>
> 19She lulled him to sleep with his head in her lap, and they brought in a barber and cut off his hair. Delilah began to hit him, but she could see that his strength was leaving him.
>
> 20Then she screamed, "The Philistines are here to capture you, Samson!" And he woke up and thought, "I will do as before: I'll just shake myself free." But he didn't realize that the Lord had left him.
>
> Judges 16: 15–20

Samson is an iconic figure standing for the symbolism of male hair. The Biblical story of Samson and Delilah, recorded in Judges 16, has enchanted countless writers, artists, composers, and ultimately the movie screens of Hollywood throughout the centuries. It is a story of love, seduction, betrayal, and redemption.

Some Bible critics have interpreted Samson as an archetypical folklore hero, modelled after Herakles from Greek Mythology and Enkidu from the Mesopotamian Gilgamesh epos. Both, Herakles and Samson bore down a lion barehanded, both had a favorite blunt weapon (in the case of Samson an ass's jawbone), and both were betrayed by woman which led them to their ultimate doom. Finally, both heroes, champions of their respective people, died by their own hand: Herakles ends his life on a pyre, while Samson makes the Philistine temple collapse upon himself and his tormenters.

Traditional Biblical scholars disagree with these views and consider Samson to be a literal historical figure and thus reject any connections to mythological heroes of foreign cultures.

Samson was one of the last of the Judges of the ancient Israelites mentioned in the Hebrew Bible (Book of Judges chapters 13–16). According to the Biblical account, Samson was granted supernatural strength by God in order to combat his enemies and accomplish heroic deeds.

> However, Samson suffered two vulnerabilities: his liking for untrustworthy women and his long hair without which he was powerless. These vulnerabilities ultimately proved fatal for him.

Samson was born at a time when the people of Israel were being oppressed by the Philistines. Samson's parents were visited by an angel, who promised them that their son would free the Israelites, but only if he took the Nazirite vow, which required him to refrain from cutting his hair. He grew up to become a powerful fighter blessed by God with supernatural strength: he was able to kill a lion with his bare hands and defeat an entire army with nothing but an ass's jawbone.

Eventually, Samson fell in love with a Philistine woman named Delilah. The Philistines bribed her (with 1,100 silver coins each) to discover the secret of his great strength. Samson at first resisted her repeated attempts to learn the secret but eventually, in a moment of weakness, revealed the secret of his long hair to her. After putting Samson to sleep on her lap, Delilah called for a servant to shave Samson's seven locks. Since that breaks the Nazirite oath, God left him, and Samson was captured by the Philistines. Rather than killing him, the Philistines preferred to humiliate him by blinding him and subjecting him to hard labor grinding grain in a Gaza prison. As he slaved, his hair began to grow, but the careless Philistines paid no attention. And in spite of his failures and sins of great consequence, Samson's heart now turned humbled to the Lord. During a pagan sacrificial ritual, the Philistines had gathered in Gaza to celebrate. As was their custom, they paraded their prized enemy prisoner into the temple of Dagon to entertain the mocking crowds. Samson braced himself between the two central support pillars of the temple and pushed them with all his might. Down came the temple, killing Samson and all of the people trapped in it.

The familiar Biblical story of Samson and Delilah implies that a man's loss of hair erodes his masculine strength or power. At the same time, Samson's hair was a symbol of his pact with God. By allowing Delilah to cut his hair, Samson was breaking a sacred vow, and so God punished him by removing his great strength. Later, broken and humiliated by the Philistines, Samson repented and God restored with the hair his strength long enough for Samson to redeem himself by destroying the temple of his enemies. Through his death, Samson killed more of his enemies in this one sacrificial act than he had previously done in all the battles of his life.

> Desmond Morris observed cross-cultural and historical consistency in the meaning of hair and its loss: head shaving is customarily imposed upon military recruits, criminals, and prisoners of war, reflecting removal of individuality and subjugation to authority.

7.1.3 Absalom

> 25 Now no one in Israel was such a handsome specimen of manhood as Absalom, and no one else received such praise.
>
> 26 He cut his hair only once a year – and then only because it weighed three pounds and was too much of a load to carry around!
>
> 2 Sam. 14:25–26

> 9 During the battle Absalom came upon some of David's men and as he fled on his mule, it went beneath the thick boughs of a great oak tree, and his hair caught in the branches. His mule went on, leaving him dangling in the air.
>
> 10 One of David's men saw him and told Joab.
>
> 11 "What? You saw him there and didn't kill him?" Joab demanded. "I would have rewarded you handsomely and made you a commissioned officer."
>
> 12 "For a million dollars I wouldn't do it," the man replied. "We all heard the king say to you and Abisai and Ittai, 'For my sake, please don't harm young Absalom."
>
> 13 And if I had betrayed the king by killing his son (and the king would certainly find out who did it), you yourself would be the first to accuse me.
>
> 14 "Enough of this nonsense," Joab said. Then he took three daggers and plunged them into the heart of Absalom as he dangled alive from the oak.
>
> 15 Ten of Joab's young armor bearers then surrounded Absalom and finished him off.
>
> 2 Sam. 18:9–15

Absalom was the third son of David, King of Israel (1 Chronicles 3:2, 2 Samuel 3:3). He moved at an early age, with the transfer of the capital, to Jerusalem, where he spent most of his life. He was noted for his personal beauty and for the extraordinary profusion of the hair of his head (2 Sam. 14:25–26). He was a great favorite of his father and of the people as well. His charming manners, his personal beauty, his insinuating ways, together with his love of pomp and royal pretensions captivated the hearts of the people from the beginning. He lived in great style, drove in a magnificent chariot, and had fifty men run before him. Such magnificence produced the desired effect upon the hearts of the young aristocrats of the royal city. To the pleasing exterior, the youth Absalom joined a temperament which, while fond of display, was nevertheless reserved, bold, and thoughtful. These character traits were enough to fuel the desire to be one day the representative of that magnificent power created by his father, from the prospective enjoyment of which his minority of birth alone seemed to exclude him. Despite his ambition, there appears to have been in the youth a generous instinct of honor which inspires noble impulses where these do not clash with the more alluring prospects of self-interest. Under such circumstances, it is not extraordinary that Absalom, idolized his surroundings, while his natural sense of gratitude and filial duty became gradually blunted, was led to cultivate that species of egotism which grows cruel in proportion as it counts upon the blind affection of its friends.

The troubles started after Absalom's full sister Tamar is raped by their half brother and David's eldest son, Amnon. After waiting for 2 years, Absalom avenged the rape of Tamar by sending his servants to murder Amnon after he was drunk on the occasion of a feast to which he had invited all the king's sons. After this deed, he fled to join Talmai, the king of Geshur who was his maternal grandfather, and only 3 years later was he fully reinstated in his father's favor and returned to Jerusalem. While at Jerusalem and restored to his former princely dignity and the apparent confidence of his father, Absalom now entered upon the course of secretly plotting to which his ambition and opportunity seemed to urge him and which has stamped his name as a synonym of unnatural revolt. Absalom built support for himself among the populace by promising justice for all and by showing humility by kissing those who approached him rather than accepting supplication. By integrating himself in the good will of the people, and at the same time fostering discontent with the conditions of his father's reign, he succeeded in preparing the minds of the disaffected for a general uprising. After 4 years, Absalom decided to announce himself king, raped his father's concubines, and then raised a revolt at the former capital Hebron. All Israel and Judah flocked to his side, and David, supported only by the Cherethites and Pelethites and his former bodyguard, took refuge from Absalom's forces beyond the Jordan River. However, David took the precaution of instructing a servant, Hushai, to infiltrate Absalom's court and subvert it. Hushai convinced Absalom to ignore the advice of Ahithophel, former counselor of David whom had espoused the cause of Absalom, to attack his father while he was on the run and instead prepare his forces for a major attack. This gave David critical time to prepare his own troops for the coming battle. A decisive battle was fought in the Woods of Ephraim where Absalom's army was completely routed. Absalom himself was caught by his hair in the branches of an oak-tree as the mule he was riding ran beneath it, an irony given that he was previously celebrated for his abundant hair and handsome head. He was discovered hanging there still alive by one of David's men, who reported the matter to Joab, the king's commander, whom finally avenged David by fatally striking and killing Absalom, by the use of three spears, followed by a group of swordsmen (2 Sam. 18:9–15).

Besides male strength and virility, flowing hair is a symbol for freedom and looseness. Because of these features and the praise he received from them, Absalom gave into vanity, as becomes apparent from the fact that he liked to display his hair by letting it grow long, cutting it only once a year, and then broadcasting the impressive weight of the shorn hair (three pounds). His addiction to admiration and adulation ultimately contributed to his plot to usurp the throne of Israel. It is thus interesting poetic justice that his hair plays a key part in his ultimate downfall.

7.1.4 Elisha and the Two Bears

> 23From Jericho he (Elisha) went to Bethel. As he was walking along the road, some young boys from the city began mocking and making fun of him because of his bald head.
>
> 24He turned around and cursed them in the name of the Lord: and two female bears came out of the woods and killed forty-two of them.
>
> 2 Kings 2: 23–24

Elisha is a prophet and a wonder-worker mentioned in the Hebrew Bible and also in the Islamic Quran. Elisha was the attendant and disciple of the prophet Elijah, and after Elijah was taken up into the whirlwind, he was accepted as the leader of the sons of the prophets and became noted in Israel. He possessed, according to his own request, "a double portion" of Elijah's spirit and from 892 to 832 BC held the office of "prophet" in Israel. That Elisha inherited the wonder-working power of Elijah is shown throughout the whole course of his life. One wonder-working of particular interest to dermatologists is the cure of Syrian general Naaman from his leprosy (2 Kings 5–19). Naaman, at first reluctant, obeyed Elisha and washed seven times in the Jordan. Finding his flesh "restored like the flesh of a little child," the general was so impressed by this evidence of God's power and by the disinterestedness of His Prophet, as to express his deep conviction that "there is no other God in all the earth, but only in Israel."

When a group of youths from Bethel taunted the prophet for his baldness, Elisha cursed them in the name of Yahweh, and two female bears came out of the forest and tore 42 of them (2 Kings 2: 23–24). 42 is a large number of people, and they were probably an organized group who had gone out to challenge Elisha. Their mockery implied a malicious intent, especially when the culture of the time insisted on showing respect to their elders. Furthermore, the epithet "baldhead" was one of contempt in the region at the time, applied to a person even with a bushy head of hair. Given the challenge of the youths, their intimidating number which could constitute the threat of a mob, the contemptuous attitude, and the fact that Elisha was the prophet of God, the Lord allowed the youths to be destroyed.

> In survey studies on the social effects of androgenetic alopecia, balding men reported frequent peer teasing about their condition.

In a nonclinical sample, such teasing was reported by 45 % of men with modest hair loss and by 79 % of men with more extensive baldness. In a study of men seeking treatment for androgenetic alopecia, 60 % reported being teased. While some men may regard such remarks as benevolent, other may find them stressful and take them as evidence of diminished social worth.

7.2 New Testament

The New Testament is the second major part of the Christian biblical canon. Its contents deal explicitly with first-century Christianity. Therefore, the New Testament has frequently accompanied the spread of Christianity around the world and reflects and serves as a source for Christian theology.

7.2.1 1 Corinthians 11:14

> [14,15]Doesn't even instinct itself teach us that women's heads should be covered?
>
> For women are proud of their long hair, while a man with long hair tends to be ashamed.
>
> 1 Corinthians 11:14,15

Corinth was the meeting point of many nationalities because the main current of the trade between Asia and Western Europe passed through its harbors. Apostle Paul's (5–67 AD) first visit lasted nearly 2 years and his converts were mainly Greeks. Paul wrote the Epistles to the Corinthians to correct what he saw as erroneous views in the Corinthian church. Several sources informed Paul of conflicts within the church at Corinth. Paul then wrote his letters to the Corinthians, urging uniformity of belief and clarifying Christian doctrine. In general, divisions within the church at Corinth seemed to be a problem, and Paul made it a point to mention these conflicts from the beginning. Specifically, pagan roots still held sway within their community. Paul wanted to bring them back to what he saw as correct doctrine, stating that God had given him the opportunity to be a "skilled master builder" to lay the foundation and let others build upon it (1 Corinthians 3:10). Later, Paul wrote about immorality in Corinth, how to resolve personal disputes, and sexual purity. The Corinthian church was in the middle of a controversy about the roles of men and women and the proper order of authority within the church. In Corinthian society, women showed submission to their husbands by wearing a veil. It seems that some of the women in the church were discarding their veils, something that only pagan temple prostitutes or other rebellious women would do. For a woman to come to church without her veil would be dishonoring to her husband, as well as culturally confusing. By the same token, for a man to wear a veil or to somehow have his head covered during worship was not culturally acceptable. In a passage that mentions hair length (1 Corinthians 11:3–15), Paul appeals to nature to illustrate the appropriateness of following the cultural standards: women naturally have longer hair than men, and men are much more prone to baldness. That is, God created women with a "natural veil" and men with an "uncovered head." If a woman spurns the mark of her submission (the veil), then she may as well shave her head (verse 6). His point is that if the culture says a woman should not be bald (going without her natural covering), then why would she reject that same culture's standard of wearing a veil (going without her cultural covering)? For the man's part, it is unnatural for him to have "long hair" (verse 14). His hair is naturally shorter (and thinner) than the woman's. This corresponds to the Corinthian tradition of men not wearing a head covering during worship. Paul urged the church to conform to the generally held ideas of male and female appearance.

> Ultimately, a man's hair is by nature not designed to grow long. It is not very manageable – notice this in those who do wear long hair – and tends to fall out altogether in the later years of life.

7.2.2 The Error of the Long-Haired Jesus?

There have been arguments with strong points that the traditional depiction of Jesus Christ with long hair in Christian iconography, the arts, and – more recently – modern cinematography is erroneous.

Of course, Hollywood, the Dream Factory, does not pretend to display the truth, but it is noteworthy that in the latest film "The Passion of the Christ" (2004) covering the final 12 h of Jesus' life, Mel Gibson claims having referred to the New Testament Gospels of Matthew, Mark, Luke, and John for authenticity reasons. Neither of the Apostles refers to Christ's hair, but it has been less known to the public that Gibson drew on the visions of the Blessed Anne Catherine Emmerich (1774–1824) as a key source for his movie. Emmerich was a Roman Catholic Augustinian Canoness Regular of Windesheim, a mystic, and a visionary. During her bedridden years, the German Romantic poet Clemens Brentano (1778–1842) interviewed her at length and wrote "The Dolorous Passion of Our Lord Jesus Christ" based on his notes of her visions of the Christ's Passion. A careful reading of the book shows the film's high level of dependence on it. Gibson allegedly carried a piece of cloth with blood from Emmerich's stigmata as a charm during the production of the film. In 1813, Emmerich was confined to bed, and (the Christ's) stigmata were reported on her body. The claims regarding her miraculous signs were examined by an Episcopal commission, which came to the conclusion that the stigmata were genuine. Emmerich was beatified on October 3, 2004 by Pope John Paul II. However, the Vatican focused on Emmerich's own personal piety and set the book written by Brentano aside while analyzing the cause for her beatification, since the authenticity of Brentano's writings had been questioned and critics had characterized the books as "conscious elaborations by a poet" and a "well-intentioned fraud" by Brentano.

Nevertheless, it is astonishing that since the time of Roman Emperor Constantine the Great (272–337), almost all the visionary experiences of people who believed they saw a personage they thought to be Jesus have seen a long-haired Jesus.

In 313, Constantine issued the Edict of Milan legalizing Christian worship. He set the foundations for the position of the Christian emperor within the church and the notion of orthodoxy, Christendom, ecumenical councils, and the state church of the Roman Empire declared by edict in 380. He and his mother, Saint Helen, were great patrons of the Christian Church. Saint Helen is traditionally credited with finding the relics of the True Cross (and others), with which she is often represented in Christian iconography.

Most intriguing is the image of Christ's face passed down by the *Turin Shroud* and the *Sudarium* (Latin for sweat cloth), both of which are referred to in John 20:6, 7:

> 6Then Simon Peter came along behind him and went straight into the tomb. He saw the strips of linen lying there, 7as well as the cloth that had been wrapped around Jesus' head. The cloth was still lying in its place, separate from the linen.

In both Holy relics, with a striking resemblance to each other, Christ's face is depicted, though scourged, in repose, with hair extending to shoulder length and a bifurcated beard.

While the origins of the Sudarium remain obscure and have later been connected with the legend of Saint Veronica (also called Saint Berenice), there is at least some scientific evidence to support the authenticity of the Turin Shroud.

According to Catholic tradition, Veronica moved with pity when she saw Jesus carrying his cross to Golgotha and gave him her veil that he might wipe his forehead. Jesus accepted the offering, held it to his face, and then handed it back to her with the image of his face miraculously impressed upon it. This piece of cloth therefore also became known as the *Veil of Veronica*.

The Turin Shroud is a length of linen cloth bearing the image of a man who appears to have suffered physical trauma in a manner consistent with crucifixion and believed by some to be the burial shroud of Jesus Christ. Joseph Kohlbeck from the Hercules Aerospace Company in Utah and Richard Levi-Setti of the Enrico Fermi Institute examined dirt particles from the Shroud surface and found them to be travertine aragonite limestone. Using a high-resolution microprobe, the spectra of samples taken from the Shroud were compared with samples of limestone from ancient Jerusalem tombs. The chemical signatures of the Shroud samples and the tomb limestone were found identical. Danin and Uri Baruch reported on pollen grains on the cloth samples, stating that they were appropriate to the spring in Israel, and Max Frei, a Swiss police criminologist who obtained pollen from the Shroud, stated that of the 58 different types of pollens found, 45 were from the Jerusalem area. A number of studies on the anatomical consistency of the image on the Shroud and the nature of the wounds on it have been performed. Among many others, Pierluigi Baima Bollone, a professor of forensic medicine in Turin, stated that the forensic examination of the wounds and bloodstains on the Shroud indicates that the image was that of the dead body of a man who was whipped, wounded around the head by a pointed instrument, and nailed at the extremities before dying. Finally, Adler studied the dark red stains on the Shroud and identified hemoglobin. Working independently, forensic pathologist Pier Luigi Baima Bollone confirmed Adler's findings and identified the blood as the AB blood group, a relatively rare blood group that is more frequently encountered in the Near East.

The mode by which Christ's face became imprinted on the respective tissues (sea silk and linen, resp.) remains a mystery, but it is clear that it has not been painted, a phenomenon regarded to be miraculous and for which the term *Acheiropoieton* (Byzantine Greek for "made without hand") has been coined.

Another striking phenomenon is the similarity of the Holy relics and the subsequent depictions of Christ's face (with long flowing hair) in Christian iconography and the arts from Jesus Christ Pantocrator in the Hagia Sophia to Albrecht Dürrer's last of three self-portraits (1500) stylizing himself with resemblance to early representations of Christ.

The critics who challenge the iconic picture of a Christ with long flowing hair as a product of Hollywood and Sunday School produce some historical arguments and refer to Biblical text passages to make their point.

In the fourth century AD, many Gentiles who had long worshiped pagan deities began identifying them with the newly worshiped Jesus, Mary, and the twelve Apostles. One particular deity that seemed to combine the features of several gods into a unified portrayal of deity was the Graeco-Egyptian god *Serapis*. Serapis was devised during the third century BC on the orders of Ptolemy I Soter I of Egypt as a means to unify the Greeks and Egyptians in his new kingdom. The god was depicted as Greek in appearance, but with Egyptian accessories, and combined iconography from a great many cults, signifying both abundance and resurrection. Serapis continued to increase in popularity during the Roman period until all forms of religion other than Nicene Christianity were suppressed under Roman Emperor Theodosius I in 391. In his book *"Backgrounds of Early Christianity,"* Everett Ferguson from the Abilene Christian University in Abilene, Texas, shows an example that statues of the Greek god of healing Asclepius were images that were modelled after the Greek chief god Zeus and that his portraiture again influenced artists in depicting Serapis and later the Christ.

In the New Testament, the apostle Paul said it was a shame for a man to have long hair (I Corinthians 11:14, 15), and long feminine-type of hair on a man is how evil spirits are portrayed in the Book of Revelation (Revelation 9:8).

In the time of Jesus, it was a common characteristic of Jewish men to wear their hair short. The respective command of God was given in the time of Ezekiel (Ezekiel 44:20):

> [20]They must not let their hair grow too long, nor shave it off. Regular, moderate haircuts are all they are allowed

Ezekiel grew up as a priest and was carried off with the Jewish exiles deported in 597 BC to Babylon, where he became a prophet of God. His message was one of coming judgement for those remaining in Jerusalem, but his preaching was not well received by the Jews who were with him in captivity. Only when his dire prediction came true in 586 BC with the destruction of Jerusalem, the people listened from then on with great earnestness. Only when Jewish men were under a Nazirite vow or during periods of mourning did Jewish men refrain from cutting their hair. As for lifetime Nazirites, it was common for them to braid the hair, like the seven braids on Samson (Judges 16:13), and to wind the braids around the head under a headgear. Since Samson was a warrior and knew that cutting off his braided hair meant his strength was gone, he would never have allowed his braids to reach below his neck lest they be grasped by his enemies and cut off. Some have mistakenly assumed that Christ was under a Nazirite vow. This was not the case, since he consumed wine (Matthew 11:19) and, on occasion, touched a dead body (Matthew 9:25), which was absolutely forbidden to anyone under a Nazirite vow (Numbers 6:3, 6). Jesus Christ came from Nazareth. The early Christians were sometimes called Namrenes. But neither of these words has anything to do with a Nazirite vow. This suggests that Jesus had short hair like any other Jewish man at the time. Indeed, when Judas pointed out who Jesus was in the moment of his betrayal, he kissed him on the cheek (Luke 22:48) rather than pointing out the man with the long hair.

Whether Jesus Christ had long hair or not, most essential is the fact that – in contrast to today's other great religions – Jesus Christ gave God a face, which has contributed to the concept of the *person* in Western Culture. This concept is a gift of Christianity to the World, thanks to the fact that God himself had become *Person* from a nameless and faceless Being.

Further Reading

The Catholic Living Bible (1971) Tyndale House Publishers, Wheaton

Old Testament

Cash TF (1992) The psychological effects of androgenetic alopecia in men. J Am Acad Dermatol 26:926–931
Cash TF (1999) The psychosocial consequences of androgenetic alopecia: a review of the research literature. Br J Dermatol 141:398–405
http://en.wikipedia.org/wiki/Absalom
http://en.wikipedia.org/wiki/Elisha
http://en.wikipedia.org/wiki/Samson
http://en.wikipedia.org/wiki/Tzaraath
Morris D (1985) Bodywatching: a field guide to the human species. Crown, New York

New Testament

Badde P (2006) Das Göttliche Gesicht. Die abenteuerliche Suche nach dem wahren Antlitz Jesu. Pattloch, München
De Wesselow T (2012) The sign. The Shroud of Turin and the secret of the resurrection. Viking, London
Everett F (1987) Backgrounds of early Christianity. Eerdmans, Grand Rapids
http://en.wikipedia.org/wiki/Anne_Catherine_Emmerich
http://en.wikipedia.org/wiki/Constantine_the_Great
http://en.wikipedia.org/wiki/Saint_Veronica
http://en.wikipedia.org/wiki/Serapis
http://en.wikipedia.org/wiki/Shroud_of_Turin
http://en.wikipedia.org/wiki/The_Passion_of_the_Christ
http://en.wikipedia.org/wiki/Veil_of_Veronica
www.askelm.com/secrets/sec103.html

Name Index

R.M. Trüeb, W.-S. Lee, *Male Alopecia*,
DOI 10.1007/978-3-319-03233-7, © Springer International Publishing Switzerland 2014

Subject Index

I

K

L

U

V

W

Z

MIX
Papier aus verantwortungsvollen Quellen
Paper from responsible sources
FSC® C105338

If you have any concerns about our products,
you can contact us on
ProductSafety@springernature.com

In case Publisher is established outside the EU,
the EU authorized representative is:
Springer Nature Customer Service Center GmbH
Europaplatz 3, 69115 Heidelberg, Germany

Printed by Libri Plureos GmbH
in Hamburg, Germany